Facts and Comparisons Publishing Group:

Executive Vice President	Kenneth H. Killion
Publisher	Cathy H. Reilly
Senior Managing Editor	Teri H. Burnham
Managing Editor	Renee M. Wickersham
Associate Editors	Lindsay D. Harmon Sara L. Schweain
Cover Design	Mark Wickersham
Manufacturing Services Manager	Susan L. Polcyn

A Therapeutic Guide to Common Problems in Gastroenterology

Chandra Prakash, MD, MRCP
Assistant Professor of Medicine
Division of Gastroenterology
Washington University School of Medicine
St. Louis, MO

Joyce A. Generali, MS, RPh, FASHP
Director, Drug Information Center
Clinical Associate Professor
University of Kansas Medical Center
Kansas City, Kansas

Co-Authors

Matthew Ciorba, MD
Department of Internal Medicine
Washington University School of Medicine
St. Louis, MO

Marc A. Fallah, MD
Assistant Professor of Medicine
Division of Gastroenterology
Washington University School of Medicine
St. Louis, MO

Lafaine Grant, MD
Division of Gastroenterology
Washington University School of Medicine
St. Louis, MO

Gregory Sayuk, MD
Department of Internal Medicine
Washington University School of Medicine
St. Louis, MO

Aaron Shiels, MD
Division of Gastroenterology
Washington University School of Medicine
St. Louis, MO

Michael Zerega, MD
Division of Gastroenterology
Washington University School of Medicine
St. Louis, MO

A Therapeutic Guide to Common Problems in Gastroenterology

ISBN 1-57439-182-8

Printed in the United States of America

Published by
Facts and Comparisons®
A Wolters Kluwer Company
111 West Port Plaza, Suite 300
St. Louis, Missouri 63146-3098
314-216-2100
Toll free customer service 1-800-223-0554
www.drugfacts.com

Table of Contents

Preface

As the field of medicine continues to expand, keeping up with newer management options and knowing enough about medications to use them safely becomes increasingly difficult and daunting. The field of gastroenterology encompasses an especially diverse spectrum of diagnoses that have varying management strategies using a wide array of pharmacotherapeutic agents. This handbook was conceived to help the reader keep up to date with management options and pharmacotherapeutic agents in gastroenterology by providing the most pertinent information in a clear and concise format.

This handbook essentially has two sections: a text section outlining common presentations, investigations, and management options for common gastroenterological conditions, followed by monographs on the pharmaceutical agents used to treat these conditions, alphabetically ordered by class or drug name. The short synopses in the text section will help acquaint users with the diseases commonly treated by gastroenterologists. Users of this handbook also can access indications, administration and dosage, contraindications, warnings, interactions, and adverse reactions of the pharmaceutical agents that affect the GI system in the drug monograph section. Additionally, an appendix provides tables for quick reference of important aspects regarding some of these agents.

The handbook is not intended to be a comprehensive reference, but it does cover the most common conditions encountered in clinical gastroenterology. The authors of the chapters have worked hard to incorporate the most up-to-date information on the diagnosis and management of these common gastroenterological disorders while maintaining brevity and clarity in the presentation. The drug monographs clearly and concisely present the most clinically relevant information. It is hoped that the handbook will allow easy access to vital information on-the-go for busy practitioners as well as students of medicine and pharmacology.

Chandra Prakash, MD, MRCP

CHAPTER 1

GASTROESOPHAGEAL REFLUX DISEASE AND ACID PEPTIC DISORDERS

GASTROESOPHAGEAL REFLUX DISEASE (GERD)

Gastroesophageal reflux disease (GERD) is an extremely common condition, and an estimated 60 million Americans have symptoms at least monthly. Heartburn is the classic symptom of GERD. Untreated, GERD can lead to more severe medical complications, including erosive esophagitis, esophageal strictures, Barrett's esophagus, and even esophageal adenocarcinoma. Given its prevalence and the cost of agents used to manage GERD, particularly the proton pump inhibitors, the treatment of GERD consumes a significant portion of the nation's health care expenditures.

Clinical features

GERD classically presents as heartburn, a burning pain in the midsternal region often occurring after eating, on bending forward, or when lying down. Other typical symptoms include regurgitation and belching. Atypical "extraesophageal" symptoms include chronic cough, asthma, chronic hoarseness/laryngitis, oral aphthous ulcers, and hiccoughs. GERD also is a cause of atypical or noncardiac chest pain, accounting for almost 50% of those with chest pain and an unremarkable cardiac evaluation. Dysphagia or odynophagia in patients with GERD may signify a more serious diagnosis such as erosive esophagitis or a peptic stricture. Large meals or foods that relax the lower esophageal sphincter (including chocolate, spices, citrus fruits, fatty foods, and alcohol) may worsen GERD symptoms. Some patients with GERD, particularly elderly patients, may not have any symptoms and subsequently do not present until they develop a complication. Conversely, patients with severe, debilitating symptoms may not have any evidence of pathologic consequences of GERD on further investigation.

Investigation

The evaluation and diagnostic approach to an individual with GERD depends on the presentation. In patients with classic symptoms of heartburn and regurgitation, an empiric treatment trial is appropriate. The presence of certain alarm symptoms should prompt early endoscopy. These alarm symptoms include weight loss, dysphagia, odynophagia, GI bleeding, and anemia. Older age (more than 45 to 50 years of age) at presentation and symptoms for more than 5 years are also indications for endoscopy to exclude Barrett's esophagus. Patients with atypical symptoms and symptoms not responding adequately to acid suppression also need endoscopic evaluation.

Endoscopy is the most sensitive test for the detection of mucosal injury from GERD and for Barrett's screening. However, esophagitis is only seen in about 60% of patients with typical symptoms undergoing endoscopic evaluation. Barium esophagograms may provide evidence of esophageal strictures, rings, webs, and hiatal hernias in addition to reflux. Provocative maneuvers, such as rolling, lying supine, or coughing, improve the detection of reflux on barium studies to about 80%. Esophageal pH monitoring allows for the assessment of the degree and duration of acid reflux, and is considered the gold standard for quantitation of esophageal acid reflux. Its utility lies in patients with suspected GERD and normal endoscopy, patients not responding to adequate acid suppressive therapy, and patients with atypical symptoms in whom GERD is suspected as the underlying problem.

Management

GERD is a chronic, relapsing condition and, therefore, long-term management strategies are essential. Lifestyle modifications are important nonpharmacologic approaches to management initiated in conjunction with pharmacologic therapy. Smoking cessation is encouraged; large meals, caffeine, alcohol and high-fat foods known to decrease lower esophageal sphincter (LES) tone are discouraged. Patients are advised not to eat 2 to 3 hours before lying supine, and are encouraged to elevate the head end of their bed 6 to 8 inches on bricks or blocks. Certain medications, particularly theophylline, calcium-channel blockers, nitrates, tricyclic antidepressants, and anticholinergics can lower LES tone and promote reflux. Additionally, drugs that may exacerbate esophagitis such as bisphosphonates, doxycycline, and NSAIDs should be substituted for other medications where appropriate.

Over-the-counter (OTC) medications are widely available for the treatment of mild or infrequent GERD symptoms, and include antacids (calcium carbonate, magnesium/aluminum hydroxide) and H_2 receptor blocking agents in reduced doses (famotidine, ranitidine, nizatidine, and cimetidine). Antacids serve to neutralize acid, effectively decreasing symptoms for a short time. OTC H_2 receptor blocking agents are all equivalent in their ability to provide relief of GERD symptoms. Proton pump inhibitors or prescription strength H_2 receptor blocking agents are recommended when symptoms are more frequent or not completely relieved with OTC medications. H_2 receptor blocking agents are not considered first-line agents if erosive esophagitis is present, as healing rates of esophagitis only approach 60% on high dose H_2 antagonists, as compared with more than 80% with proton pump inhibitors. Proton pump inhibitors (omeprazole, esomeprazole, lansoprazole, rabeprazole, pantoprazole) act by inhibiting the H^+-K^+ ATPase in the parietal cells of the stomach, blocking the final common pathway of acid secretion, and are thus extremely effective at diminishing gastric acid secretion. Accordingly, they have shown to be consistently superior to high dose H_2-antagonists in alleviating reflux symptoms and promoting the healing of erosive esophagitis, with most patients experiencing complete relief of GERD symptoms within 4 weeks.

Prokinetic agents have a limited role in the treatment of GERD. Metoclopramide is a dopaminergic agent that improves gastric emptying and may alleviate heartburn symptoms but does not promote healing in esophagitis. Cisapride also was used commonly in this setting but has now been recalled due to difficulties with life-threatening cardiac arrhythmias. A limited-access program is available for compassionate use of cisapride for patients with refractory GERD, gastroparesis, pseudo-obstruction, or chronic constipation.

Because GERD is a chronic condition, recurrence of symptoms and esophagitis are common when medications are discontinued. Antireflux surgery is an option in patients with significant GERD requiring long-term or high-dose proton pump inhibitor therapy for symptom relief. It is important to objectively document GERD prior to surgical intervention, using 24-hour esophageal pH monitoring. Esophageal manometry helps document adequate esophageal peristalsis prior to surgery. Antireflux surgery involves wrapping the proximal stomach around the distal esophagus, called fundoplication. Fundoplication can be performed laparoscopically and generally has good to excellent success rates with minimal complications when performed by expert surgeons.

Complications

In the setting of longstanding GERD, the normal squamous epithelial lining of the esophagus may change to columnar epithelium, with intestinal metaplasia and goblet cells on microscopy. This abnormal epithelium is termed Barrett's esophagus and represents a premalignant condition, with a small percentage of patients progressing on to esophageal adenocarcinoma. Acid suppression may slow the progression of Barrett's esophagus but does not reverse this metaplastic change. Regular endoscopic surveillance is recommended to look for histopathologic evidence of dysplasia. When high-grade dysplasia is diagnosed, distal esophagectomy may be recommended in patients who are good surgical candidates. Newer ablative therapies (eg, photodynamic therapy, endoscopic mucosal resection) in conjunction with high dose proton pump inhibitors are being used to manage dysplasia in Barrett's esophagus with some success when surgery is not an option.

Other complications of severe esophagitis include esophageal ulceration and peptic strictures. Both require aggressive acid suppression with high-dose proton pump inhibitors. Esophageal ulcers need to be biopsied to exclude malignancy. Strictures may present as dysphagia in patients with chronic GERD and may require intermittent esophageal dilation for symptom relief.

PEPTIC ULCER DISEASE (PUD)

Peptic ulcer disease (PUD) is characterized by mucosal breaks in the gastric or duodenal mucosa when the corrosive effects of gastric acid and pepsin overwhelm mucosal defense mechanisms. Common causes of PUD are *Helicobacter pylori* infection and NSAID use. *H. pylori* is a Gram-negative bacillus that colonizes the gastric mucosa and is strongly associated with PUD. Cigarette smoking doubles the risk of peptic ulcers. Less common causes include extreme physiologic stress in critically ill patients (resulting in stress ulcers) and acid hypersecretion in Zollinger-Ellison syndrome. Treatment focuses on acid suppression, *H. pylori* eradication, and avoidance of NSAIDs for ulcer healing as well as to prevent potential complications. Peptic ulcers are a significant cause of morbidity, accounting for annual health care costs of more than $5 billion in the US alone.

Clinical features

Dyspepsia is a common presenting symptom. Patients may experience this as a "burning" or "gnawing" sensation, with occasional radiation to the left or right upper quadrants or to the back. Classically, duodenal ulcers are described to be symptomatic 2 to 3 hours after a meal or in the early morning hours, when circadian variation in acid secretion is at its peak. Symptoms from gastric ulcers may be exacerbated by food. Other symptoms include "indigestion" or heartburn, bloating, belching, cramping, nausea, vomiting, and abdominal fullness. A small number of patients can be completely asymptomatic, especially patients with NSAID-related ulcers. Approximately 10% present with complications of the disease, including GI bleeding, perforation, penetration into adjacent organs, and gastric outlet obstruction. Some ulcers heal spontaneously while others persist despite aggressive medical therapy.

A careful history is important to exclude "alarm symptoms" such as weight loss, early satiety, GI bleeding, anemia, and lack of appropriate response to acid suppression. The presence of alarm symptoms warrant a more aggressive approach to exclude malignancy or a bleeding lesion. Patients with gastric outlet obstruction may present with nausea and vomiting. Penetration into the pancreas may result in focal pancreatitis, presenting as more persistent pain radiation to the back. A careful medication history helps determine if the patient is taking NSAIDs or aspirin, risk factors for PUD. Physical examination is usually nonspecific but may provide limited diagnostic information. Hypotension and tachycardia are suggestive of significant blood loss from bleeding ulcers. When ulcers perforate, the presence of abdominal rigidity, guarding and rebound tenderness may suggest peritonitis.

Investigation

Endoscopy is the gold standard for the diagnosis of PUD, with a diagnostic accuracy of over 95%. In addition to direct visualization of the ulcer, biopsies can be taken to exclude malignancy in gastric ulcers.

Tissue specimens also can be used for the rapid urease test and histopathologic examination for the detection of *H. pylori*. Costs may limit upper endoscopy as an initial diagnostic tool in all patients with dyspepsia. Endoscopy should be considered in dyspeptic patients with 'alarm symptoms' including weight loss, early satiety, GI bleeding, anemia, and lack of appropriate response to acid suppression. Older patients with dyspepsia of recent onset and short duration should also undergo endoscopic evaluation to exclude malignancy.

Barium upper GI x-ray series have good sensitivity for the detection of PUD, although small lesions less than 5 mm are notoriously difficult to detect. The addition of gas as a double contrast and compression technique may further increase the sensitivity. Certain radiographic characteristics may suggest malignancy in a gastric ulcer. The main disadvantage of barium studies is the inability to obtain tissue for histopathology.

H. pylori may be present in as many as 80% of duodenal ulcers and 70% of gastric ulcers. Given this strong association with PUD, looking for this organism is an important consideration. Assessment for serum IgG antibodies against *H. pylori* is the most economical noninvasive test that can be used to detect exposure to this organism in dyspeptic patients. The test may remain positive even after successful eradication of the organism and, therefore, cannot be used to evaluate for persistence of the organism after treatment. Stool antigen tests assess for the presence of *H. pylori* bacterial proteins in the stool. When endoscopy is indicated, the rapid urease test is easily performed on a biopsy specimen. However, this test may be falsely negative in patients with recent GI bleeding or in patients taking proton pump inhibitors. Histopathologic examination or serology are alternatives in these situations. The urea breath test is the most accurate noninvasive test for the diagnosis of H. *pylori* infection; this test can be used to document successful eradication in patients with persistent symptoms. If these screens are positive, it is reasonable to treat the patient for *H. pylori* infection (see below).

Patients with refractory or persistent PUD may have underlying acid hypersecretory states; although, persistent *H. pylori* infection and surreptitious NSAID use need to be excluded. A fasting serum gastrin level more than 1000 pg/mL in a patient not on a proton pump inhibitor is diagnostic of Zollinger-Ellison syndrome. In patients with lower elevations of serum gastrin, secretin infusion results in a paradoxical increase of the serum gastrin level by at least 20 Zollinger-Ellison syndrome. Imaging studies including CT octreotide scans may help localize the gastrin-secreting tun surgery.

Management

Regardless of etiology, acid suppression is the cornerstone of PUD management. H_2 receptor antagonists heal 70% to 80% of duodenal ulcers in 4 weeks. Once daily bedtime dosing of famotidine, ranitidine, nizatidine, or cimetidine provides adequate acid suppression for the treatment of PUD. H_2 receptor antagonists also are utilized in the prophylaxis and treatment of stress ulcers. In recent years, proton pump inhibitors have replaced H_2 receptor antagonists in the therapy of PUD. Proton pump inhibitors (omeprazole, esomeprazole, lansoprazole, rabeprazole, and pantoprazole) heal more than 90% of peptic ulcers in 4 weeks. They provide better daytime acid suppression compared with H_2 receptor antagonists and are an integral part of regimens for *H. pylori* eradication. Intravenous proton pump inhibitors are now available for short-term use in patients who cannot tolerate oral medications in the acute setting, for example, in acute GI bleeding.

When present, eradication of *H. pylori* is essential to the management of PUD. Not only does *H. pylori* eradication help heal the ulcer, but relapse after successful ulcer treatment is much less frequent when this organism is eradicated. Duodenal ulcers recur less than 20% of the time when *H. pylori* is successfully eradicated, in contrast to 70% to 90% with persistent infection. Several *H. pylori* treatment regimens have been developed that can effectively eradicate the organism in around 75% to 80% percent of cases. These regimens are generally triple agent therapies and include acid suppression (a proton pump inhibitor) and 2 antibiotics (amoxicillin, clarithromycin, metronidazole, bismuth subsalicylate, tetracycline) continued for 10 to 14 days. In refractory situations, 4 drug regimens (proton pump inhibitor, bismuth subsalicylate, metronidazole, and tetracycline) are preferred. In addition to its bacteriostatic activity against *H. pylori*, bismuth subsalicylate may also form a protective coating on ulcer craters.

Cytoprotective agents have a role in management and prophylaxis of certain peptic ulcers. Sucralfate coats gastric mucosa, and therefore, forms a protective barrier. It has been used in the treatment and prophylaxis of stress ulcers. Misoprostol is a prostaglandin E_1 analog used for the prophylaxis and treatment of NSAID-related ulcers. Diarrhea is a significant side effect that may limit its use.

Duodenal ulcers typically heal completely with 8 weeks of therapy, while gastric ulcers may need to be treated for 12 weeks. Follow-up evaluation (using endoscopy or barium studies) is necessary to document healing of some gastric ulcers at the end of the treatment period, and non-healing ulcers need to be biopsied to exclude malignancy. Large or complicated ulcers may require prolonged courses of acid suppression. NSAIDs should be discontinued if possible; maintenance acid suppression with a proton pump inhibitor is necessary if the NSAID is continued due to substantial risk of ulcer recurrence. COX-2 selective anti-inflammatory agents carry a much lower risk of PUD-related complications compared with conventional NSAIDs. Cigarette smoking has been associated with increased likelihood of ulcer recurrence; therefore, smoking cessation should be emphasized.

In critically-ill patients with stress ulcers, treatment is largely supportive with optimization of hemodynamic, ventilatory, and nutritional status while providing acid suppression IV or through a nasogastric tube. H_2 receptor antagonists are first line agents for therapy and prophylaxis of stress ulcers. Sucralfate may be used as an alternative agent. Intravenous proton pump inhibitors also can be considered; although, data documenting efficacy are not yet available. Surgical removal of the gastrin-secreting tumor, if identified, is indicated for patients with Zollinger-Ellison syndrome. High doses of proton pump inhibitors are required before surgery and in patients in whom the tumor cannot be localized.

With the advent of potent acid-blocking medications, the need for surgery for routine treatment of peptic ulcer disease has declined dramatically. However, surgery remains a useful treatment option in refractory ulcers and when complications such as perforation, bleeding, or gastric outlet obstruction occur.

Complications

The major complications of PUD are GI bleeding, gastric outlet obstruction, perforation, and penetration into adjacent organs. The most common complication is bleeding, accounting for more than 150,000 hospitalizations annually. This can present with overt bleeding (hematemesis and/or melena), but some patients may present with occult blood loss and anemia. Most ulcers stop bleeding spontaneously, but overt bleeding warrants urgent endoscopic evaluation. Gastric outlet obstruction can occur from ulcers in the pyloric channel or proximal duodenum. Patients with this complication may experience bloating, nausea, and vomiting. Standard PUD therapies should be implemented, and surgical intervention is reserved for refractory cases. Rare patients with pyloric strictures from healed pyloric ulcers may benefit from endoscopic balloon dilation.

Patients who develop sudden onset of severe abdominal pain with rigidity, guarding, and rebound tenderness in the setting of PUD should be evaluated promptly for ulcer perforation. Definitive management is surgical, though supportive management is initiated with intravenous fluids, antibiotics, and acid suppression therapy. Ulcer penetration is rare and can occur into the pancreas, colon, and liver. Despite improvements in acid suppression and identification of *H. pylori* as an associated pathogen, the incidence of life-threatening complications due to PUD has not declined over the years. This observation may reflect the trend towards increased NSAID use, particularly in elderly patients. Patients with complications of PUD are more likely to develop recurrence of complicated PUD in the future.

CHAPTER 2

INFLAMMATORY BOWEL DISEASE

CROHN DISEASE

Crohn disease is 1 of the 2 major types of inflammatory bowel disease. Crohn disease is distinct from ulcerative colitis, the other major inflammatory disease, in that it can affect any portion of the bowel from mouth to the perianal region. Its transmural inflammatory pattern is also unique, accounting for a multitude of clinical presentations. Disease manifestations range from diarrhea with abdominal cramping to perforation and fistulae. Systemic symptoms include fever and weight loss as well as involvement of the eyes, skin, and joints.

Incidence in the US approximates 6 to 7 per 100,000 population. The incidence rate for Crohn disease is bimodal with the first, and most significant peak, occurring between the ages of 15 and 30. A minor peak is seen between 50 and 80 years of age. Prevalence is higher in ethnic Jews, and it shows preference to white over black and Hispanic populations.

Genetic and environmental factors are thought to play a role in the etiology of Crohn disease. Patients with a family history have an increased chance of developing the disease and frequently develop it at a younger age. Twin studies reveal a high concordance rate. Environmental factors have been implicated in contributing to disease expression in susceptible individuals. Cigarette smoking has been associated with increased risk of flares. Other factors such as infectious agents (including intestinal flora), nutritional deficiencies, and oral contraceptives have been studied as etiologic factors but remain unproven.

Clinical features

Crohn disease has a variety of clinical presentations. The onset is typically insidious with nonspecific digestive symptoms frequently dating years before frank presentation. Sometimes symptoms resemble irritable bowel syndrome. Diarrhea, fever, abdominal pain, and weight loss are typical symptoms for patients with ileo-colonic disease. Diarrhea is secondary to the combined effects of decreased fluid absorption, increased secretion and even fat malabsorption in extensive ileal disease. Abdominal pain is very common and is sometimes related to inflammation-induced fibrotic strictures causing bowel obstruction. Gross GI bleeding is less frequent than with ulcerative colitis.

The transmural inflammatory pattern of Crohn disease often leads to the development of sinus or fistulous tracts, which can present as perianal disease (perirectal abscesses, anorectal fistulae), pneumaturia (fistula to the urinary system), female genital tract (rectovaginal fistula), or indolent bowel perforation, resulting in localized abdominal mass and fever. Fistulae to the urinary bladder, retroperitoneum, skin, or other loops of bowel are common.

Symptoms can also arise from the various locations where Crohn disease occurs. These can include mouth pain from aphthous ulcers, odynophagia or dysphagia with esophageal involvement, nausea and vomiting from gastroduodenal involvement or gastric outlet obstruction, and malabsorption symptoms from small bowel disease. Weight loss can result from anorexia due to ongoing inflammation, malabsorption, or protein loss from inflamed bowel mucosa. Fevers result from the inflammatory aspect of the disease itself and from infectious complications.

Extraintestinal manifestations include involvement of the eyes, skin, joints, and hematologic and hepatobiliary systems. Episcleritis and uveitis of the eye, and skin manifestations, such as cutaneous erythema nodosum and pyoderma gangrenosum, are common. Ankylosing spondylitis and peripheral arthritis of large joints also have been described. Finally, hypercoagulable states resulting in venous thrombosis, and sclerosing cholangitis presenting with features of biliary obstruction also have been seen.

Investigation

A careful history and physical examination may identify features suspicious of Crohn disease. The choice of initial testing depends on the suspected location of disease. In patients presenting with a diarrheal illness, stool studies for microscopic examination and culture may help exclude infectious colitis. Other conditions in the initial differential diagnosis include irritable bowel syndrome, lactose intolerance, ulcerative colitis, and microscopic colitis. Other presentations may resemble intra-abdominal neoplasia, endoemetriosis, diverticulitis, appendicitis, and other inflammatory conditions.

Endoscopic evaluation is a very effective diagnostic tool. Crohn disease often demonstrates rectosigmoid sparing and involvement of the ileocecal region. Focal or serpininous ulcers and erosions may be separated by normal appearing segments of mucosa, the so called 'skip lesions'. Other abnormalities include strictures and bleeding. Biopsies may demonstrate granulomas that are typical of Crohn disease. Focal acute and chronic inflammation with accompanying ulceration are commonly seen.

Air contrast barium enema and small bowel follow through studies are useful radiologic exams. Barium enemas detect aphthous ulcers, disease extent and severity of colonic strictures. Perforations with fistulae also may be demonstrated. Upper GI x-ray series and small bowel follow through may demonstrate extent of involvement in the proximal gut. A "string sign" from lumenal narrowing, cobblestone pattern, fistulae, and bowel wall thickening also may be seen.

In a select group of patients who are highly suspected to have Crohn disease, but for whom further confirmation is sought, adjunctive autoantibody testing may be pursued. These typically analyze the relation of P-ANCA vs ASCA (anti-*Saccharomyces cerevisiae* antibodies) positivity and are more specific than sensitive.

Management

Crohn disease has a variety of clinical presentations, and the magnitude and variety of individual organ involvement differs between patients. The following is a generalized approach to managing the main GI syndromes.

The 5-aminosalicylate (5-ASA) compounds are lumenal and systemic anti-inflammatory agents and first line agents in therapeutic choice. Sulfasalazine is a combination of 5-ASA and sulfapyridine and is metabolized to the active 5-ASA compound by colonic bacteria; therefore, it can be used for Crohn disease involving the colon. Mesalamine is an oral slow release 5-ASA agent formulated for release either in the distal ileum and colon (*Asacol*) or throughout the GI tract (*Pentasa*). The location of disease often determines the choice of agent. Response is typically seen in 3 to 4 weeks. These agents can be used in the acute setting for mild to moderate disease as well as for maintenance therapy.

Antibiotics covering a broad range of aerobic and anaerobic enteric bacteria also are used as therapeutic agents in Crohn disease. Ciprofloxacin may be as effective as 5-ASA compounds in Crohn ileitis. Metronidazole also may be used alone or in combination with ciprofloxacin. Other antibiotics less frequently used include trimethoprim-sulfamethoxazole, clarithromycin, tetracycline, and cephalexin.

Use of systemic steroids for short periods, alone or in combination with 5-ASA agents, is appropriate for inducing remission in moderate to severe disease. Starting doses at 40 to 60 mg/day prednisone induces remission in 60 to 80% of patients. Long-term use is discouraged because of side effects, but is sometimes necessary in patients who are steroid dependent. Alternatives include synthetic steroids, such as budesonide, that are now available for ileocolonic disease. Infliximab *(Remicade)* is a monoclonal antibody against tumor necrosis factor alpha that helps curb the inflammatory response, particularly in patients with fistulous Crohn disease and refractory inflammation.

Crohn disease that is steroid dependent or refractory to anti-inflammatory medication may be responsive to immunosuppressive therapy. Azathioprine, its active metabolite 6-mercaptopurine, and methotrexate are the immunosuppressive agents available. Response time is often slow at 3 to 6 months, but these medications are useful in 60% to 70% of patients with disease of the small bowel or colon. Steroid doses may be tapered starting 1 to 2 months after immunosuppressive therapy is initiated in patients with steroid-dependent disease.

Surgery is sometimes necessary when medical management is unsuccessful in controlling symptoms or when acute complications or noninflammatory processes such as fibrous strictures are the cause for symptoms. The following are some situations in which surgery may be needed and the appropriate concurrent or antecedent medical therapy:

- Microperforation and frank bowel perforation may present with signs of localized peritonitis. Bowel rest and broad-spectrum antibiotics (third generation cephalosporins, metronidazole) are indicated. Surgery is generally required for frank perforation, but microperforations can heal with medical management alone.
- Intra-abdominal abscesses can be treated with broad spectrum antibiotics and/or percutaneous drainage successfully in 50% of cases, surgery being reserved for failures.

- Obstruction can result from stricture formation in longstanding disease, or from an acute inflammatory process. Nasogastric tube decompression and intravenous fluids are often sufficient therapy, especially when acute inflammation is the culprit. Tight fibrous strictures often require surgery.

Symptomatic therapy is recommended in certain patients with Crohn disease. Patients with ongoing diarrhea despite adequate anti-inflammatory treatment may be treated with antidiarrheal medication. While loperamide is generally effective, diarrhea resulting from inadequate bile salt resorption may be more appropriately treated with cholestyramine. Pain associated with oral aphthous ulcers can be eased with topical hydrocortisone or sucralfate. Supplementary control of gastroduodenal mucosal disease can be achieved with acid suppression or sucralfate.

Many factors contribute to loss or poor absorption of iron, calcium, vitamins A, D, E, K, B_{12}, and folate, as well as protein and fat. Deficiencies need to be adequately repleted orally or parenterally. Bone mineral density should be checked periodically particularly if patients require prolonged or frequent steroid use.

Complications

Fistula formation, perianal disease, perforation, and intra-abdominal abscesses and strictures are complications frequently seen, and have been discussed in sections above. Other complications include malabsorption and the risk for cancer.

Malabsorption in Crohn disease is related to small bowel disease. Absorption of vitamin B_{12}, as well as enterohepatic circulation of bile acids, occurs in the terminal ileum. With severe ileocecal disease or if the terminal ileum has been resected, bile acids and vitamin B_{12} cannot be absorbed adequately. Mildly inadequate reabsorption causes colonic irritation and results in watery diarrhea, while more severe degrees impair fat absorption and cause steatorrhea and subsequent malnutrition. Significant bile acid malabsorption along with altered bilirubin metabolism can predispose Crohn disease patients to pigmented gallstones. Finally, alterations in absorption and diarrhea also increase the risk of developing calcium oxalate and uric acid stones.

Patients with Crohn disease involving the colon are at increased risk for colon cancer, although the risk for colonic neoplasia may be less than with ulcerative colitis. An increased incidence of other cancers, including duodenal cancer, small bowel cancer, lymphoma, and squamous cell carcinoma of the anus also have been reported.

ULCERATIVE COLITIS

Ulcerative colitis is an inflammatory bowel disease involving the colonic mucosa. Symptoms vary by extent and severity of disease. Cramping abdominal pain and bloody diarrhea are typical, and systemic symptoms such as fever and weight loss may occur. Like Crohn disease, extraintestinal manifestations involving the eyes, joints, skin, and other organs may co-exist.

The incidence of ulcerative colitis in North America and Europe is similar to that of Crohn disease and averages 6 to 10/100,000 population. Geographic and ethnic patterns are roughly equivalent between the 2 diseases. Interestingly, cigarette smoking can help induce remission in flares of ulcerative colitis while it worsens Crohn's disease flares. Some reports suggest that appendectomy may be protective against the development of ulcerative colitis.

Clinical features

Because ulcerative colitis is limited to the colon, the clinical presentation is less variable. Symptoms depend on severity of disease and extent of the colon involved. If affecting only the rectum and distal colon, mild diarrhea and abdominal pain of insidious onset may be the only manifestations. Usually, onset is gradual with involvement of the distal third of the colon or a mildly severe pancolitis. Less commonly, an extensive inflammatory process may be present, with severe abdominal cramping and multiple loose, bloody bowel movements and systemic signs such as fevers, weight loss, and anemia. As with Crohn disease, extraintestinal manifestations may provide additional clues to the diagnosis.

Investigation

The diagnosis of ulcerative colitis is dependent on a thorough history and physical examination followed by endoscopic evaluation. Other causes of colitis, infectious and otherwise, need to be ruled out prior to initiating therapy, especially in immunocompromised patients in whom infectious causes may be more likely. Medications, particularly NSAIDs and antibiotics, also may contribute to colitis and need to be excluded with a careful history.

Endoscopy is the most effective investigative tool to determine extent of disease. Flexible sigmoidoscopy is usually sufficient for initial diagnosis in patients with severe disease. Mucosal inflammation starting at the rectum and extending proximally in a contiguous fashion are typical. The mucosa appears erythematous and sometimes friable, showing loss of vascular markings. Exudate, petechiae, hemorrhage, and large ulcerations may be present. Pseudopolyps indicate chronic inflammation. Histopathology demonstrates chronic inflammation with crypt abscesses and glandular atrophy. These results, in the setting of an appropriate clinical picture, confirm the diagnosis of ulcerative colitis. In patients initially investigated with flexible sigmoidoscopy, a full colonoscopy to determine extent of disease is performed when acute symptoms resolve. Patients with disease duration of 10 to 15 years or longer need a yearly surveillance colonoscopy to exclude histologic evidence of dysplasia, as patients with ulcerative colitis are at increased risk for colon cancer.

Radiologic exams, including the barium enema, are less useful in the diagnosis of ulcerative colitis. In long-standing disease, pseudopolyps, colonic shortening, loss of haustra, and a narrowed lumen may be present.

Management

Choice in treatment is typically dependent on the severity of symptoms and the location and extent of colonic involvement. Commonly used medications include oral and topical anti-inflammatory agents, steroids, and immunomodulators. Surgery may be necessary in severe, complicated, or medically nonresponsive disease.

In mild to moderate colitis, aminosalicylates (mesalamine, sulfasalazine, and olsalazine) are the initial drugs of choice. Disease limited to the distal colon may be treated topically with 5-ASA enemas and suppositories, while diffuse disease is typically treated with oral agents. Topical steroids in the form of hydrocortisone enemas or cortisone foam are also effective as adjunctive agents but need to be replaced with oral agents if response is inadequate. Overall, oral prednisone at 40 to 60 mg/day can induce remission in approximately 70%

of patients not responding to aminosalicylate therapy. When response is attained, prednisone is tapered slowly and other agents used for maintenance. In refractory situations, immunosuppressive therapy should be initiated. Azathioprine and its active metabolite 6-mercaptopurine are the agents most frequently used. A slow onset of action, often 3 months or greater, limits the utility of these agents in some settings. Weekly dosing of methotrexate also may be used but is less effective in ulcerative colitis than Crohn disease.

Severe colitis often requires the patient to be hospitalized for intravenous steroids and bowel rest. In refractory situations, intravenous cyclosporine may induce remission in almost 80% of patients with severe colitis within 1 week. If response is achieved, maintenance therapy is initiated or resumed with 5-ASA compounds and/or immunosupressive agents. If response is inadequate, total colectomy needs to be considered, taking the patient's comorbid illnesses, prognosis, and quality of life issues into consideration.

Complications

Extensive inflammation can lead to fulminant colitis, which in turn can progress to toxic megacolon and possible perforation. Toxic megacolon, a condition of colonic dilatation in the setting of an acute flare of colitis, is a real and serious risk. Management consists of bowel rest and broad spectrum antibiotics. If the medical condition deteriorates or there is no improvement within a few days, total colectomy may be necessary.

Chronic inflammation also predisposes to stricture formation that can lead to obstruction. Strictures are most common in the rectosigmoid colon. All strictures need to be investigated carefully, as malignancy or Crohn disease, may be the culprit. The relative risk of colon cancer increases starting 7 to 10 years after disease onset and is highest in patients with pancolitis. Yearly surveillance colonoscopy with 4 quadrant biopsies at 5 to 10 cm intervals is recommended starting at 10 to 15 years of disease onset.

Extraintestinal manifestations also may result in complications. Eye involvement may present as uveitis and episcleritis, causing significant pain sometimes requiring topical steroids. Inflamed tender nodules on the lower extremities termed erythema nodosum, as well as pyoderma gangrenosum, occur in some patients and run parallel in activity with the colitis. Acute arthropathy, usually affecting large joints, occurs in 10% to 15% of patients. Ankylosing spondylitis is less common. A serious related disorder is primary sclerosing cholangitis, a cholestatic liver disease resulting from ductal inflammation and strictures.

MICROSCOPIC COLITIS

Microscopic colitis is a condition clinically characterized by chronic nonbloody diarrhea. Although the colon appears normal on endoscopic or radiographic (barium enema) examination, inflammation is evident on histopathologic examination. Two variants have been described: collagenous colitis, with a conspicuous thickened subepithelial collagen band on light microscopy, and lymphocytic colitis. Both variants have inflammatory cell infiltration of the epithelium. The etiology is unknown. The annual incidence of microscopic colitis ranges from 1 to 3 per 100,000 population. Microscopic colitis is diagnosed in 10% of normal appearing colonoscopic examinations in patients with watery diarrhea.

While speculation of an autoimmune and/or infectious process exist, the etiology of this inflammatory condition remains unclear. Proposals of a dietary, self, or microbiologic antigen all have support. Drugs such as NSAIDS, simvastatin, ticlopidine, and proton pump inhibitors have each been implicated in some cases. Microscopic colitis also has been inconsistently linked with other autoimmune diseases such as rheumatoid arthritis or thyroid diseases. An observed link between celiac disease and microscopic colitis makes testing for gluten enteropathy a reasonable step. The diagnosis of microscopic colitis prior to a diagnosis of Crohn disease or ulcerative colitis likely represents an early presentation of 1 of the latter 2 rather than true disease progression.

Clinical features

Patients typically present in middle age. While female predominance exists for lymphocytic and collagenous colitis, this predominance is greater in the collagenous variety (this may be secondary to estrogen effects). Individuals typically have 4 to 9 loose stools each day producing up to 2 liters of watery diarrhea. Nocturnal diarrhea is common. The course is usually chronic, with intermittent bouts of diarrhea; continuous symptoms are less common. Accompanying symptoms may include weight loss, nausea, non-specific abdominal pain and urgency.

Investigation

There are no specific laboratory markers. A mild anemia, an elevated erythrocyte sedimentation rate, or autoantibodies (rheumatoid factor, antinuclear antigen, or antinuclear cytoplasmic antigen) may be present. Stools studies are nonspecific, fecal leukocytes being identified in over 50% of cases. Endoscopic and radiographic examination typically reveal normal appearing colonic mucosa. However, in some cases of collagenous colitis the mucosa can appear granular or even friable. Mild edema or erythema also may be present.

Careful microscopic examination of multiple biopsies is necessary to make the diagnosis. Samples should be taken from the proximal colon (ascending or transverse) as the severity of inflammation typically decreases distally. An inflammatory intraepithelial infiltrate of predominately mononuclear cells is the histologic hallmark. Scattered neutrophils and eosinophils also are frequently present. Distortion of crypt architecture is unusual. The subepithelial collagen band in collagenous colitis measures greater than 7 mcm in diameter. An inadequate histologic evaluation may lead the clinician to mistake microscopic colitis for diarrhea-predominant irritable bowel syndrome.

Management

A comprehensive, evidence-based treatment protocol for microscopic colitis has yet to be developed. Antidiarrheal medication may suffice in patients with mild symptoms. NSAIDS should be stopped and a gluten-free diet initiated for patients who test positive for celiac disease. Bismuth subsalicylate has resulted in clinical and histological improvement with continued benefit after treatment is stopped. Aminosalicylates (sulfasalazine, mesalamine) may be used in patients with more persistent symptoms. Patients may improve on smaller doses of these medications compared with established inflammatory bowel disease. When symptoms respond, the medications can be weaned off after 6 to 12 months of therapy, reserving long-term therapy for patients whose symptoms recur off medication. Cholestyramine can be a useful adjunct in some patints with persistent diarrhea. For nonresponders, systemic or topical steroids (prednisone, budesonide) may be used. Small uncontrolled studies indicate that therapies ranging from metronidazole to octreotide to verapamil may be of use in steroid resistant diarrhea. Surgery to create an ostomy is very rarely needed. Diarrhea may resolve within weeks with or without treatment. Symptomatic improvement does not necessarily correspond to histologic resolution.

Complications

Complications are unusual. The rare patient with significant secretory diarrhea can develop significant dehydration or electrolyte disturbance. Resolution or significant improvement of symptoms is more common in the lymphocytic variety vs collagenous. No increase in mortality has been described, and serious complications are rare.

CHAPTER 3

IRRITABLE BOWEL SYNDROME AND FUNCTIONAL BOWEL DISEASE

IRRITABLE BOWEL SYNDROME

Irritable bowel syndrome (IBS) is a condition characterized by abdominal discomfort in the setting of altered bowel function. With an estimated incidence of 15% to 20% in the general population, IBS is the most common disorder treated by gastroenterologists. Altered motility, visceral hypersensitivity, psychosocial factors, and an imbalance in neurotransmitters have been implicated in the pathogenesis, while infection may play a role in triggering symptoms.

Clinical features

As defined by the Rome II criteria, IBS consists of abdominal discomfort or pain for at least 3 months (which need not be consecutive) in the previous 12 months associated with 2 of the following 3 features: relief with defecation, onset associated with a change in stool frequency, onset associated with a change in appearance of stool. IBS can be subcategorized into pain predominant, diarrhea predominant, and constipation predominant, depending on the predominant symptom reported by the patients. Patients can have diarrhea or constipation, and in some instances, alternate between diarrhea and constipaton. Other associated symptoms include abnormal stool passage with straining, urgency, or feeling of incomplete evacuation, passage of mucus, and bloating, or feeling of abdominal distension.

Investigation

IBS is suspected when symptoms conform to the Rome II criteria, and only limited investigation is necessary in most instances. Alarm symptoms prompting further evaluation include evidence of occult or overt GI bleeding, anemia, anorexia, weight loss, fever, persistent diarrhea, severe constipation or fecal impaction, family history of GI cancer, celiac sprue or inflammatory bowel disease, and onset of symptoms after the age of 50 years. After a careful history and physical examination, routine testing includes a complete blood count; metabolic profile, including liver function tests, electrolytes, and kidney function; and thyroid stimulating hormone level. In the absence of alarm symptoms, no further testing is required. In the presence of alarm symptoms, further evaluation can include stool studies, endoscopy including biopsies, serology to exclude celiac disease, and imaging of the abdomen. These tests also can be considered if a patient suspected to have IBS does not respond appropriately to symptomatic measures. The diagnosis of IBS should not be made in older individuals developing bowel symptoms prior to exclusion of organic pathology, including colorectal cancer by appropriate diagnostic testing.

Management

Establishment of a sound physician-patient relationship is crucial in the management of IBS. Education with emphasis on a benign nature of the condition helps reassure the patient. Avoidance of food items that precipitate symptoms is reasonable; other patients report improvement in symptoms from limiting intake of caffeine, alcohol, dairy products, or gas-producing vegetables. Invasive testing should be minimized and repetitive testing avoided.

Diarrhea predominant IBS

For patients with mild or intermittent diarrhea, treatment with antidiarrheal agents, such as loperamide or diphenoxylate, on an as needed basis may be adequate. Other patients with more persistent symptoms may need to use antidiarrheal agents on a more regular basis. Cholestyramine also has been used with benefit in certain patients. Tincture of belladonna or tincture of opium is reserved for more refractory diarrhea associated with IBS. Tricyclic antidepressants (amitriptyline, nortriptyline, desipramine) in low doses also may be beneficial in this subgroup of patients. Finally, alosetron, a 5-HT_3 receptor antagonist, may improve colonic symptoms in women with diarrhea-predominant IBS. Severe side effects including constipation and ischemic colitis have been reported; therefore, its use is reserved for women with symptoms refractory to other medications.

Constipation predominant IBS

Increasing the fiber content of the diet or fiber supplementation (*Metamucil, Citrucel, Fibercon*) may relieve symptoms of constipation in mild cases. Osmotic laxatives (lactulose, sorbitol, magnesium citrate, milk of magnesia) are safe for intermittent use. Polyethylene glycol preparations (*Miralax, Golytely*) can be used on a regular basis for patients with more persistent symptoms. Tegaserod, a $5HT_4$ agonist, acts as a promotility agent and may improve symptoms predominantly in women with constipation-predominant IBS. Stronger laxatives such as senna, cascara, castor oil, and mineral oil can be reserved for more refractory cases of constipation. Anecdotal reports suggest that certain selective serotonin receptor inhibitors (SSRIs, eg, sertraline, paroxetine) may be beneficial.

Pain predominant IBS

Antispasmodic agents (hyoscyamine, dicyclomine, nitrates) may improve abdominal cramping and bloating by relaxation of intestinal smooth muscle, either directly or through anticholinergic effects. Tricyclic antidepressants in low doses may be particularly useful in these patients. Coexisting diarrhea or constipation may need symptomatic management as outlined above. In refractory situations, SSRIs and opioid agents (tincture of opium) may be needed.

Complications

Complications are rare. Patients with severe constipation can rarely develop anal fissures, stercoral ulcers, and fecal impaction. Patients with significant diarrhea can become dehydrated, but this should prompt evaluation for an organic cause of diarrhea. Patients requiring analgesic medication stand the risk of drug dependence and narcotic addiction.

FUNCTIONAL DYSPEPSIA

Functional dyspepsia consists of persistent or recurrent upper abdominal symptoms (epigastric discomfort or pain, bloating, early satiety, nausea) in the absence of metabolic abnormalities and mucosal pathology in the upper GI tract. Nonulcer dyspepsia is another term used to describe this condition. This condition may follow successful treatment of acid peptic disease, and the symptom spontaneously resolves in 30% of patients over time. Unrecognized *Helicobacter pylori* infection or gastroesophageal reflux, visceral hypersensitivity, and less commonly, abnormal gastric motor activity may contribute to symptoms.

Clinical features

Patients complain of episodic or intermittent discomfort or pain in the epigastric area. A sense of fullness, typically after meals, is another common symptom. Other associated symptoms include bloating, early satiety, nausea, and sometimes vomiting or retching. Heartburn or regurgitation may coexist.

Investigation

Peptic ulcer disease may be the cause of symptoms in about 15% of dyspeptic patients. Endoscopy is the gold standard for excluding peptic ulcer disease or neoplasia, especially in patients with alarm symptoms (see below). Barium studies also may detect peptic ulcer disease with good sensitivity although subtle mucosal lesions may not be visualized and biopsies are not possible. Metabolic and other systemic disorders can be ruled out with laboratory tests, including liver and kidney function tests, thyroid hormone levels, and serology to exclude collagen vascular diseases. Gastric emptying scans can exclude gastroparesis in the appropriate clinical scenario. Imaging studies (ultrasound, CT scans) have a low yield but may be useful in excluding biliary and pancreatic disorders in selected patients.

Treatment

Because history recording alone may be inaccurate in excluding peptic ulcer disease or malignancy, older patients with alarm symptoms, including new onset dyspepsia, concurrent GI bleeding, early satiety or weight loss, and symptoms unresponsive to empiric proton pump inhibitor therapy, need further investigation with upper endoscopy. Young patients without the above alarm symptoms can undergo empiric acid suppressive therapy using proton pump inhibitors or H_2 receptor antagonists. Serologic tests for *Helicobacter pylori* can be performed and the organism eradicated, although *H. pylori* eradication probably will not resolve symptoms in the absence of peptic ulcers. Metoclopramide may improve symptoms in selected patients but is associated with significant side effects. Likewise, anticholinergic agents may afford relief in some patients. Low dose tricyclic antidepressant therapy for visceral hypersensitivity can be considered when acid suppression is unsuccessful in resolving symptoms. Formal psychiatric assessment is recommended when overt psychiatric disorders are identified.

Complications

Specific complications are unusual. Frequent and severe retching may lead to Mallory-Weiss tears. Patients rarely lose weight from anorexia and inability to eat, in which instance other organic etiologies need to be excluded. Nausea and vomiting is rarely severe enough to result in fluid and electrolyte disturbance. Patients treated with narcotic analgesics may develop drug addiction and dependence.

ATYPICAL CHEST PAIN

Atypical chest pain consists of recurrent midline or substernal chest pain that may mimic angina after significant coronary artery disease has been excluded by reasonable cardiac evaluation. Approximately 33% of coronary angiograms are negative for cardiac disease, and medical expenses in patients with chest pain and normal coronary arteries runs close to a billion dollars every year. Although mortality is low, morbidity remains high because of significant health care utilization and inability to work. Gastroesophageal reflux disease (GERD) may account for symptoms in as many as 50% of patients. Other etiologies include esophageal motility disorders (diffuse esophageal spasm, nonspecific spastic disorders) and visceral hypersensitivity. Patients with chest wall tenderness to palpation may have musculoskeletal pain or costochondritis.

Clinical features

Esophageal pain can be indistinguishable from cardiac pain, and clinical history may not be very useful in distinguishing the two. Both can result in burning or pressure, like chest pain in the midline with radiation to back, shoulders, neck, or arms. Nitrates can relieve cardiac and esophageal pain. The presence of concurrent regurgitation or dysphagia may help localize the pain to the esophagus. Esophageal pain, especially when due to acid reflux, can result in prolonged episodes of nocturnal pain, often waking the patient up from sleep, and may respond promptly to antacids.

Patients with atypical chest pain may have evidence of concurrent psychiatric disorders, including panic disorder, anxiety, and depression. Somatization disorder and fibromyalgia may be associated. Patients are often young women.

Investigation

A comprehensive history and physical examination followed by limited laboratory tests (blood count, liver function tests, chest x-ray, hepatobiliary ultrasound) helps exclude musculoskeletal conditions, hepatobiliary disease, and pulmonary disease. In the appropriate clinical scenario, significant coronary disease needs to be excluded, preferably with coronary angiography in consultation with a cardiologist. Empiric proton pump inhibitor therapy is useful as a therapeutic test at the outset. Endoscopy and 24-hour pH monitoring help further explore the diagnosis of GERD, while esophageal manometry looks for esophageal motility disorders. Formal psychiatric evaluation helps identify psychiatric disorders that are frequently associated with atypical chest pain from visceral hypersensitivity.

Treatment

Empiric acid suppression with a proton pump inhibitor is usually the first step, as GERD is the most common cause of this condition. If symptoms improve, treatment needs to be continued over the long term. If a spastic esophageal motor disorder is diagnosed after esophageal manometry, smooth muscle relaxants, such as calcium channel blockers or nitrates, can be tried. Anticholinergic agents (hyoscyamine, dicyclomine) and low dose tricyclic antidepressants (amitriptyline, nortriptyline, desipramine, imipramine) also may be useful. Patients with visceral hypersensitivity also respond to low dose tricyclic antidepressants or trazodone. Narcotic analgesics should be avoided as long as possible. When anxiety or panic disorder is a prominent part of the symptomatology, formal psychiatric consultation is recommended. In patients with mild anxiety symptoms, benzodiazepines (alprazolam, lorazepam) in small doses may be beneficial while awaiting formal psychiatric consultation.

Complications

Complications are unusual, and the overall mortality is reported to be less than 1% over a 10-year follow up. However, despite the benign prognosis, patients remain concerned about a cardiac etiology for their chest pain, leading to anxiety, lost work, and increased utilization of health care resources. In patients treated with narcotic analgesics, drug dependence can be a problem.

CHAPTER 4

VIRAL AND DRUG-INDUCED LIVER DISORDERS

VIRAL HEPATITIS

Viral hepatitis results from infections that cause diffuse hepatic inflammation and variable degrees of hepatic necrosis, and can be acute, chronic, or fulminant. Hyperbilirubinemia, elevated serum levels of liver transaminases (aspartate aminotransferase or AST, and alanine aminotransferase or ALT), and alkaline phosphatase are hallmarks of hepatic damage. Acute hepatitis involves significant inflammation followed by either recovery, progression to chronic hepatitis, or fulminant liver failure from severe hepatocyte necrosis. Chronic viral hepatitis is defined as persistent hepatic inflammation lasting at least 6 months, and can progress further to cirrhosis, hepatocellular carcinoma, and/or liver failure. Fulminant hepatitis occurs when altered mental status (encephalopathy) ensues within 8 weeks of the onset of hepatitis in an otherwise healthy individual. Rapid progression to multisystem organ failure and death can occur without adequate supportive care and timely referral to a liver transplant center.

Although the number of potential viruses that can cause hepatitis are numerous, the most well known are hepatitis A (HAV), hepatitis B (HBV), and hepatitis C (HCV). Other viruses such as hepatitis E virus, cytomegalovirus, Epstein-Barr virus, and herpes virus are less common causes.

HEPATITIS A

Hepatitis A is a single stranded RNA virus transmitted through the oral-fecal route or person-to-person contact, particularly in the setting of poor hygiene, overcrowding, and poor sanitation. HAV exposure is almost universal in developing countries during the first decade of life. In industrialized countries, infections occur at an older age through either water-borne or food-borne exposures.

Clinical features

HAV has an incubation period of 2 to 4 weeks and can present with a wide spectrum of clinical symptoms. Silent disease (mild constitutional symptoms) may be overlooked, especially when exposure occurs at a younger age. Symptoms can range from self-limited jaundice to prolonged cholestasis (icterus, dark urine, acholic stools, pruritis) lasting 2 to 3 months. Other symptoms include arthralgias, myalgias, nausea, vomiting, abdominal pain, and fevers. Recovery occurs within 6 to 12 weeks in the majority. Although relapsing infection can occur, chronic hepatitis does not develop. Less than 1% progress to fulminant liver failure, most frequently older patients with comorbid illnesses.

Investigation

Serology is the ideal method to diagnose HAV in the setting of elevated liver enzymes. The presence of IgM-anti-HAV is diagnostic of acute hepatitis A. The IgM antibody can persist for 3 to 6 months and up to a year with relapsing infection. IgG-anti-HAV develops after vaccination or recovery from an acute infection and provides life-long immunity.

Management

Because spontaneous resolution of HAV infection is the norm, no pharmacologic intervention is indicated. Active immunization prevents acquisition of infection, and administration of HAV immunoglobulin (0.02 mL/kg) to family members or close contacts prevents transmission from known exposure.

Complications

Other than the rare cases of fulminant liver failure, there are no chronic sequelae once recovery has occurred.

HEPATITIS B

HBV is a circular, partially double stranded DNA virus that consists of an outer envelope (comprised of hepatitis B surface antigen or HBsAg) and an inner core (comprised of hepatitis B core antigen or HBcAg). There are approximately 300 million people infected with HBV worldwide. In Africa and Asia, it is spread predominantly through vertical transmission (mother-to-infant) as well as horizontally between children. Chronic infection develops in 90% of newborns and 25% of young children with HBV. In the US and Europe, HBV is associated with sexual transmission, IV drug use, blood transfusions, and needle stick injury. Chronic infection after an acute exposure develops in 5% to 10% of adults.

Clinical features

Acute HBV occurs after an incubation period of 40 to 180 days. Nonspecific constitutional symptoms including fatigue, malaise, anorexia, nausea, vomiting, abdominal pain, and fevers are common. Approximately 30% develop jaundice a week later. The vast majority recover from the acute infection, and only 5% to 10% develop chronic HBV. Chronic HBV is often an asymptomatic disease although patients may have mild nonspecific constitutional symptoms as well as abnormal liver enzymes and develop exacerbations resembling an acute infection. Fulminant hepatitis B can occur in 1% to 2% with acute HBV due to a vigorous immune response to the virus.

Investigation

Active HBV infection is documented by the presence of serum HbsAg, which develops within 2 months of exposure. Anti-HB antibody is associated with the disappearance of HBsAg and indicates recovery from acute infection. It also is seen after active immunization. Persistence of HBsAg for more than 6 months indicates chronic infection.

Acute HBV is diagnosed by the presence of IgM-anti-HBcAb, which appears 4 weeks after HBsAg. IgG-anti-HBc indicates recovery or chronicity and develops after the IgM-HBcAb disappears. Therefore, the presence IgG-HBcAb and HBsAb indicate recovery from acute HBV infection. IgG-HBcAb and HBsAg indicate chronic infection with either latent virus (chronic carrier) or actively replicating virus (chronic active). Active replication is diagnosed by the presence of HBeAg and detectable serum HBV-DNA. These markers indicate infectivity and also identify patients who are potential candidates for therapy.

Management

No pharmacologic intervention is indicated for adults, children, or infants with acute HBV as the majority will spontaneously recover. However, newborns of mothers who have chronic HBV should receive hepatitis B immunoglobulin and undergo immunization to prevent transmission.

Pharmacologic therapy is available to patients who have chronic active viral replication as indicated by the presence of HBeAg and/or serum HBV-DNA for more than 6 months. Although the presence of liver injury is important in determining therapy, liver biopsies are not always needed. The goal of treatment is to stop liver injury by either suppressing replication or eradicating the infection. In general, the loss of HBeAg and the development of HBeAb is associated with the loss of HBV-DNA, indicating biochemical and histologic remission. However, in some cases, a mutation in the HBV genome leads to the loss of HBeAg production despite active viral replication. These patients with "precore" mutations have active viral replication with detectable serum HBV-DNA despite the development of HBeAb.

Interferon α2b (IFN α 2b) has antiviral and immunomodulatory activity and has been used in the treatment of chronic HBV since 1992. The recommended dose is 5 million units SC daily for 16 weeks. The goal of therapy is sustained response with loss of detectable HBV-DNA and HbeAg, seen in 33% of patients taking IFN α 2b. Response is often associated with acute elevation of serum transaminases secondary to an effective immune-mediated clearance of the HBV infected virus, followed by normalization of biochemical and histologic parameters. Factors that predict a higher chance of successful therapy include low pretreatment serum HBV-DNA levels (less than 200 pg/mL), high ALT levels (more than 100 U/L), necroinflammation on biopsy, female sex, duration of disease less than 4 years, acquisition of infection after age 6, no concomitant HIV infection, and horizontal rather than vertical transmission. Side effects from interferon therapy are ubiquitous and include flu-like symptoms, bone marrow suppression, hypothyroidism and depression. Underlying autoimmune disease, poorly controlled depression, and severe cardiac dysfunction are contraindications for interferon use.

Lamivudine is a nucleoside analog that inhibits viral reverse transcriptase activity by competitive inhibition of nucleosides, thereby suppressing HBV-DNA levels, although DNA reappears with discontinuation. It decreases HBV replication to undetectable levels in 93% to 100% of patients within 12 weeks of starting therapy, with histologic improvement in 50% after 1 year. Lamivudine therapy is associated with loss of HbeAg in 17% to 33% and development of HBeAg in 16% to 18%. It is not effective in "precore" mutant infections. Lamivudine is administered orally at 100 mg/day for a year, but continued use may result in viral resistance in as many as 30%, rendering the drug ineffective. In contrast, resistance is not seen with interferon. Lamivudine is very well tolerated with little to no side effects. Stopping therapy can lead to flares related to the resumption of viral replication in some patients. Due to the favorable tolerability and safety profile compared with interferon, lamivudine has gained more acceptance as first-line therapy in patients with chronic HBV.

Other nucleoside analogs include famciclovir, tenofovir, and adefovir. Famciclovir inhibits HBV-DNA polymerase and suppresses viral replication, but the rate of seroconversion is lower compared with lamivudine. It also is associated with development of viral resistance. Tenofovir may be effective in patients with lamivudine resistant strains. Tenofovir and adefovir have loss of HBV-DNA and seroconversion rates similar to lamivudine, and may be effective in lamivudine resistant strains. Both are well tolerated, and no resistance has been reported with adefovir. There is no evidence that combination therapy with interferon and a nucleoside analog is more effective than either therapy alone in chronic hepatitis B.

Complications

Extrahepatic manifestations are the result of deposition of immune complexes in the microcirculation, which occurs in 15% of patients with chronic infection. Symptoms include rash, arthralgias, fevers, vasculitis, cryoglobulinemia, glomerulonephritis, aplastic anemia and possibly idiopathic thrombocytopenic purpura. Patients with chronic infection are at risk for cirrhosis and hepatocellular carcinoma.

HEPATITIS C

Hepatitis C is a single stranded RNA virus with a worldwide distribution. There are an estimated 3 million people in the US with chronic HCV, predominantly adults 30 to 50 years of age. Screening has drastically decreased transmission through blood product transfusions, and intravenous drug use is now the most common mode of transmission. Chronic HCV is prevalent in 60% to 90% of intravenous drug users. Other risk factors are hemodialysis, high risk sexual behavior, and health care workers exposed to needle-stick injuries. Sexual transmission with a monogamous partner carries a very low rate of transmission (1% to 2%).

Clinical features

The average incubation period after acute infection is 7 to 8 weeks. Patients may be asymptomatic (more than 70%) or have minor symptoms such as fatigue, malaise, and mild jaundice. The natural history of HCV infection is not yet fully defined. The chance of developing chronic HCV after acute infection is 80%. Chronic HCV is indolent in nature, with the most common complaint being fatigue. The reason why some clear the acute infection is not known but may be related to the host immune response. Approximately 20% to 25% of patients with chronic HCV develop cirrhosis. Of these, 20% develop end-stage liver disease and liver failure 10 to 20 years later, and 1% to 3% develop hepatocellular carcinoma. Chronic HCV is currently the most common indication for liver transplantation in the US.

Investigation

Screening for HCV involves antibody testing (anti-HCV antibody) using the enzyme immune assay (EIA), which tests for antigens against various structural and nonstructural viral proteins. The EIA test is sensitive in patients with known risk factors for HCV but can be insensitive in those without risk factors, in whom a subsequent confirmatory test is indicated. One such confirmatory test is the Recombinant Immuno Blot Assay (RIBA), which detects several antigens related to the HCV virus. The presence of 2 or more antigens is considered positive and confirms the presence of infection in lower risk populations.

The most definitive test for chronic HCV infection is the detection of HCV-RNA. Because of its cost, it is only used as a confirmatory test after a positive antibody result, or when the antibody test is suspected to be falsely negative in immunosuppressed patients. HCV-RNA detection also is useful in patients with recent needle stick injuries before they develop antibodies to the virus. The HCV-RNA measured by PCR can provide qualitative and quantitative information. The qualitative test is very sensitive and can effectively rule out the presence of viremia when negative. The quantitative test provides measurement of viral load and is utilized for monitoring patients on therapy. There are 6 genotypes of HCV, with genotypes 1, 2, and 3 most common in the US. Genotype determination plays an important role in determining treatment duration and success.

Elevated serum ALT levels can predict viral activity. However, normal ALT levels do not necessarily reflect quiescent disease. The best tool to determine disease activity is a liver biopsy. This can provide histologic evidence of inflammatory and fibrotic activity. Liver biopsies also play an important role in determining treatment plans.

Management

Avoidance of alcohol consumption is a very important intervention thought to be beneficial in chronic HCV. Pharmacologic therapy should be considered in patients with chronic HCV with persistent viremia lasting more than 6 months and absence of substantial fibrosis on liver biopsy.

Previously, therapy consisted of interferon alone or in combination with oral ribavirin. Ribavirin is a nucleoside analog that inhibits viral replication but also has antiviral activity. More recently, the concomitant use of ribavirin with interferon and the addition of a polyethylene glycol (PEG) moiety to the standard interferon molecule has increased the efficacy of treatment. Because of its increased size, PEG-interferon has an extended half life as it is not readily cleared by the kidneys, allowing for once a week dosing. The increased efficacy of pegylated-interferon has made combination therapy with PEG-interferon and ribavirin the treatment regimen of choice for patients with chronic HCV. After 52 weeks, there is a 54% sustained-response rate indicated by persistent clearance of viremia. Patients with genotype 1 HCV infection (the most common) require 52 weeks of treatment with a sustained-response rate of 42%. Patients with genotype 2 and 3 require 26 weeks of treatment and have an 80% sustained-response rate. Limited studies on a few of the other genotypes indicate that they respond in a fashion similar to genotype 1. Patients not responding to pegylated interferon and ribavirin at 12 weeks are unlikely to achieve a response, and discontinuation of thearpy should be considered.

Patients with well-compensated cirrhosis have a lower response rate compared with those with mild to moderate fibrosis. Patients treated unsuccessfully in the past with standard interferon monotherapy or combination standard interferon and ribavirin tend to have lower sustained response rates as well. Interferon α-2b is available in the US and Europe, while interferon α-2a is still awaiting approval in the US. The optimal dose of PEG-interferon has not yet been determined. Side effects with PEG-interferon are similar to standard interferon, with similar rates of bone marrow suppression, psychiatric side effects and worsening of underlying cardiomyopathy. The dose needs to be adjusted for renal failure.

Ribavirin is well tolerated and is administered orally either by weight-base dosing (10.6 mg/kg/day) or 800 to 1200 mg/day. There is a significant association with hemolytic anemia, which is dose dependent. Patients also need to have their blood counts monitored on therapy and have their dose adjusted if significant anemia occurs. Ribavirin is contraindicated in patients with severe coronary artery disease and/or severe pulmonary disease, chronic renal failure, and pregnancy. Male and female patients of child-bearing age must practice some form of contraception while they are on treatment. If ribavirin cannot be used, PEG-interferon monotherapy can be used with a lower rate of response (40% after 52 weeks).

Complications

Chronic HCV is associated with immune-mediated extrahepatic manifestations. Mixed cryoglobulinemia develops from the deposition of viral-immunoglobulin complexes that lead to small vessel damage. Joint pain, rashes, and renal failure can occur. Membranous glomerulonephritis, porphyria cutanea tarda, and nonHodgkin lymphoma are other illness associated with chronic HCV infection. Treating the underlying HCV infection can frequently lead to the resolution of some of these other extrahepatic diseases.

DRUG-INDUCED LIVER DISEASE

The incidence of drug-induced hepatotoxicity has been increasing because of the greater number of available medications. Drug-induced liver disease is very common in the elderly and in hospitalized patients. Hepatotoxicity can occur from either direct or immune-mediate mechanisms of injury. Detoxification of medications through either the cytochrome P450 system or conjugation produces toxic by-products. Drugs or their metabolites can cause direct hepatocyte damage by altering plasma cell membranes, cellular enzyme activity, or mitochondrial function. Immune-mediate injury occurs when the drug or its metabolites induce a host immune response and cause hepatocyte damage from the production of inflammatory mediators.

Drug hepatotoxicity can be either intrinsic or idiosyncratic in nature. Intrinsic hepatotoxicity is predictable and uniform in presentation and is dose-dependent. Close serum drug monitoring is often required. In idiosyncratic reactions, the damage is variable and unpredictable and not dose-dependent.

Clinical features

Drug-induced hepatotoxicity is frequently either mild or subclinical. On less frequent occasions, the presentation can be severe, and medication use accounts for up to 25% of cases of fulminant hepatic failure. Chronic liver disease can develop in patients who are continuously or repeatedly exposed to the offending agent. The 2 patterns of drug hepatotoxicity are the following: 1) hepatitis (elevated transaminases) and 2) cholestasis (elevated bilirubin and alkaline phosphatase), although a mixed pattern can develop at times. In both cases, complete hepatic recovery can occur within 6 months of having the medication discontinued.

Elevations in serum transaminases are typically mild and are found frequently in asymptomatic patients. These abnormalities are seen a few days after the initiation of therapy and usually resolve without any residual effect. When transaminase elevations are significant, the patients are usually no longer asymptomatic. They may develop fatigue, myalgias, and rash as a result of the underlying hepatocyte damage. On very rare occasions, progressive hepatocyte damage can lead to hepatic failure and/or death from submassive necrosis.

Drug-induced cholestasis occurs with the development of elevated serum bilirubin, alkaline phosphatase, and gamma-glutamyl transpeptidase. Patients can be either asymptomatic or develop jaundice, fevers, arthropathy, myalgias, and rash. A bland cholestasis is seen when clinical jaundice develops without the associated systemic symptoms. Hepatic necrosis does not develop with cholestatic drug reactions and complete recovery will occur after the offending medication has been removed.

Hepatic congestion resulting from veno-occlusive disease is a rare presentation of drug toxicity. The damage to the small hepatic venules from the use of antineoplastic agents leads to significantly abnormal hepatic blood flow. Patients can develop symptoms of ascites, abdominal pain, and hepatomegaly. The course is variable with definitive treatment available.

Investigation

The key to the diagnosis of drug-induced hepatotoxicity is careful history taking. Once a timeline of symptoms and any new medications or overdoses is established, appropriate therapy can be initiated. Liver biopsy can be helpful at times, as there may be evidence of eosinophil infiltration or cholestasis typical of certain medication reactions. However, the histologic findings can be very nonspecific as well. A right upper quadrant ultrasound to rule out obstruction and viral hepatitis serologies are helpful in ruling out other causes of elevated transaminases or cholestasis.

Management

Most cases of drug-induced hepatotoxicity do not require any specific intervention other than identifying and removing the causative agent. If hepatotoxicity progresses to the point of hepatic failure, liver transplantation may be the only life-saving intervention available. The use of antidotes has been proven to be effective in the management of acetaminophen toxicity. N-acetylcysteine (NAC) is potentially life saving when administered early. The usual hepatotoxic dose of acetaminophen is 10 to 15 g. Early recognition of acetaminophen toxicity can lead to a 95% survival if treated with NAC within 24 hours of acute ingestion. NAC repletes serum glutathione that has been used to detoxify the hepatotoxic metabolite of acetaminophen, N-acetyl-p-benzoquinone imine. This toxic metabolite is produced from the metabolism of acetaminophen through the cytochrome P450 system. By replenishing glutathione, subsequent tissue hypoxia and damage can be averted, and hepatocyte recovery can proceed without sequelae.

Complications

Because liver function recovers completely after hepatotoxicity has resolved, long-term complications do not occur except in rare cases where chronic liver disease develops. As mentioned above, fulminant hepatic failure can occur as a rare complication.

FULMINANT HEPATIC FAILURE

Acute liver failure may develop in patients with no history of underlying chronic liver disease. The hallmark of fulminant hepatic failure (FHF) is the rapid development of encephalopathy and coagulopathy within 8 weeks after the onset of illness or within 2 weeks after the onset of jaundice. Over 50% of cases of fulminant hepatic failure in the U.S. are due to drug or supplement toxicity, with acetaminophen being the most common medication. Acute hepatitis B, acute hepatitis A, autoimmune hepatitis, Wilson disease, ischemic hepatic injury, and pregnancy-related diseases (acute fatty liver of pregnancy, HELLP [hemolysis, elevated liver enzymes, low platelets]) are other less common causes of FHF. Women appear to develop FHF more frequently than men.

When acute hepatic failure occurs, manifestations are multisystemic and dramatic. Because of the life-threatening nature of this disease process, rapid evaluation and aggressive supportive care are imperative. Timely transfer to a liver transplant center is also crucial. For many of these patients, liver transplantation is the only available cure but only 40% of patients at liver transplant centers receive a transplant. Without transplantation, only 25 % of patients will survive with supportive care alone. The 1-year survival after transplantation is 75%, and the overall prognosis depends on the cause of liver failure.

Clinical features

Prognostic factors have been proposed to help determine outcome and identify those who would benefit from liver transplantation. The King's Hospital criteria and the Acute Physiology and Chronic Health Evaluation (APACHE) II are commonly used but may not be as reliable as once thought. The common clinical features of FHF are hepatic encphalopathy, cerebral edema, coagulopathy, cardiac failure, respiratory failure, renal failure, and sepsis.

Hepatic encephalopathy and cerebral edema affect patients with FHF to a varying degree. The spectrum ranges from subclinical confusion (Grade 0) to coma (Grade 4). The progression to worsening encephalopathy can be very rapid. The most feared complication of cerebral edema is brainstem herniation and immediate death. Because of unrecognized factors, cerebral edema develops as water accumulates in the brain cells. As a result, cerebral perfusion is greatly compromised and subsequent herniation can occur. Severe coagulopathy can develop as hepatocyte function is lost during FHF. Because the proteins required for effective blood clotting are produced by the liver, hepatocyte loss leads to ineffective coagulation. As a result, intracranial, GI, pulmonary or other vital organ hemorrhage may develop spontaneously. Cardiovascular complications caused by increased cardiac output, decreased peripheral oxygen extraction, and decreased peripheral vascular resistance are commonly seen in FHF. Pulmonary failure results from cardiogenic or noncardiogenic pulmonary edema, pneumonia, or intra-alveolar hemorrhage. Renal failure is a poor prognostic indicator and may develop from direct nephrotoxicity (acetaminophen), hypotension, or the underlying liver disease itself (hepatorenal syndrome). The metabolic abnormalities that arise from acute renal failure further complicate management. Lactic acidosis and sepsis can develop due to persistent hypoperfusion and a severely compromised immune system, respectively. The most common sources of infection are the lungs, the urinary tract, and the skin. Multisystem organ failure may eventually develop despite aggressive supportive care, and patients will no longer be eligible for transplant once this occurs.

Investigation

The most important initial evaluation of patients who develop FHF is a thorough history. Investigation should be aimed at finding any potential medications that may have been taken as well as the amount. The timing of symptoms is also important, as this may predict the rate of progression of liver failure. Any history of sick contacts or travel may be indicative of a viral etiology. Once the cause of the hepatic failure has been determined, the subsequent work up should concentrate on the extent of organ failure present and the need to monitor any progression. Close monitoring of mental status for signs of progressive encephalopathy is very important. Adequate evaluation is best performed by avoiding sedatives and neuromuscular blocking agents, if possible. The development of hyperreflexia, pupillary changes, and sudden signs of systemic hypertension can indicate impending brain stem herniation. Unfortunately, clinical signs of neurologic impairment may present too late in the course of cerebral edema. Computed tomography can help if there is a sudden change in mental status in order to rule out intracranial hemorrhage. Intracranial pressure monitors (ICP) can be placed to determine cerebral perfusion pressures by subtracting the intracranial pressures from the mean arterial pressures. Cerebral perfusion should be maintained at 40 mm Hg in order to minimize neurologic damage. ICP monitors are associated with significant risk because of the underlying coagulopathy present in the setting of FHF. As a result, the significant risks of bleeding and infection associated with ICP monitors limit their routine use, and they are not currently felt to be imperative. A central venous catheter or pulmonary artery catheter can help determine volume status, cardiac function, and renal function. Urine output can help determine whether oliguric (less than 300 mL/day) renal failure has developed.

Management

Patients with low-grade encephalopathy should be treated with lactulose and/or neomycin. Despite these interventions, progressive encephalopathy may ensue and intubation may be required. Elevating the head of the bed 30 degrees can help by improving cerebral venous drainage. Hyperventilation (goal PCO2 25 to 30 mm Hg) also may help by inducing intracranial vasoconstriction and lowering pressures. Mannitol (100 mL of 20% solution given IV at 0.5 to 1 mg/kg) can osmotically draw water from brain cells and reduce pressures as well. Using corticosteroids or decreasing cerebral metabolism (hypothermia or barbiturates) has been shown to be of limited benefit. Administration of vitamin K may help the underlying coagulopathy if there is an associated vitamin K deficiency. Fresh frozen plasma and platelets are helpful only in the setting of active bleeding. Hypotension may be treated with vasoactive medications (eg, dopamine, norepinephrine), but their use is associated with a poor outcome. Supplemental oxygen and intubation are frequently required because of hypoxemia and the obtunded patient's inability to protect his/her airway. Renal failure requires close monitoring and management of volume status, serum creatinine, electrolytes, and urine output, as well as avoiding nephrotoxic medications. Hemodialysis can be offered as a supportive modality in some cases. If sepsis is suspected, blood cultures should be obtained and broad-spectrum antibiotics should be initiated.

In some cases of FHF, treatment is available beyond supportive care. In cases of mushroom toxicity, antidotes are available. In pregnancy-related liver failure, inducing delivery is therapeutic if performed in a timely fashion. Acetaminophen overdose can be treated with N-acetylcysteine as described in the previous section "Drug-Induced Liver Disease." Liver transplant offered in a timely fashion is curative. Because of the shortage of cadaveric liver donors, studies are underway to investigate the use of living donors as well as bioartificial liver-assist devices that consist of human or porcine hepatocyte cultures. Some of these supportive modalities may ultimately provide an effective bridge to transplantation. It is too premature to determine if these interventions will have any clinical applicability.

Complications

Complications discussed above include coagulopathy and hemorrhage into vital organs, cardiac failure, pulmonary failure, hepatorenal syndrome, sepsis, cerebral herniation, multiorgan failure, and death. Persistent neurologic deficits can be present after transplant and/or recovery if significant brain damage occurred. Recovery of other organ function is variable. Unfortunately, mortality rates remain high despite the best supportive care available.

CHAPTER 5

CIRRHOSIS AND END-STAGE LIVER DISEASE

CIRRHOSIS

Cirrhosis is characterized by irreversible pathological changes from repeated hepatocyte destruction and regeneration, with connective tissue deposition that results in irreversible scarring leading to abnormal hepatic architecture, blood flow, and function. Abnormal architecture manifests as nodularity, while abnormal blood flow increases the resistance of portal blood flow leading to portal hypertension. Hepatocyte dysfunction can be metabolic or excretory. Metabolic dysfunction presents as hypoalbuminemia leading to ascites and edema, clotting abnormalities such as an elevated prothrombin time and thrombocytopenia, and ineffective mobilization of hepatic glycogen stores resulting in hypoglycemia. Excretory dysfunction presents as jaundice caused by abnormal bilirubin excretion, itching due to poor bile salt excretion, and encephalopathy caused by abnormal detoxification of endogenous products. Other complications of cirrhosis are life-threatening variceal bleeding caused by portal hypertension, spontaneous bacterial peritonitis caused by infection of ascitic fluid, gynecomastia and cutaneous changes (spider nevi, palmar erythema) caused by abnormal estrogen breakdown, and hepatocellular carcinoma.

Hepatorenal syndrome occurs in advanced end-stage liver disease and is associated with a high mortality. Abnormal arterial circulation and systemic vasoactive substance activity present in end-stage cirrhosis can lead to oliguric renal failure without underlying renal disease. Hepatorenal syndrome can develop over a period of hours to days and is associated with a median survival of only 2 weeks. Patients can be supported with hemodialysis but can only be cured with liver transplantation.

Etiologies of cirrhosis are numerous, but the most common causes are alcohol use/abuse, chronic viral hepatitis, chronic autoimmune hepatitis, chronic biliary damage, and genetic diseases related to abnormal hepatocyte metabolism. The course of cirrhosis is variable and treatment options are limited once end-stage disease occurs.

Although liver transplantation is the best cure available, many patients die while still on the waiting list.

ASCITES

Ascites is the increased accumulation of fluid in the peritoneum frequently caused by underlying liver disease. Abnormal reabsorption of lymph caused by hypoalbuminemia and portal hypertension occurs in conjunction with increased renal sodium absorption because of arterial vasodilation and decreased glomerular perfusion, promoting accumulation of fluid in the peritoneal space. This, in turn, leads to intravascular volume depletion and further sodium reabsorption. Abnormal levels of vasoactive substances such as angiotensin, vasopressin, and antidiuretic hormone further exacerbate ascites accumulation. As the underlying liver disease progresses, these abnormalities are exacerbated leading to further fluid accumulation. In fact, the development of ascites is an indicator of decompensated cirrhosis and predicts higher mortality.

Clinical features

Although frequently caused by underlying liver disease, ascites also can develop in patients with heart failure, renal failure, malignancy, or intra-abdominal infection. Clinically significant ascites can be barely detectable, although most patients present with significant abdominal distension. Portal hypertension is an integral factor in the development of ascites and primarily is due to abnormal portal venous return to the heart. The abnormal portal venous return seen in liver disease can be prehepatic (portal vein thrombosis), intrahepatic (cirrhosis) or posthepatic (Budd-Chiari syndrome, veno-occlusive disease).

Investigation

Ascites can often be readily identified on physical examination. In patients with a minimal amount of ascites or in the obese, ultrasonography may be needed to identify ascites. In new onset ascites, albumin level, cell count with differential, and cultures are performed on ascitic fluid obtained after paracentesis to determine the cause. Cytology, amylase, and triglyceride levels also can be obtained if clinically indicated. The serum-ascites albumin gradient (SAAG) is calculated by subtracting the albumin value in ascitic fluid from the serum albumin.

A SAAG greater than 1.1 indicates the ascites is due to portal hypertension. If the SAAG is less than 1.1, other causes of ascites accumulation such as heart failure, malignancy, or intra-abdominal inflammation are more likely. The fluid can be bloody from malignancy or tuberculosis. An elevated white cell count suggests peritonitis.

Management

Initial therapy for ascites involves dietary sodium restriction to 500 mg/day. Free water restriction is not indicated unless there is evidence of hyponatremia. Sodium restriction is combined with diuretic therapy, which is the mainstay of treatment for persistent ascites. Diuretics that act on the distal nephron and/or loop of Henle are preferred because these are the sites of avid sodium retention in cirrhotic patients. The potassium-sparing aldosterone antagonists (spironolactone, amiloride, triamterene) target the distal nephron and impair sodium reabsorption. Spironolactone is very effective, but its use is associated with hyperkalemia and painful gynecomastia. The addition of loop diuretics (furosemide, bumetanide) is an important adjunct to therapy as it targets another segment of the nephron. Although furosemide is an effective diuretic, it is not very effective in managing ascites when used alone. Patients on diuretics need to have their electrolytes and renal function monitored.

Large volume paracentesis (LVP) can remove a significant amount of ascitic fluid (4 to 10 L) in patients whom are refractory to medical therapy. Patients with respiratory compromise from ascites frequently require LVP. The use of albumin in the setting of LVP is somewhat controversial because of its short half-life and high cost. However, intravenous albumin infusion (6 to 8 g/L removed) can lower the incidence of hypotension and renal impairment and may be particularly useful in renal insufficiency, hyponatremia, or bacterial peritonitis, and progressive protein depletion due to multiple LVPs.

A transjugular intrahepatic portosystemic shunt (TIPS) is a potential option for patients who have failed medical therapy and repeated LVP. Although surgical portosystemic shunts are effective, their use is limited because of the risks of surgical intervention in patients with advanced liver disease. TIPS can effectively relieve the underlying portal hypertension by providing a conduit for the portal venous blood flow through the liver. Because of the subsequent bypassing of the liver, hepatic encephalopathy can occur but is usually readily treatable.

Because shunt stenosis is a frequent occurrence (30% over 1 year), follow up Doppler ultrasound imaging is required to help monitor shunt patency. TIPS is contraindicated in patients with untreated infections and those with severe liver failure because of the risk of precipitating further hepatic decompensation.

Complications

As the ascites worsens, patients can develop shortness of breath because of impaired ventilation. The respiratory compromise can either occur from increased intra-abdominal pressure or the development of pleural effusions as a result of ascites. Abdominal pain, anorexia, and umbilical hernias, which run the added risk of causing an acute intestinal strangulation, can also develop. The most serious complication of ascites is the development of spontaneous bacterial peritonitis.

SPONTANEOUS BACTERIAL PERITONITIS

Because of the low protein levels in cirrhotic ascites, bacterial infections can develop and result in spontaneous bacterial peritonitis (SBP). The low level of bacterial opsins in the ascites is felt to promote susceptibility to infections.

Clinical features

Many patients will have abdominal pain, fevers, and/or encephalopathy. However, SBP can be easily missed because some patients have very subtle symptoms or no symptoms at all. Up to 30% of patients with ascites who are admitted to the hospital for any indication have clinical or subclinical SBP. Timely intervention is important in patients with SBP given the high mortality (up to 70%) related to the acute infection.

Investigation

A diagnostic paracentesis is required to diagnose SBP. Any patient with new onset ascites or a patient with cirrhosis requiring hospitalization or developing clinical deterioration should be evaluated for SBP. Ascitic fluid should be sent for a cell count with differential as well as cultured in blood culture bottles. Although blood culture bottles can significantly increase the yield of isolating an organism, less than 50%

of cultures are positive. Therefore, the cell count is much more helpful as it provides an immediate, reliable result. If the ascitic fluid has a polymorphonuclear (PMN) count of greater than 250 cells/mm^3, a leukocyte count of greater than 500 cells/mm^3, and/or positive cultures, the diagnosis of SBP can be made.

Management

Antibiotic therapy is the only treatment for SBP. The most common organisms that cause SBP are gram-negative bacteria, and adequate coverage should be initiated as soon as possible. *Escherichia coli* and *Klebsiella* account for 55% of the organisms that cause SBP. Other gram-positive and anaerobic organisms comprise another 25% of cases. If more than 1 organism is identified, the possibility of secondary bacterial peritonitis because of intra-abdominal infection or perforation needs to be strongly considered. The ideal antibiotic should have gram-negative and enteric organism coverage without nephrotoxicity. Intravenous third generation cephalosporins, ampicillin/sulbactam, or ciprofloxacin are very effective therapies. Aminoglycosides should be avoided. Intravenous therapy needs to be administered for 5 days and follow up paracentesis is indicated only when patients are not responding to therapy. If patients are not responding, antibiotic coverage should be broadened.

Complications

Because of the risk of precipitating acute renal failure, renal perfusion should be optimized. Avoidance of diuretics and/or large volume paracentesis is important during the acute infection period. Intravenous albumin (1.5 g/kg on day 1, 1 g/kg on days 2 and 3) can help maintain renal perfusion in some cases as well.

Because patients who survive the initial episode of SBP have a 70% chance of recurrent infection, secondary prophylaxis is frequently used. Patients should be maintained on prophylactic therapy after their first episode using a quinolone daily or trimethoprim-sulfamethoxazole every other day. There is no clear role for primary antibiotic prophylaxis against an initial infection other than in patients with upper GI bleeding or those with very low ascites protein levels. Patients with ascites who develop an acute gastrointestinal bleed should be evaluated for SBP and treated empirically to prevent infection.

The median survival for patients who develop their first episode of SBP is 9 months. These patients should be considered for transplantation following successful treatment of infection if they are potential candidates.

HEPATIC ENCEPHALOPATHY

Chronic portosystemic encephalopathy develops as hepatic function deteriorates. Encephalopathy results from the inability to remove certain toxins that affect CNS function because of the development of portosystemic collaterals that effectively bypass the liver. The failure to detoxify these endogenous compounds is the underlying cause of encephalopathy. However, no specific toxin or toxic byproduct has been identified as the causative agent.

Clinical features

Encephalopathy can present with a wide variety of presentations. It can range from very mild behavioral or sleep pattern disturbances to frank confusion or obtundation. Its course can also wax and wane. Encephalopathy can be precipitated by acute events such as increased nitrogen load (GI bleeding, excess dietary intake, azotemia, constipation), infection (SBP, pneumonia, urinary tract infection), electrolyte abnormalities, medications (narcotics, sedatives, diuretics), or progression of underlying liver disease.

Investigation

Identifying the precipitating event is the key to treating encephalopathy. Metabolic abnormalities, hypovolemia, bleeding, infection, or medical noncompliance should be investigated and treated as soon as possible. Although serum ammonia levels are frequently used as a marker for encephalopathy, they are not very reliable in following clinical symptoms.

Management

After the precipitating event has been treated, much of the therapy for encephalopathy is targeted at decreasing endogenous nitrogen production and nitrogen delivery to the liver. Excess dietary protein intake should be avoided, as should severe protein restriction due to the catabolic effects of protein avoidance on chronic liver disease. Lactulose is frequently the initial treatment for patients with encephalopathy. Lactulose is a non-absorbable, disaccharide that creates an osmotic diarrhea as well as an acidic colonic environment. The overall effect of lactulose is to decrease the amount of nitrogen absorbed from the colon. The dose can be titrated to produce 3 to 4 loose stools a day. For patients who become refractory to lactulose, neomycin can help with management. Neomycin (500 to 1000 mg twice daily) is a minimally absorbed antibiotic that alters colonic bacterial flora and reduces nitrogen production, but chronic exposure may result in ototoxicity. Metronidazole also can be used as an adjunct to lactulose therapy.

Complications

Successful treatment of encephalopathy rarely is associated with complications. Neomycin is associated with ototoxicity as well as renal failure, and its chronic use should be avoided in patients, especially those with renal insufficiency. Long-term metronidazole use is associated with peripheral neurotoxicity. Intractable encephalopathy despite aggressive medical therapy is an indication for transplantation.

VARICEAL BLEEDING

Variceal bleeding is a life-threatening complication of portal hypertension seen in patients with cirrhosis. Bleeding can occur spontaneously from esophageal or gastric varices that develop from increased portal venous pressures. Approximately 40% of patients with cirrhosis will suffer from a variceal bleed, and the bleeding episode itself is associated with 30% to 50% mortality. Prompt recognition and treatment are key interventions in managing patients with acute variceal bleeding. Because two thirds of patients with an initial variceal bleed will have recurrent bleeding, prevention of the initial and recurrent bleeding episodes is of utmost importance.

Clinical features

Patients with variceal bleeding will present with symptoms consistent with a rapid, large volume upper GI bleed. Gross hematemesis and melena are frequent presenting symptoms. However, patients may not develop hematemesis but may present with only melena or hematochezia if bleeding is brisk. Patients usually become hypotensive and tachycardic and can develop syncope or presyncope, depending on the degree of bleeding. Variceal bleeding also can present with an acute worsening of encephalopathy. Patients with signs or symptoms of chronic liver disease and portal hypertension, such as jaundice, ascites, spider angiomas, thrombocytopenia, or encephalopathy, in the setting of GI bleeding should be suspected of having a variceal bleed.

Investigation

Determining the rate and amount of blood loss are important factors in investigating patients who present with upper GI bleeding. The degree of hemodynamic instability is a reliable marker for assessing the extent of blood loss. A nasogastric tube lavage helps determine if bleeding is brisk or ongoing. Patients should have a complete blood count and clotting times measured to determine if any platelets or fresh frozen plasma are required to help control the bleeding.

Management

The patient with a variceal bleed needs to be rapidly evaluated, stabilized, and treated. Establishment of venous access and initiation of aggressive volume resuscitation with normal saline or packed red blood cells should be the first steps in treatment. Patients can be admitted to the intensive care unit once hemodynamic stability has been achieved. Thrombocytopenia or coagulopathy should be corrected with platelet and/or fresh frozen plasma administration. Protective intubation to prevent pulmonary aspiration may be needed in some cases if the bleeding is massive.

The somatostatin analog, octreotide, also should be started as soon as intravenous access has been established. Octreotide effectively decreases splanchnic blood flow and thereby rapidly decreases portal venous pressures. Octreotide is administered IV with a 50 to 100 mcg bolus followed by a continuous drip at 50 mcg/hr. Octreotide is most effective in the initial 24 to 48 hours of use and has no systemic effects. Intravenous vasopressin also can help decrease portal venous pressures in a fashion similar to octreotide. However, vasopressin use has fallen out of favor because of the rather significant and at times fatal systemic side effects such as cardiac ischemia associated with its use. Acid suppression has no proven benefit in treating an acute variceal bleed. Endoscopic therapy is the preferred intervention in controlling acute variceal bleeding. Endoscopic variceal band ligation (EVL) or sclerotherapy can control bleeding in the majority of cases. EVL involves placement of rubber bands on the varices that inhibit blood flow and promote thrombosis, thereby leading to the obliteration of the varices. EVL is associated with significantly less complications when compared with sclerotherapy, which involves injecting an irritating sclerosant into the bleeding varices that subsequently leads to thrombosis and scarring. Because of the inflammatory response seen with the use of sclerosants, patients may develop chest pain, fevers, esophageal ulcers, strictures, or perforations. In cases that are refractory to endoscopic therapy, other interventions such as balloon tamponade, surgical portosystemic shunting, or transjugular intrahepatic portosystemic shunting (TIPS) are required. TIPS has become the preferred intervention in these cases because of the high mortality associated with balloon tamponade and surgical intervention. TIPS is also the only definitive treatment for gastric variceal bleeding.

Prevention of the initial (primary) or recurrent (secondary) variceal bleeding episode relies on treatment aimed at reducing portal pressures and obliterating the varices. Nonselective beta-blocker therapy with or without nitrates can be effective medical therapy for primary and secondary prophylaxis. Propranolol (20 mg PO BID) can be titrated up to a dose that decreases the resting heart rate. Oral nitrates also can be used but are sometimes limited by their side effects (headaches, hypotension). Elective endoscopic obliterative therapy in conjunction with medical therapy is effective as secondary prophylaxis and may be helpful for primary prophylaxis, as well. TIPS placement is effective in patients who have failed medical and endoscopic therapy for their varices.

Complications

Patients with ascites can develop SBP in the setting of an acute variceal bleed. Significant bleeding also can lead to acute renal failure in some cases. The major complications for those who survive a variceal bleeding episode are recurrent bleeding and death. One year mortality after an initial bleeding episode is 40% to 50%. As a result, patients should be referred for transplantation if they are candidates.

CHAPTER 6

CHOLESTATIC, AUTOIMMUNE, AND METABOLIC LIVER DISORDERS

PRIMARY BILIARY CIRRHOSIS

Primary biliary cirrhosis (PBC) is an autoimmune liver disease that results from destruction of the small intrahepatic bile ducts. Persistent damage to the small bile ducts leads to impaired biliary drainage and cholestasis. PBC is a common cause of chronic liver disease and a frequent indication for liver transplantation. The estimated prevalence of the disease is 2 to 24 per 100,000 people, mostly of Western European origin. Although the exact etiology of PBC is unknown, an abnormal immune response to environmental factors is thought to precipitate the disease. Family studies indicate that PBC occurs at a higher rate between related individuals when compared with the general population. This suggests a strong role for genetic susceptibility to unknown triggering event(s).

Clinical features

Women constitute 90% of the patient population with PBC. There is also an increased incidence of other autoimmune diseases such as Sjogren syndrome, sicca syndrome, systemic lupus erythematosus, and myasthenia gravis. Patients with PBC display a wide spectrum of symptoms depending on the stage of the disease. Early symptoms may include fatigue, severe itching, abdominal pain, and mild jaundice. As the disease progresses, the jaundice may worsen and signs and symptoms of cirrhosis or liver failure may develop. The rate of progression of PBC is extremely variable with no markers available to help predict the course of the disease. The development of significant jaundice and liver failure are poor prognostic indicators.

Investigation

Hepatic transaminases reflect a cholestatic pattern with predominantly elevated serum alkaline phophatase and total bilirubin levels.

As the disease progresses, other laboratory abnormalities consistent with cirrhosis, such as low serum albumin and elevated prothrombin time, may develop. The diagnosis of PBC can be made by the presence of antimitochondrial antibody (AMA). AMA is targeted against mitochondrial enzymes such as pyruvate dehydrogenase but is not directly responsible for the bile duct damage. Approximately 95% of patients with PBC are positive for AMA, with the remainder having "AMA-negative PBC" or autoimmune cholangiopathy. Despite its name, not all patients with PBC have cirrhosis. Therefore, a liver biopsy is often helpful in diagnosing and staging the disease. Liver biopsy may have classic findings of bile duct destruction and granulomas in the early stages. With worsening disease, liver biopsy can reveal significant fibrosis and possibly cirrhosis. Liver biopsies are staged from I to IV depending on the histologic findings and the disease activity. Stage IV PBC is consistent with cirrhosis and associated with a poorer prognosis.

Management

No definitive cure for PBC has been discovered. However, the use of urso dexoycholic acid (UDCA) has been shown to slow disease progression. The accumulation of intrahepatic bile is thought to contribute to hepatic injury. UDCA is a water-soluble bile acid that increases the solubility of intrahepatic bile and leads to decreased hepatic damage caused by improved bile flow. UDCA can be dosed at 8 to 10 mg/kg and is associated with very little side effects. Methotrexate has been used in the treatment of PBC and its efficacy has yet to be elucidated.

The exact cause of the severe pruritis seen in PBC is also not clear. Treatment targeted at decreasing bile acids has proven to be effective. UDCA can help patients with mild itching. Bile acid binding resins, such as cholestyramine, have a variable effect on symptoms. As the pruritis worsens, the treatment options become more limited. Rifampin and naltrexone are used in refractory cases with variable success. Once cirrhosis and its complications develop, liver transplant is the only curative intervention. Recent evidence has shown that PBC can recur in approximately 20% to 25% of the transplanted livers.

Complications

The complications seen in PBC are frequently the result of cholestasis. Impaired bile flow can lead to steatorrhea and subsequent fat malabsorption. As a result, fat soluble vitamin (A, D, E, K) deficiency and their sequelae develop. There is also a very high prevalence of hypercholesterolemia (over 50%) in patients with PBC as a result of the cholestasis. Patients can form xanthelasmas that are seen on physical examination around the eyes and extensor tendon surfaces. Despite the elevated total cholesterol levels, patients with PBC are not at increased risk of coronary artery disease because of higher HDL levels (good cholesterol) and relatively lower LDL levels (bad cholesterol). Osteoporosis is also a frequent complication of PBC. Osteomalacia from vitamin D deficiency also occurs but is less common. Renal tubular acidosis develops in 30% of patients with PBC possibly because of reduced excretion of hepatic agents (copper, bile acid) that accumulate in the distal tubules and impair their function. The complications of cirrhosis also develop with severe PBC. Patients can develop portal hypertension with the associated complications of variceal bleeding and ascites. Hepatocellular carcinoma also can occur but at a much lower incidence than in other forms of chronic liver disease.

PRIMARY SCLEROSING CHOLANGITIS

Primary sclerosing cholangitis (PSC) is a cholestatic liver disease that involves progressive destruction of the intrahepatic and extrahepatic bile ducts. The damage is characterized as an obliterative fibrosis that can lead to cirrhosis with an indolent and variable course. The cause of PSC is not known, but there is thought that the disease process may be immune mediated. The fact that PSC is closely associated with inflammatory bowel disease (IBD), especially ulcerative colitis, suggests that inflammatory mediators may play an important role in pathogenesis. The increased awareness of the link between PSC and IBD has led to more aggressive screening and diagnosis of PSC. The estimated prevalence of PSC in the US is 1 to 6 per 100,000 people, with a higher incidence in patients with IBD. At least 70% of patients with PSC have ulcerative colitis. PSC can occur in all races and in any age group. Approximately two thirds of the patients are men, and most are young with the mean age at diagnosis being 32 to 42 years of age. The reason why young men appear to be most affected is not clear.

Clinical features

Patients who are symptomatic usually develop fatigue, pruritis, abdominal pain, or jaundice. Fevers related to cholangitis can occur if an intrahepatic stricture impairs biliary flow and sets up a nidus for infection. However, many patients can be asymptomatic and have abnormal liver enzymes or a history of concomitant IBD. In patients with IBD, the course of PSC progression does not parallel the underlying colitis activity. In some cases, PSC can present with complications related to cirrhosis such as variceal bleeding, ascites, or encephalopathy. These patients need to be considered for liver transplant. Patients with PSC are also at increased risk of developing cholangiocarcinoma and can present with symptoms ranging from nonspecific complaints to acute decompensation of liver disease. The estimated mean time from diagnosis of PSC to death or liver transplant is 12 years.

Investigation

The diagnosis of PSC is based on cholangiographic findings on endoscopic retrograde cholangiopancreatogram (ERCP). Recent advances in magnetic resonance imaging have lead to the increased use of magnetic resonance cholangiopancreatography (MRCP) as a diagnostic tool. The finding of multiple, small intrahepatic, and extrahepatic duct strictures are characteristic of the disease. If a large dominant stricture is present, there may be focal dilation of the biliary tree related to poor drainage. A liver biopsy can be helpful but is usually nondiagnostic. The biopsy may show evidence of biliary obstruction indicated by bile duct proliferation. The classic finding of concentric fibrosis (onion-skinning) around the intrahepatic ducts is not always present. There are no markers for the rate of disease progression or the risk of developing cholangiocarcinoma. Patients with PSC should be followed with annual imaging of the hepatic parenchyma and bile ducts to monitor disease progression and evaluate any lesions suggestive of malignancy. Biannual or annual assessment of tumor markers for cholangiocarcinoma (carcinoembryonic antigen, CA 19-9) and hepatocellular carcinoma (alphafeto protein) should be performed.

Management

Nonpharmacological management is focused on correcting any symptomatic and dominant stricture that may be present. Because a focal stricture presents with obstructive symptoms (fever, pain, jaundice), an ERCP can be performed as a therapeutic intervention in this case. Through balloon dilation and subsequent placement of a stent across the stricture, the obstruction can be effectively relieved. There is evidence that resolving the obstructive process in PSC may slow down disease progression. Unfortunately, the small peripheral strictures are not amenable to therapy. In cases with cholangitis, adequate drainage and antibiotic therapy are life-saving interventions. Because cholangiocarcinoma can often present as a focal stricture, tissue diagnosis can be attempted by obtaining brushings during ERCP.

There is no medical therapy available to cure PSC. The use of anti-inflammatory agents such as methotrexate and steroids has not been shown to be beneficial. Studies have indicated that urso deoxycholic acid (UDCA) (10 to 15 mg/kg/day) can improve liver biochemistries but not necessarily halt the progression of liver damage. Because of the relatively safe side effect profile of UDCA, it is used frequently despite the lack of evidence that it clearly prevents complications or death related to cirrhosis. The only curative intervention for PSC is liver transplantation. PSC has been noted to recur in 20% to 25% of transplanted livers. Because many patients with PSC have IBD, they should undergo colonoscopy for colon cancer screening as indicated.

Complications

Complications of cholestatic liver disease similar to PBC can develop in PSC. Fat-soluble vitamin deficiency, steatorrhea, and osteoporosis are common. Episodes of recurrent cholangitis can be life threatening and eventually lead to further stricturing and hepatic damage. Patients who have cirrhosis in the setting of PSC are at risk for developing the usual complications of end-stage liver disease. The most feared complication of PSC is the development of cholangiocarcinoma. Cholangiocarcinoma is associated with a very poor prognosis as there are no curative interventions available unless diagnosed very early. The diagnosis of cholangiocarcinoma is a contraindication to liver transplantation.

AUTOIMMUNE HEPATITIS

Autoimmmune hepatitis is characterized by persistent immune mediated hepatocyte damage. The immune response is felt to be secondary to the abnormal recognition of autoantigens found on hepatocytes. The triggering event has yet to be elucidated, but there is evidence of a genetic predisposition to the disease. The disease has been shown to predominantly affect young women with a female to male ratio of 4:1. There is an association with other autoimmune processes involving other organs such as diabetes mellitus, hypothyroidism, Addison disease, and systemic lupus erythematosus. Approximately 10% of chronic hepatitis in the US is due to autoimmune hepatitis, and end-stage liver disease can develop if not treated adequately.

Clinical features

Patients with autoimmune hepatitis are usually asymptomatic. Fatigue is the most common complaint along with anorexia and malaise. Abnormalities in serum liver enzymes can vary depending on the disease activity. The disease is progressive and indolent. If untreated, cirrhosis frequently develops. Acute liver failure is a potential but unusual presentation of autoimmune liver disease. Along with other autoimmune diseases, autoimmune hepatitis is commonly associated with acne and amenorrhea in young women. Overlap syndromes of autoimmune hepatitis and PBC, PSC, as well as autoimmune cholangiopathy can be seen.

Investigation

Autoimmune hepatitis can be diagnosed by the presence of auto antibodies. Type 1 autoimmune hepatitis is the most common and is associated with positive serum antinuclear antibody (ANA) and anti-smooth muscle antibody. Type 2 autoimmune hepatitis is much less common and is diagnosed by the presence of antiliver kidney microsomal antibodies (anti-LKM). Type 3 hepatitis has been poorly described but is felt to be associated with the presence of soluble liver antigen. Hypergammaglobulinemia is also frequently seen in patients with autoimmune hepatitis. Histologic findings on liver biopsy are very characteristic. There is evidence of portal tract infiltration with plasma cells and mononuclear cells that spill into the surrounding hepatocyte parenchyma. This "interface hepatitis" is very consistent with autoimmune hepatitis. Sparing of the bile ducts distinguishes this disease from other autoimmune liver diseases such as PBC and PSC. The extent of fibrosis and scarring can be evaluated on biopsy and may help with prognosis.

Management

Therapy is based on pharmacological intervention with immunosuppressive therapy. The recommended regimen is a combination of prednisone and azathioprine. Prednisone is dosed at 40 to 60 mg/day and tapered to 2.5 to 5 mg/day maintenance therapy. Azathioprine is started at 50 to 75 mg/day with maintenance therapy at 75 to 100 mg/day. Treatment is usually life-long, but some advocate a trial of withdrawal of medications after 1 to 2 years. If treatment is stopped, closely following with a possible repeat biopsy is indicated due to the high rate of relapse after withdrawal (60%). In patients with end-stage liver disease because of autoimmune hepatitis, liver transplantation is indicated. There is a 25% chance of recurrent disease in the new transplanted liver.

Complications

Complications of autoimmune liver disease are predominantly related to chronic immunosuppressive therapy. Long-term prednisone therapy is associated with moon facies, weight gain, osteoporosis, diabetes, psychiatric changes, and easy bruisability. Azathioprine use is associated with pancytopenia and pancreatitis. Patients with chronic autoimmune hepatitis are at risk for the same complications of cirrhosis seen with other chronic liver diseases.

HEMOCHROMATOSIS

Hereditary hemochromatosis (HH) is an autosomal recessive genetic disease that leads to hepatic parenchymal iron overload. The underlying cause of HH is excessive iron absorption from the GI tract. As a result, excess iron deposition occurs in the liver, heart, pituitary gland, skin, and pancreas. HH is the most common genetic disorder in Caucasians (1 in 250 to 400 people) and has a high incidence in patients of Northern European decent. Secondary hemochromatosis can occur in the setting of multiple blood transfusions, oral iron supplementation, chronic alcohol intake, and hemodialysis. The degree of hepatic damage that is seen in HH is not seen in secondary causes of iron overload.

Clinical features

Iron accumulation in HH correlates with age. The clinical tetrad of hepatomegaly, bronzed skin, diabetes mellitus, and CHF develops over time as a result of the oxidative damage caused by iron to the end organs. Cirrhosis develops in older patients and is rare in patients younger than 45 years of age. Concomitant alcohol use increases the rate of progression of the disease and can lead to cirrhosis at an earlier age. Most patients with early HH are asymptomatic. Some patients may have abnormal liver enzymes depending on the degree of iron accumulation. Complications of cirrhosis such as portal hypertension and hepatocellular carcinoma frequently occur in end-stage disease. There is a 100-fold increased risk of developing hepatocellular carcinoma in patients with cirrhosis and hemochromatosis.

Investigation

The diagnosis of hemochromatosis was previously made by performing a liver biopsy and measuring the patient's hepatic iron concentration (HIC) and hepatic iron index (HII). The HII is calculated by measuring the quantitative iron level on a biopsy, multiplying it by the molecular weight of iron (56) and dividing it by the age of the patient. The diagnosis of HH could be established with HIC more than 4000 mcg/g and/or HII more than 1.9. Identifying the presence of the HFE gene mutation through genotype analysis can now reliably make the diagnosis of HH. The HFE gene is located on chromosome 6 and encodes the protein that regulates receptor-mediated endocytosis of dietary iron. Mutations in this gene lead to abnormal iron absorption and transport in the intestinal villi. The discovery of the HFE mutation has precluded the need to biopsy all patients in order to make the diagnosis of HH. A biopsy is helpful in assessing the extent of liver damage in patients with HH who are over 40 years of age, drink alcohol, and have elevated liver enzymes, elevated serum ferritin levels more than 1000 ng/mL or other liver diseases (hepatitis C virus [HCV]). Young patients with normal liver enzymes, low serum ferritin levels, and no signs of cirrhosis do not need to undergo a liver biopsy. A liver biopsy may be needed if the HFE genotype evaluation is negative, but a clinical suspicion for the disease remains. Histologic evidence of iron accumulation in the periportal hepatocytes rather than sinusoidal cells may differentiate HH from other causes of hepatic iron accumulation.

All patients with a family history of hereditary hemochromatosis should undergo HFE-genotype analysis, and subsequent serum iron studies if positive. Elevated iron studies (fasting serum transferrin saturation more than 45%, ferritin more than 300 ng/mL) with a positive HFE analysis indicate the need to start therapy. Again, a liver biopsy may be pursued at this time to assess prognosis as indicated. Evaluating young children of patients with HH is debatable, although assessing the other spouse's HFE status is usually recommended. HFE analysis can be pursued if the parents have either one or both of the mutations.

No screening tests are recommended for the general population. However, further evaluation is warranted if there is clinical suspicion that the disease is present. An elevated fasting serum transferrin (more than 45%) indicates the need to pursue further evaluation through genetic testing or other iron studies. If the gene analysis is negative, other causes of iron overload should be evaluated. If the analysis is positive, the diagnosis can be made and the need for subsequent biopsy and treatment should be made as described above.

Management

Therapy is aimed at decreasing iron stores. Nonpharmacological therapy is the mainstay of treatment and involves phlebotomy. Phlebotomy can increase survival by decreasing the risk of developing cirrhosis, hepatocellular carcinoma, and progressive end-organ damage. Phlebotomy should be initiated in patients with HH who have abnormal iron studies and/or develop end-organ damage. One unit of blood should be removed every week until serum ferritin levels are less than 50 ng/mL or serum hemoglobin is less than 10 g/dL. Oral iron chelators such as desferroxamine can help decrease intestinal iron absorption. Iron chelation therapy is a good adjunctive therapy for those who cannot tolerate adequate phlebotomy. Screening for hepatocellular carcinoma with annual alphafeto protein and imaging study is very important in managing patients with HH. Liver transplant is indicated in those patients with complications of cirrhosis and/or small (less than 3 to 5 cm), resectable hepatomas. HH is a systemic disease, which makes liver transplantation a noncurative intervention. As a result, patients who undergo liver transplant for HH need to continue with life-long phlebotomy but still have a lower survival rate.

Complications

The complications in hemochromatosis are related to end-organ damage from iron accumulation. Patients can develop cardiac arrhythmias because of conduction system damage as well as heart failure from myocardial damage. Diabetes mellitus can develop with progressive destruction of the pancreas. Pancreatic exocrine function such as malabsorption and steatorrhea is very rare in HH. The hyperpigmentation and atrophy of the skin that can be present is the reason that HH has been labeled "bronze diabetes." Pituitary damage leads to decreased libido and testicular atrophy in men. Arthritis and pseudogout are caused by destruction of peripheral joints. Patients with cirrhosis have a 100-fold increased risk of developing hepatocellular carcinoma.

WILSON DISEASE

Wilson disease is a genetic disorder of copper metabolism that can lead to hepatic dysfunction. It is an autosomal recessive disorder with an incidence of 1 in 30,000 Caucasian people. The underlying abnormality is related to a mutation in the gene that regulates copper transport out of the liver. The transporter protein associates copper with ceruloplasmin in order to promote adequate excretion of copper. Copper is normally excreted by the liver into the bile. Abnormal excretion leads to copper accumulation in the liver as well as other organs. Cellular damage occurs as a result of the excess copper leading to free radical formation and cellular membrane oxidation.

Clinical features

Clinical symptoms are related to the degree of damage that occurs secondary to copper accumulation. Copper accumulates in the liver first but is then released into the bloodstream. Extrahepatic organs such as the CNS, joints, kidneys, cornea, heart, and pancreas then begin to accumulate copper. Patients usually present with either hepatic or neurologic symptoms between the ages of 10 to 22 years of age. Symptoms developing before age 5 and after age 40 are extremely rare. Hepatic symptoms tend to occur at an earlier age and include chronic hepatitis, cirrhosis, or fulminant hepatic failure. Neurologic symptoms present later in adolescence with behavioral or cognitive abnormalities or autonomic or motor neuropathy, but never with sensory neuropathy. The deposition of copper into Decemet's membrane of the cornea leads to the classic finding of Kaiser-Fleischer (K-F) rings around the pupils. K-F rings are seen in almost all patients with neurologic symptoms and in some patients with predominant hepatic symptoms. Hemolytic anemia may develop in acute Wilson as a result of the sudden systemic release of copper that damages the red blood cell membrane. Patients may develop proteinuria, hypercalcuria, or a renal tubular acidosis because of renal tubule damage. Bone demineralization, cardiac arrhythmias, amenorrhea, and glucose intolerance can all develop as a result of ongoing organ damage.

Investigation

There is no single confirmatory test for Wilson disease. Genetic testing for the detection of the abnormal copper transport protein is not available because there are a number of mutations that can cause the defect. Low serum ceruloplasmin levels (less than 20 mg/dL) can be consistent with Wilson disease. Elevated urine copper (more than 100 mg/24 h) and hepatic copper concentration (more than 250 mcg/g) on liver biopsy are more specific, but not necessarily diagnostic of Wilson disease. Slit lamp evaluation of the eyes for K-F rings or "sunflower cataracts", peripheral smear evaluation to detect hemolysis, and liver biopsy to measure and stain for copper can help establish the diagnosis. There are no histologic findings that are specific to Wilson disease. However, diagnosis needs to be made on clinical findings as well as supportive laboratory results as described.

Management

Treatment of Wilson disease is aimed at decreasing intestinal copper absorption and increasing hepatic copper excretion. Oral D-penicillamine (1 g BID) can chelate iron and increase hepatic excretion. Its use is associated with hypersensitivity reactions, vitamin B6 deficiency, ulcers, and lupus-like symptoms. Trientine HCl works in a similar fashion to D-penicillamine but is less potent. Oral zinc acetate therapy also can chelate copper and inhibit absorption. Patients with end-stage liver disease or fulminant hepatic failure caused by Wilson disease can be treated by liver transplantation. Because the underlying defect is primarily hepatic in origin, liver transplant is a curative intervention.

Complications

Complications of cirrhosis and hepatocellular carcinoma can be seen in patients with end-stage liver disease. The rate of progression of damage to various organs dictates the array of complications that can be seen as described above. Fulminant liver failure is a rare complication.

NONALCOHOLIC STEATOHEPATITIS (NASH)

NASH is part of a spectrum of fatty liver disease that includes bland, noninflammatory fat infiltration (nonalcoholic fatty liver disease), and fat infiltration with nonspecific inflammation. Hepatic inflammation identical to alcoholic hepatitis occurs but is associated with no significant alcohol intake. Patients with NASH drink little to no alcohol (less than 20 g/day for women, less than 40 g/day for men) but have the same hepatic histologic changes that are seen in the setting of alcohol use. In contrast to the other fatty liver diseases, patients with NASH often have progressive disease. Approximately 20% of Americans have nonalcoholic fatty liver disease and 2% to 3% have NASH. The prevalence is higher in patients who are obese and diabetic. As the rate of obesity increases in the US, the incidence of NASH is expected to rise, as well. The pathogenesis of NASH is not known. Abnormalities involving lipid metabolism, hepatic lipid peroxidation, and cytokine production are felt to be key factors leading to NASH in some patients.

Clinical features

Patients with NASH are usually obese females with diabetes but the disease can occasionally be seen in males as well as the nonobese. Progressive disease can evolve from steatosis to steatohepatitis to fibrosis and finally to cirrhosis. Patients are usually asymptomatic but may complain of fatigue and malaise. In addition to obesity and diabetes, patients also may present with other conditions associated with NASH, including dyslipidemia (elevated triglycerides and/or cholesterol), medications (steroids, estrogens, amiodarone), obesity-related surgical procedures (jejunoileal bypass, gastroplasty), and the use of total parenteral nutrition.

Investigation

Patients with NASH often have liver enzyme abnormalities. The aminotransferases are usually twice the upper limit of normal with the ALT:AST ratio more than 1. Although unreliable for making a diagnosis, this ratio can sometimes distinguish NASH from alcohol-related disease as it is usually less than 1 in alcoholic steatohepatitis. NASH is diagnosed after all the other potential causes of liver disease have been ruled out. Therefore, patients need to be evaluated for any potential viral, autoimmune, metabolic, drug-related, or obstructive cause of their hepatitis. Abdominal imaging with either a CT or ultrasound frequently reveals fatty infiltration. A liver biopsy can be helpful in making the diagnosis in some cases, although the diagnosis can frequently be made without one. The biopsy usually reveals findings also seen in alcoholic hepatitis. There is fatty infiltration with inflammatory cells, sinusoidal fibrosis, ballooning degeneration of the hepatocytes, and Mallory hyaline bodies seen on histology. The liver biopsy plays a more prominent role in assessing the risk of disease progression and prognosis. Some have recommended that patients over 45 years of age who are obese (body mass index more than 30), diabetic, and have an AST:ALT ratio more than 1 undergo a liver biopsy to assess their risk of disease progression.

Management

There is no definitive therapy for NASH. Medications that can cause NASH need to be discontinued. Treating the associated conditions should be aggressively pursued. Weight loss, tight diabetic control, and lipid management are key interventions in improving the enzyme abnormalities and histologic changes seen in NASH. Other agents such as antioxidants (vitamin E), ursodeoxycholic acid, betaine, and N-acetylcysteine have been investigated, but their efficacy has yet to be determined.

Complications

Disease progression can be seen in 20% of patients with NASH over 10 to 20 years. As a result, cirrhosis and its complications may develop. Patients with progressive NASH also are at increased risk of mortality, need for liver transplantation, and hepatocellular carcinoma.

CHAPTER 7

BILIARY AND PANCREATIC DISORDERS

GALLSTONE DISEASE AND BILIARY COLIC

Gallstones form within the gallbladder from crystallization of cholesterol, bilirubin, or a variety of calcium salts. Approximately 20 million Americans have gallstones, although the majority are asymptomatic. Nevertheless, over 700,000 cholecystectomies are performed each year, making this one of the most common surgeries performed in the United States.

Gallstones can be classified into cholesterol or pigmented stones, with cholesterol stones accounting for up to 75% of all gallstones in Western countries. Cholesterol stones form in the setting of biliary supersaturation with cholesterol. Stone formation begins with the process of nucleation, encouraged by several factors, including gallbladder mucin and certain biliary proteins. Defective biliary acidification and gallbladder stasis also play a role. Pigmented gallstones, on the other hand, are formed from a variety of bilirubin and calcium salt precipitants. They also may include small amounts of cholesterol, fatty acids, glycoproteins, and mucins. Black stones primarily form from bilirubin polymers and are seen in hemolytic diseases (eg, sickle cell disease) and cirrhosis. Brown stones primarily are formed from calcium bilirubinate and are associated with infected bile. They are seen most commonly in Asia and can form within the bile ducts.

Epidemiologically, gallstones occur more frequently with age and are more common in females. Other predisposing factors include diet, obesity, and use of hormone replacement therapy or oral contraceptives. Rapid weight loss can increase mobilization of tissue cholesterol, and small bowel diseases or surgery may interfere with bile salt recycling. Genetic factors play a role through alterations in the handling of bile salts and cholesterol.

Biliary sludge is composed of mucin, calcium bilirubinate granules, and cholesterol monohydrate crystals. It can be detected by gallbladder bile aspiration (after administration of cholcystokinin) endoscopically or ultrasound-guided, transabdominal or endoscopic. Biliary sludge can precipitate acute pancreatitis or biliary colic. Frank gallstones can develop in 14% of patients with biliary sludge.

Clinical presentation

The majority of patients with gallstones are asymptomatic and require no therapy. Up to one-third will eventually develop symptoms, the majority presenting with uncomplicated biliary colic. However, 20% to 30% of symptomatic patients may present with complications such as cholecystitis, cholangitis, or pancreatitis.

The term biliary colic is used to describe the pain associated with uncomplicated gallstone disease. It most frequently results from transient obstruction of the cystic duct, leading to tonic spasms around the duct. Occasionally, transient obstruction of the common bile duct may occur. Symptoms are usually episodic and may be precipitated by a large meal. Though described as a colic, the pain is usually constant, developing over approximately 15 minutes and lasting up to 3 hours. Pain longer than 6 hours raises the possibility of complications. Pain is most frequently epigastric, although it may center in the right upper quadrant. Radiation may occur to the interscapular region or less commonly to the right shoulder. Nausea, vomiting, and diaphoresis are other associated symptoms. Though the differential diagnosis for epigastric pain is broad, important conditions to rule out include ischemic heart disease, cholecystitis, pancreatitis, peptic ulcer disease, and other intraabdominal catastrophies.

Physical examination during an episode may demonstrate epigastric or right upper quadrant tenderness. Peritoneal signs are uncommon, and suggest an intra-abdominal inflammatory process, including cholecystitis and pancreatitis. Jaundice may occur from transient biliary obstruction.

Investigation

Routine laboratory studies usually are normal in uncomplicated biliary colic, although transient elevation of bilirubin and liver function tests may occur if the patient has passed a gallstone through the bile duct. Plain x-rays reveal gallstones in 13% to 17% of cases. The initial imaging test of choice is an ultrasound, which has sensitivity and specificity of approximately 95% for stones within the gallbladder. CT scanning is less sensitive for stones as they are usually radiolucent. It is difficult to demonstrate transient obstruction of the cystic duct on imaging studies in patients with biliary colic; therefore the diagnosis is made on the basis of appropriate clinical findings in the presence of gallstones.

Management

Patients with asymptomatic gallstones most frequently remain asymptomatic, with 18% to 50% developing biliary colic over 20 years. Complications develop in 2% to 20% and are frequently preceded by episodes of biliary colic. Therefore, asymptomatic gallstones are best left untreated unless symptoms develop.

After any episode of biliary colic, recurrent attacks and complications are frequent and elimination of gallstones becomes a therapeutic goal. Treatment strategies include medical dissolution, extracorporeal shock wave lithotripsy, and cholecystectomy. Though nonsurgical methods frequently can eliminate stone disease, high rates of recurrence and the development of laparoscopy have made cholecystectomy the standard of care.

Medical dissolution therapies include bile acids administered orally or chemical solvents delivered percutaneously into the gallbladder under radiologic guidance. Bile acids alter the composition of bile and decrease the amount of biliary lipid secretion, thereby decreasing the biliary cholesterol saturation index. Ursodeoxycholic acid has a more favorable side effect profile than chenodeoxycholic acid. When used at 8 to 12 mg/kg/day, it has up to a 70% success rate in selected patients with small, cholesterol based stones and normal gallbladder function. However, stones larger than 1cm have only a 35% response rate. Given the mechanism of action, there is little success with pigmented or calcified stones.

Methyl-*tert*-butyl ether (MTBE) can be used as a contact solvent through a catheter placed into the gallbladder under radiologic guidance. MTBE can achieve dissolution within hours in up to 90% of selected patients with small, non-calcified cholesterol stones. However, its utility is limited by complications from the percutaneous introduction, as well as complications of hemolytic anemia, duodenitis, aspiration pneumonia, and somnolence if MTBE drains into the duodenum. MTBE is also an explosion risk. Given these risks and the advent of laparoscopic cholecystectomy, oral or contact dissolution rarely is used.

Extracorporeal shock wave lithotripsy (ESWL) uses focused energy waves to fragment gallstones. This technique usually is used in conjunction with oral ursodeoxycholic acid. Success rates very from 34% to 90%, depending on patient selection. Complications include post-procedure biliary colic in 20% and pancreatitis in 1% as well as local complications from the lithotriptor. This technique also has been used in combination with dissolution agents.

Nonsurgical methods of gallstone management result in a high rate of recurrence, ranging from 15% at 2 years to 50% at 10 years. Cholecystectomy, on the other hand, is curative and is the treatment of choice in good surgical candidates. Greater than 90% of cases can be performed laparoscopically. Possible limitations include morbid obesity or the so-called "hostile" abdomen after multiple prior intrabdominal surgeries or episodes of peritonitis.

Complications

The major complications of gallstones include cholecystitis, cholangitis with stones migrating to the common bile duct, and acute pancreatitis. Potential problems after cholecystectomy include retained bile duct stones and rare formation of primary bile duct stones. Bile duct injuries occur infrequently at cholecystectomy, although there is clearly a learning curve for laparoscopic techniques. Bile duct injuries include biliary leaks, which can present as biliary peritonitis. The injuries may be amenable to endoscopic biliary stenting or may require T-tube placement or surgical correction if more severe. Ischemic injury can cause biliary strictures which may present as jaundice or cholangitis. Treatment options include dilation with endsocopic biliary stent placement over the stricture or choledochoenterostomy. Large, retrospective, population-based studies of laparoscopic cholecystectomy report a 0.5% incidence of biliary injuries, with a 2% complication rate and a mortality rate of 0.05%.

CHOLEDOCHOLITHIASIS

Choledocholithiasis refers to the presence of biliary stones within the common bile duct. This occurs most frequently after passage of a gallbladder stone through the cystic duct and into the bile duct. Rarely, primary biliary stones can develop in the setting of bile infection or obstruction. These stones most commonly are the brown pigment type.

Clinical presentation

Choledocholithiasis may present with biliary colic, or more frequently with cholangitis or pancreatitis. These entities are described in other sections in this chapter. Patients also may be asymptomatic with choledocholithiasis detected at the time of cholecystectomy.

Investigation

Jaundice and abnormal liver function tests are frequent. Isolated elevation of the alkaline phosphatase may occur. Criteria predicting the presence of a common bile duct stone include jaundice and elevated bilirubin, and ultrasonography demonstrating a common duct stone or a common duct greater than 7 mm in diameter. These criteria have a sensitivity of 88% and specificity of 67% with a negative predictive value of 92% and positive predictive value of 55%. The diagnostic gold standard is cholangiography. This frequently is performed intraoperatively at the time of elective cholecystectomy, though endoscopic or percutaneous cholangiography may be necessary for therapy in the setting of complications.

Management

Several treatment strategies have been proposed. Routine pre-operative endoscopic retrograde cholangio-pancreatography (ERCP) appears to add significantly to the cost and complications of management of gallstones because of frequent normal exams. Other strategies include routine intra-operative cholangiography or selective intra-operative cholangiography with intra-operative laparosocpic bile duct exploration or postoperative ERCP as treatment options if a stone is present. The choice between these options is based on local expertise. In most situations, open bile duct exploration cannot be justified given a significant increase in morbidity compared to endoscopic or laparoscopic techniques. Selective pre-operative ERCP is another reasonable alternative where area expertise favors endoscopic management.

Endoscopic management of bile duct stones generally consists of sphincterotomy and bile duct clearance with a balloon or basket. Large or impacted stones may require endoluminal mechanical or shock wave lithotripsy. Extracorporeal shock wave lithotripsy also has been used. Biliary stenting allows drainage while awaiting definitive therapy of difficult stones. The stent also may cause mechanical disruption over time. Long-term results with biliary stenting as primary therapy have not been promising. Finally, laparoscopic or open choledochotomy may be necessary for difficult stones.

Complications

Complications include cholangitis and pancreatitis. Urgent bile duct decompression, endoscopically or percutanteously, is performed concurrent with broad spectrum antibiotics in patients with cholangitis.

CHOLECYSTITIS

Cholecystitis is characterized histologically by inflammation of the gallbladder wall. It can be defined as calculous (gallstone related), or acalculous. Approximately 90% of cases are associated with gallstones. More permanent obstruction of the cystic duct by a gallstone damages the gallbladder mucosa and initiates an inflammatory reaction. Bacterial infection frequently occurs as a secondary process.

Repeated attacks of cholecystitis can lead to chronic cholecystitis. This is manifested by a thickened, fibrotic gallbladder with evaginated mucosal pouches (Rokitansky-Aschoff sinuses).

Acalculous cholecystitis is a disease of critically ill patients. The underlying illness and the frequent use of narcotics, total parenteral nutrition, and positive pressure ventilation predispose the patient to biliary stasis and ischemia. Again bacterial infection is usually secondary.

Clinical presentation

Calculous cholecystitis presents most commonly as acute biliary pain in patients with a predisposition to gallstones. Pain is more persistent than the episodic pain of uncomplicated biliary colic and frequently localizes to the right upper quadrant over time. Nausea and vomiting are common, as is low grade fever.

Acalculous cholecystitis is seen in patients with other severe illnesses. Frequently, history and physical are limited by the patients underlying medical condition, and the physician must keep a high index of suspicion in patients in intensive care units with unexplained fever, leukocytosis, or other evidence of deterioration.

Localized peritoneal signs may be present on physical examination. Murphy's sign describes the abrupt arrest of inspiration caused by pain from the inflamed gallbladder. A palpable mass representing the inflamed gallbladder may be present in 30% to 40%. These signs are usually absent in chronic cholecystitis.

Investigation

Leukocytosis is a frequent laboratory finding. Mirizzi syndrome describes obstruction of the common hepatic duct by a gallstone impacted in the cystic duct and can lead to jaundice in the occasional patient.

Imaging studies are useful to confirm acute cholecystitis. Ultrasound is a useful initial test for suspected calculous cholecystitis given its sensitivity for gallstones. Pericholecystic fluid collections and gallbladder wall thickening or intramural gas are suggestive of cholecystitis. Overall sensitivity is reported to be 67% to 93% with specificity of 82% to 100%. CT also is sensitive for gallbladder wall changes and may be useful to evaluate for acalculous cholecystitis or other intrabdominal infectious process in an intensive care unit patient with unexplained deterioration.

Hepatobiliary scintigraphy is useful in patients presenting acutely and is performed using ^{99m}Tc-iminodiacetic acid. This agent is excreted into the bile with subsequent uptake by the gallbladder and excretion into the duodenum. Failure to image the gallbladder within 90 minutes despite normal images of the liver, common bile duct, and duodenum is highly suggestive of cystic duct obstruction and cholecystitis. False positives can occur in nonfasting state or after a prolonged fast. Liver disease can result in inability to excrete the radiolabeled agent into the bile ducts. False positives can be limited by delayed 4-hour images, or administration of morphine. Morphine increases contraction at the sphincter of Oddi, thereby increasing bile duct pressures. Sensitivity ranges from 95% to 100% with specificty 38% to 100%. Some of this variation may be due to inconsistencies in definition of the gold standard.

Some authors have advocated percutaneous cholecystostomy and aspiration for both treatment and diagnosis of acute cholecystitis. However, the negative predictive value of culture negative bile without leukocytes is unclear.

Management

Treatment is primarily surgical, although percutaneous drainage may be used as a bridge to surgery or in poor surgical candidates. Percutaneous cholecystotomy is a common mode of therapy for acalculous cholecystitis, especially in the critically ill patient. Broad spectrum antibiotics covering gram negative and anerobic bacteria are also mandatory. Typical agents include second-generation cephalosporins, fluoroquinolones, and broad spectrum penicillins with β-lactamase inhibitors.

Complications

Untreated cholecystitis can be complicated by pericholecystic abscess, gallbladder perforation with associated peritonitis, or cholecystoenteric fistulas (particularly involving the duodenum, hepatic flexure of the colon, stomach, or jejunum).

ASCENDING CHOLANGITIS

Cholangitis refers to inflammation of the bile ducts. Ascending cholangitis occurs in the setting of bile duct obstruction. Etiologies include choledocholithiasis, biliary strictures, or other abnormalities of biliary anatomy such as choledochal cysts. Biliary strictures can be malignant or benign, as seen in primary or secondary sclerosing cholangitis. Overall, ascending cholangitis is uncommon in choledocholithiasis. Rates of infection approximate 10% to 15% in malignant biliary strictures. The predominant organisms of infectious cholangitis include enteric organisms such as *E. coli*, *Klebsiella*, *Psuedomonas*, and enterococci. Anaerobic infection occurs in 15%.

Clinical presentation

Charcot's triad refers to the classic clinical presentation of infectious cholangitis and includes biliary pain, jaundice, and chills and rigors. The triad occurs in 70% of cases, with pain in 90%, chills and fever in 95%, and jaundice in 80%. Deterioration to hypotension and shock caused by septicemia can occur unless therapy is initiated urgently.

Investigation

Physical exam may reveal tender hepatomegaly or occasional rebound. Laboratory studies may show leukocytosis and elevated transaminases, bilirubin, and alkaline phosphatase reflective of biliary obstruction.

Ultrasound is the most useful initial imaging study. Typical findings include bile duct dilation. Gallstones also may be present. Ultrasound typically is not sensitive for distal common bile duct stones. CT also may show bile duct dilation and may be useful to exclude other pathology in atypical cases.

Endoscopic retrograde cholangiography (ERC) or percutaneous transhepatic cholangiography (PTC) may be useful to demonstrate biliary stones or strictures and have the added benefit of providing therapeutic drainage. MR cholangiograms may be useful to demonstrate biliary obstruction in difficult cases, eliminating the possible complications of ERC and PTC, although subsequent ERC or PTC will be required for decompression when obstruction is visualized.

Management

Biliary drainage and antibiotics are the mainstays of treatment. Antibiotics with gram negative and anaerobic coverage should be initiated immediately upon suspicion of infectious cholangitis. As with cholecystitis, typical agents include second-generation cephalosporins, fluoroquinolones, and broad spectrum penicillins with β-lactamase activity. Ceftriaxone can precipitate in bile and probably should be avoided.

Biliary drainage is necessary for definitive treatment, and may be performed on an urgent or emergent basis in critically ill patients. Endoscopic drainage is the treatment of choice when possible. Sphincterotomy is usually performed to facilitate drainage, and temporary stents are frequently placed. Bile duct stones are extracted if possible. Elective cholecystectomy is required to avoid repeat attacks.

Percutaneous cholangiography and drainage is useful for decompression of the biliary system if the endoscopist is unable to obtain access or if the patient is too sick to undergo conscious sedation for the endoscopic procedure.

Complications

Complications of cholangitis can include liver abscesses, shock, and multisystem organ failure. Urgent decompression and prompt antibiotic therapy often decreases the likelihood of complications.

ACUTE PANCREATITIS

Acute pancreatitis is characterized by discrete episodes of abdominal pain associated with elevated serum levels of pancreatic enzymes. Histologic features include parenchymal inflammation, disruption of pancreatic acini, and in severe cases necrosis and hemorrhage.

Acute pancreatitis occurs in 1 to 5 of 10,000 people per year. Gallstones and alcohol are responsible for 70% to 80% of cases in the West, but a variety of other insults can lead to pancreatitis, including medications, trauma, infections, and surgical procedures or ERCP. The number of cases characterized as idiopathic decreases as more is learned about rare causes of pancreatitis such as microlithiasis, sphincter of Oddi dysfunction, and hereditary pancreatitis.

Events initiating acute pancreatitis include pancreatic duct obstruction, pancreatic ischemia, and premature activation of zymogens within pancreatic acinar cells. These events lead to release of cytokines such as platelet-activating factor, TNF, and IL-1, which perpetuate the injury. Further damage occurs with secondary vascular damage and ischemia and through inflammatory pathways. The end result is local damage through pancreatic enzyme activation and ischemia, and systemic effects from both enzyme release and inflammatory mediators.

Clinical presentation

Pancreatitis presents with pain in 95% of patients. The pain is usually epigastric with radiation to the low thoracic region of the back. The pain peaks from 30 minutes to several hours and can last hours to days. Precipitating factors include eating, and relieving factors may include sitting or leaning forward. Nausea and vomiting are seen in up to 85% of patients and do not relieve the pain.

On physical examination, low grade fevers are seen in 60% of patients, while tachycardia or hypotension are seen in 40%. The abdominal exam reveals epigastric pain and guarding is frequently present. Bowel sounds may be decreased or absent. Pleural effusions may be present, particularly on the left. Jaundice may be present, but bilirubin greater than 4 suggests extrahepatic obstruction. Turner's sign (dark discoloration of the back/flank) and Cullen's sign (dark discoloration of the periumbilical region) may be seen with retroperitoneal hemorrhage.

Patients also may present with shock or respiratory failure or coma. Intestinal ileus and its complications are common. These symptoms may predominate in severe pancreatitis and can lead to missed diagnosis.

Investigation

Serum and urine levels of several pancreatic enzymes can be used to diagnose pancreatitis. The most commonly used are serum amylase and lipase. Levels may return to normal within 24 hours, making timing an issue in diagnostic sensitivity. The sensitivity and specificity also depend on the cutoff used to define disease. Using a cutoff just above normal, sensitivity is greater than 90% with specificity of 70%. Defining disease at with values 3 times normal decreases sensitivity to 60% but increases specificity to near 100%. P-isoamylase, an isomer of amylase, may be elevated in biliary tract disease and intestinal perforation, obstruction, or ischemia. Lipase also can be detected in other GI organs. Sensitivity is comparable with amylase, with improved specificity. Serum elevation also persists longer than amylase abnormalities. Lipase determination is readily available, rapid, and the preferred single serum enzyme test. Other pancreatic enzymes are elevated in pancreatitis but operating characteristics have not been defined. Urinary trypsinogen-2 has been shown to have a high sensitivity and specificity and may become more widely used.

Imaging studies are most frequently used to exclude alternative diagnosis, determine disease severity, and evaluate the presence of local complications. Abdominal plain films may help rule out viscous perforation. Ileus is frequently seen. Specific findings include the "sentinel loop," which represents an isolated dilated loop of small bowel overlying the pancreas. The "colon cut-off sign" results from colon obstruction with air in the right and transverse colon and abrupt cutoff at the splenic flexure.

Ultrasound may be useful through detection of pancreatic edema, but visualization of the pancreas can be difficult in 30% to 40% of patients secondary to intestinal gas or surrounding fat. It is the initial test of choice for the detection of gallstones.

Computed tomography (CT) also may show pancreatic enlargement, effacement of the pancreatic contour, inhomogenity of the parenchyma, or peripancreatic fat stranding. It is particularly useful because it reliably images the entire gland and can demonstrate complications such as necrosis and fluid collections. CT guided aspiration can be used to evaluate for infected necrosis or fluid collections. Helical CT also may detect duct stones.

Management

Several schemes have been developed to predict severity. Ranson used a variety of clinical and laboratory parameters to predict severity in alcoholic pancreatitis. Variations have simplified the scheme and applied it to other causes of pancreatitis. The APACHE II scoring system for critical illness has been applied, and CT scan criteria regarding the degree and extent of pancreatic changes have been developed. Supportive care and management of complications are the mainstays of therapy for acute pancreatitis.

Supportive care begins with fluid management and pain control. Pancreatitis can result in significant intravascular volume depletion secondary to third spacing of fluids. Follow measurements of fluid status including urine output, vital signs, and laboratory evidence of hemoconcentration carefully. Pain control frequently requires narcotic analgesia, typically using meperidine as IV bolus or patient-controlled analgesia (PCA). Although morphine is frequently avoided, there is no clinical evidence to support this on the basis of increased sphincter of Oddi pressure after administration of morphine. Patients should remain NPO while pain continues.

Nutrition frequently becomes an issue during severe pancreatitis. Total parenteral nutrition has been a mainstay of therapy. However, studies have shown that enteral nutrition through a tube placed distal to the ligament of Trietz leads to a decreased incidence of infection and is the route of choice. Tube feeding decreases the risk of line infection and likely reduces bacterial translocation from the intestine.

Studies have shown benefit from urgent ERCP in patients predicted to have severe gallstone pancreatitis. This benefit actually may be related to decreased incidence of concomitant cholangitis. Antibiotics are not indicated in uncomplicated pancreatitis. Several agents, including octreotide, gabexate mesylate, steroids, and several cytokines, have been investigated to prevent post-ERCP pancreatitis with variable success. Premedication using these agents is not currently standard.

Complications

Metabolic abnormalities can include hyperglycemia, hypocalcemia, and hypomagnesemia. Hyperlipidemia can be secondary to acute pancreatitis and does not need therapy in the acute phase. Other potentially severe systemic complications include respiratory failure (frequently from acute respiratory distress syndrome [ARDS]), acute renal insufficiency, and ileus. GI hemorrhage may arise from gastritis, pseudoaneurysms, or esophageal or gastric varices related to splenic vein thrombosis.

The most feared local complication of pancreatitis is infected pancreatic necrosis. Necrosis can be diagnosed by CT scan, which should be performed in the first few days in patients with predicted severe pancreatitis, slow recovery, or deterioration. Infected necrosis is frequently accompanied by increased pain, fever, marked leukocytosis, and bacteremia and occurs 1 to 2 weeks after initial presentation. If infection is suspected, CT guided aspiration samples from the areas of suspected infection should be sent for gram stain and culture. Gram stain is frequently positive. Infected pancreatic necrosis most often requires broad spectrum antibiotics and aggressive surgical debridement, although percutaneous and endoscopic drainage and lavage procedures have been used. Sterile pancreatic necrosis is commonly treated expectantly unless severe pancreatitis symptoms persist for several weeks. Prophylactic antibiotics play a role to prevent infection in patients with severe pancreatitis and pancreatic necrosis. Imipenem/cilastatin is most frequently used. Cefuroxime also has been successful. The benefit of antibiotics may relate more to decreased incidence of cholangitis than to effects on infection of pancreatic necrosis.

Fluid collections are another frequent complication. The majority of such collections resolve spontaneously over weeks. Drainage is only necessary if the collection becomes infected or is expanding rapidly. Fluid collections persisting beyond 4 weeks can be defined as a pseudocyst. Pseudocysts are present in up to 10% of patients with acute pancreatitis. They may present with abdominal pain or bloating or with gastric outlet obstruction, jaundice, or other symptoms of local compression. Hemorrhage from a pseudoaneurysm is rare.

Pseudocysts generally resolve spontaneously. If infection, rapid enlargement, or other symptoms occur, drainage may be necessary. Common drainage methods include endoscopic cystgastrostomy or cystenterostomy. Anatomy or local expertise may favor surgical drainage in some cases. Percutaneous drainage into the stomach or externally also may be successful.

CHRONIC PANCREATITIS

Chronic pancreatitis implies permanent structural or functional damage to the pancreas. The most common etiology in developed countries is alcohol, accounting for up to 70%. Other causes include primary structural problems such as trauma, pancreatic duct obstruction, and pancreatic divisum. Metabolic abnormalities such as hyperparathyroidism and hypertriglyceridemia rarely can be associated. Autoimmune pancreatitis and hereditary causes including cystic fibrosis are occasionally seen. Twenty percent of cases are idiopathic.

In the setting of alcohol, recurrent episodes of acute pancreatitis with cellular damage may lead to chronic changes. In addition, alterations in pancreatic exocrine secretions may predispose to protein precipitants and obstructive disease. Pain may be related to inflammation or obstruction. Neural inflammation also may play a role.

Clinical presentation

Pain associated with chronic pancreatitis is usually a dull, constant, epigastric pain with radiation to the back. Pain also may radiate throughout the upper abdomen. Pain may last for days or persist indefinitely. Recurrent attacks of pain early in the course must be differentiated from recurrent acute pancreatitis. Nausea, vomiting, and anorexia also are frequent.

Over time, fibrosis of the gland can lead to pancreatic endocrine and exocrine dysfunction. Malabsorption generally develops when exocrine function has decreased to 10%. Steatorrhea is the common clinical presentation, although azotorrhea also occurs. Diabetes is also a late finding, but occurs in up to 60% of patients with chronic pancreatitis.

Physical examination may reveal muscle wasting or abdominal tenderness.

Investigation

Leukocytosis and mild elevations of amylase and lipase may be present during painful episodes, although normal values do not exclude the diagnosis. Stool studies may reveal steatorrhea in more advanced cases.

The most characteristic imaging finding is pancreatic calcification on plain abdominal films or CT scan. Sensitivity of CT scan for the diagnosis of chronic pancreatitis is 80% to 90% with a specificity of 90%. CT also has the advantage of revealing pancreatic mass lesions. Ultrasound also may be used. Characteristic findings include pancreatic duct dilation greater than 4mm, reduction in echogenecity, and irregular contour.

ERCP is the current gold standard. Changes include dilation and irregularity of pancreatic duct branches in mild disease. The pancreatic duct may be dilated or stenotic in moderate disease. Cyst formation can be seen in advanced cases. ERCP also may detect pancreatic duct stones.

Newer technologies include MRCP and endoscopic ultrasound (EUS). EUS has excellent sensitivity and specificity for severe and moderate chronic pancreatitis and the normal pancreas. Operating characteristics are not as good for mild disease.

Treatment

Pain is frequently the most debilitating symptom of chronic pancreatitis. Alcohol cessation may improve pain in some patients, but the relationship between continued alcohol consumption and pain is not universal. Analgesia should begin with non-narcotic medications (acetaminophen, NSAIDs). These should be given before meals to ameliorate postprandial symptoms. Narcotic analgesics (alone or in combination with acetaminophen) frequently are necessary with time. Celiac plexus block has been used with variable success for the pain of chronic pancreatitis. However, results are temporary and potential complications limit utilization.

Several strategies attempt to decrease pancreatic secretion. Administration of pancreatic enzymes inhibits further secretion by feedback mechanisms. The role of pancreatic enzyme supplementation in pain control is controversial. Variation in results may depend on the preparation. Microsphere and buffered preparations such as *Pancrease*, *Creon*, and *Pancreacarb* may deliver more enzyme to the duodenum, where feedback occurs. Individual therapeutic trials are a reasonable approach. Octreotide has been used to inhibit CCK release with some success at 200 mcg 3 times daily. Further studies are needed, and cost may be a limiting factor.

Invasive techniques attempt to relieve obstruction, thereby reducing pain. Endoscopic therapy focuses on dilation of focal pancreatic duct strictures and the removal of pancreatic stones. Surgical procedures vary according to the anatomy of disease. Distal pancreatectomy, duodenum-preserving resection of the pancreatic head, or lateral pancreaticojejunostomy may be performed.

Complications

Pancreatic insufficiency is a late complication of chronic pancreatitis. Endocrine insufficiency manifests as brittle diabetes mellitus requiring insulin. Exocrine insufficieny can result in malabsorption of fat, protein, and carbohydrate. Steatorrhea is the most difficult to treat. Approximately 28,000 units of lipase should be delivered during a 4-hour postprandial period. A variety of pancreatic enzyme preparations are available, including several with coating mechanisms to reduce neutralization in the stomach. However, delivery mechanisms have been difficult and uncoated preparations are likely sufficient. Concurrent acid suppression is often prescribed to prevent neutralization by gastric acid.

CHAPTER 8

INFECTIOUS DISORDERS

INFECTIOUS ESOPHAGITIS

Primary esophageal infections usually are seen in the immunocompromised host, and are rare in the immunocompetent patient without an underlying condition that disturbs the balance of normal oral flora or disrupts the mucosal barrier. Patients with diabetes mellitus, an underlying malignancy, or disorders of esophageal emptying are predisposed to esophageal infections. Patients receiving therapy with antibiotics, corticosteroids, or radiation are also at increased risk. Infections are primarily fungal or viral in etiology. Infections caused by the *Candida* species are overwhelmingly the most common of the fungal infections. Cytomegalovirus (CMV) and herpes simplex virus type 1 (HSV-1) are the predominant viral agents. Bacterial pathogens rarely cause primary infectious esophagitis.

CAN*DIDA* ESOPHAGITIS

Thirteen *Candida* species are known to cause infection in humans, of which C. *albicans* remains the most common pathogen. This organism is considered a commensal in the oropharyngeal cavity, GI and genitourinary tract of humans, capable of causing disease when there is a disruption in the normal flora, mucosal barrier or host cellular immunity. Any impairment in cellular immunity (eg, AIDS) predisposes to mucocutaneous candidiasis, whereas impaired innate immunity tends to result in systemic candidiasis. Fifty percent of all esophageal infections in AIDS patients are caused by *Candida*, with increased incidence seen as the CD4 lymphocyte count falls below 200/mm^3. Organ transplant recipients are also at increased risk because of impaired function of the immune system as well as neutropenia induced by chemotherapy, radiation, and immunosuppressive drugs.

Clinical features

The hallmark of esophageal candidiasis is dysphagia, often with associated odynophagia. If odynophagia is severe and is the primary symptom, then *Candida* esophagitis is less likely and another etiology or coinfection must be investigated. Concomitant oral candidiasis (thrush) is present in two-thirds of AIDS patients with *Candida* esophagitis. In fact, the presence of oral thrush and dysphagia is highly predictive of *Candida* esophagitis in this population, with a positive predictive value of 90%. Patients with accompanying oropharyngeal candidiasis complain of a cottony feeling in the mouth, loss of taste, or pain on eating. Patients may report difficulty swallowing and substernal chest pain of varying intensity.

Investigation

The history and physical exam is insufficient for definitive diagnosis. Barium esophagram can show some typical features of *Candida* esophagitis, including nodular elevations of mucosa, discrete plaques, ulcers, and cobblestoning. A normal esophagram, however, does not exclude the diagnosis, and odynophagia may limit the ability to perform this test.

Endoscopy with biopsy remains the test of choice to establish a specific diagnosis and has been proven to be more sensitive than radiographic analysis. Characteristic white mucosal plaque-like lesions seen at endoscopy support the diagnosis. Biopsies obtained at endoscopy show the presence of yeasts and pseudohyphae invading mucosal cell. This also helps to rule out coexisting disorders, especially when ulcers are identified. Many clinicians choose empiric treatment with a systemic antifungal agents, based on the clinical presentation, reserving endoscopy and biopsy for situations where symptoms do not improve in 5 to 7 days.

Management

Topical therapy is ineffective. Systemic therapy is required for the effective treatment of esophageal candidiasis. Azoles or IV amphotericin are the mainstay of therapy. Fluconazole is superior to ketoconazole, itraconazole capsules, and flucytosine because of variable absorption of the latter. However, itraconazole capsules plus flucytosine is as effective as fluconazole and up to 80% of patients who fail therapy with fluconazole will respond to itraconazole solution.

Fluconazole 100 mg/day or itraconazole solution 200 mg/day orally for 14 to 21 days is the recommended initial therapy. Fluconazole can also be used for recurrent esophagitis. Itraconazole solution 200 mg/day orally is recommended for fluconazole refractory esophagitis. IV amphotericin B can be used for azole refractory infections. Prophylactic therapy is not generally recommended.

Complications

Severe complications are rare and include esophageal hemorrhage at the site of severe erosion and ulceration. There also have been rare cases of esophageal necrosis and perforation requiring esophagectomy. More frequently, symptoms reduce oral intake of foods and liquids, resulting in dehydration. Complications related to treatment with azoles include nausea, hepatotoxicity, and inhibition of steroid production, and are dose dependent. Adverse effect of amphotericin B is primarily acute renal insufficiency.

HERPES SIMPLEX ESOPHAGITIS

HSV-1 is the second most common cause of infectious esophagitis, after the *Candida* species (herpes simplex type 2 rarely involves the esophagus). It typically occurs in immunocompromised patients. Unlike the *Candida* species and CMV, HSV-1 is an uncommon cause of esophageal infection in HIV-infected patients. It is more frequently seen in transplant recipients receiving immunosuppressive medication. HSV-1 esophagitis is also well described in otherwise healthy people.

Clinical features

Patients typically present with odynophagia as the primary symptom with associated dysphagia. Patients may have concurrent herpes labialis (cold sores) or oropharyngeal ulcers, which may predate esophageal symptoms. In the immunocompetent host, spontaneous resolution is common in about 2 weeks even without treatment.

Investigation

Diagnosis is supported by visualizing typical lesions at endoscopy and confirmed by biopsy. The earliest manifestations are vesicles, which coalesce to form ulcers. These ulcers are described as well circumscribed lesions (usually less than 2 cm) with a "volcano" like appearance. Barium swallow may reveal this characteristic focal ulceration on a background of normal esophageal mucosa. Severe, diffuse, erosive esophagitis may be present and result in a similar cobblestone pattern as seen with *Candida* esophagitis. Biopsies or cytologic brushings should be taken from the ulcer edge where the cytopathic effect is best identified (as compared with changes seen in the ulcer base with CMV infection). Multinucleated giant cells with ground-glass nuclei and eosinophilic inclusions (Cowdry type A inclusion bodies) are typical findings. Immunohistochemical stains on biopsy samples using specific monoclonal antibodies to HSV can be helpful. Viral culture may establish the diagnosis and identify resistant isolates. Serologic tests are of little value.

Management

Spontaneous resolution usually occurs in about 2 weeks in immunocompetent hosts. However, a short course of antiviral therapy may be beneficial in patients with severe odynophagia, hastening the relief of symptoms. All immunocompromised hosts should be treated with a longer course of therapy. Recommended initial therapy is acyclovir 400 mg orally 5 times a day for 14 to 21 days. For patients unable to tolerate oral intake, acyclovir 5 mg/kg IV every 8 hours for 7 to 14 days is recommended. For acyclovir resistant strains, foscarnet 40 mg/kg IV every 8 to 12 hours for 2 to 3 weeks is effective. Valacyclovir and famciclovir generally are accepted as valid alternatives to oral acyclovir allowing more convenient twice-daily dosing, although there are limited studies with these agents in HSV esophagitis. Prophylaxis is not recommended.

Complications

Complications are rare and include bleeding from severe ulcerations. As with other causes of infectious esophagitis, odynophagia diminishes oral intake and increases the risk of dehydration and malnutrition. Acyclovir is remarkably well tolerated by most patients with rare instances of renal insufficiency and neurotoxicity (agitation, tremors, hallucinations, delirium).

CYTOMEGALOVIRUS ESOPHAGITIS

CMV is a rare cause of disease in immunocompetent hosts, and is most frequently seen in immunocompromised patients. In solid organ transplant patients, disease typically occurs when the donor is CMV-seropositive and the recipient is negative. In bone marrow transplant patients, disease results from reactivation of latent infection in the recipient 1 to 3 months after transplant. In HIV-infected patients, reactivation of CMV is the cause of disease. This usually occurs when the $CD4^+$ T lymphocyte counts are less than $50/mm^3$. CMV is the most common cause of esophageal ulcer in AIDS patients and was the cause of GI disease in up to 5% of these patients prior to the availability of highly active antiretroviral therapy (HAART).

Clinical features

CMV esophagitis presents with severe odynophagia. This is often accompanied by focal, substernal chest pain. Oral lesions often in the form of mouth sores and low-grade fever also may be present.

Investigation

Typical lesions include single or multiple, linear, deep ulcers with central umbilication, often greater than 2 cm in size. Barium esophogram may reveal these lesions, but diagnosis usually is confirmed by visualizing these ulcers at endoscopy, along with biopsies from the base of the ulcer (where the cytopathic viral effect is found). Up to 10 biopsy samples may be necessary to confirm the diagnosis. Mucosal biopsy reveals cytomegalic cells, large cells containing eosinophilic intranuclear and basophilic intracytoplasmic inclusions. Viral culture of mucosal biopsy is unhelpful as CMV shedding is neither sensitive nor specific for CMV GI disease. Likewise, serologic testing is of little value because of the high rate of seropositivity in the population. Patients with CMV GI diseases often have concurrent or previous CMV retinitis. Therefore, all patients will require an ophthalmologic evaluation.

Management

IV therapy with ganciclovir, foscarnet, or cidofovir are all equally effective and form the mainstay of therapy. Valganciclovir, the oral formulation of ganciclovir, is believed to have similar efficacy to IV ganciclovir based on treatment of CMV retinitis. Initial therapy is recommended with ganciclovir 5 mg/kg IV every 12 hours or foscarnet 90 mg/kg IV every 12 hours for 3 to 6 weeks. An additional 4 to 8 weeks of therapy is recommended in transplant patients until immunosuppressive medication may be discontinued or decreased. Patients with AIDS may benefit from instituting HAART regimen. Maintenance therapy is not usually recommended in patients with satisfactory response to therapy as it does not prevent progression of disease or decrease time to relapse. Reinduction with ganciclovir 5 mg/kg IV every 12 hours for 3 to 6 weeks and then 5 mg/kg IV daily or 1 to 2 g orally 3 times daily is recommended for relapse therapy. Foscarnet is used in patients with ganciclovir resistance. Salvage therapy with a combination of ganciclovir and foscarnet is indicated for relapse despite maintenance treatment or failure of ganciclovir. For patients intolerant of ganciclovir or foscarnet, cidofovir 5 mg/kg IV weekly for 2 weeks, then 5 mg/kg IV every 2 weeks is recommended based on treatment of CMV retinitis (decrease to 3 mg/kg IV every 2 weeks for increased serum creatinine of 0.3 to 0.4 mg/dL over baseline).

Complications

Mucosal inflammation and tissue necrosis can lead to hemorrhage (up to 5% of patients) and perforation, rarely resulting in bronchoesophageal fistula. Myelosuppression is the main toxicity of ganciclovir therapy. Neutropenia may be treated with granulocyte-colony stimulating factor. Foscarnet is known to cause acute tubular necrosis with resulting rise in serum creatinine. In contrast to foscarnet, the nephrotoxicity of cidofovir is irreversible. Cidofovir can cause a dose-dependent proximal tubular cell injury. Concomitant use of probenecid (to block the uptake of cidofovir by proximal tubular cells) and IV hydration may help to reduce the incidence of renal insufficiency. Other less frequent side effects include neutropenia, peripheral neuropathy, hypotony, anterior uveitis, and alopecia.

BACTERIAL OVERGROWTH SYNDROME

Bacterial overgrowth syndrome occurs when there is an increased number of bacteria in the upper GI tract, with resulting nutrient malabsorption. At birth, the intestine is sterile, but enteric bacteria colonize the intestinal tract within 3 weeks. The GI tract usually hosts about 500 bacterial species, the composition of which is based on host and dietary factors. Under normal conditions, the number of bacteria progressively increases from the stomach and proximal small bowel to the colon. The composition of the intestinal flora remains stable throughout life unless there is a disruption in the normal protective mechanisms that maintain a balance in the number and type of bacteria in the upper GI tract. These host defense mechanisms include the following: Antegrade peristalsis, gastric acid and bile (which destroy bacteria), integrity of bowel mucosa, a mucin layer that traps bacteria, immunoglobulins and immune cells, and an intact ileocecal valve that prevents reflux of bacteria into the small bowel. Disorders compromizing these mechanisms favor the development of bacterial overgrowth. Intestinal stasis may result from strictures due to Crohn disease or radiation treatment, surgical procedures (end-to-side enteroenteric anastomosis, jejunoileal bypass, or Billroth II anastomoses), or intestinal motility disorders (diabetic autonomic neuropathy, scleroderma, or idiopathic intestinal pseudo-obstruction). Small intestinal diverticula may serve as reservoirs for bacterial overgrowth. Immunodeficiency (common variable immunodeficiency, AIDS, severe malnutrition) and hypochlorhydria (acid suppressive medication or peptic ulcer disease surgery) are other predisposing conditions.

Clinical features

Symptoms may be nonspecific and mild. Common symptoms include abdominal pain, bloating, flatulence, diarrhea and weight loss, predominantly caused by malabsorption of bile acids, fats, carbohydrates, and protein. In more severe cases, patients may present with tetany (from hypocalcemia), night blindness (from vitamin A deficiency), arthritis, dermatitis, or peripheral neuropathy. Physical exam may reveal surgical scars and abdominal distention. Bacterial overgrowth should be suspected in patients who present with diarrhea or signs of malabsorption and have a predisposing condition that puts them at high risk. It is not always possible to establish a definitive diagnosis or a causal relationship between bacterial overgrowth and symptoms. Therefore, some clinicians favor empiric treatment with antibiotics targeted at both aerobic and anaerobic enteric flora.

Investigation

Laboratory studies will frequently reveal a macrocytic anemia from vitamin B_{12} malabsorption. Serum folate levels are normal or increased because of bacterial production of folate. An upper GI series with small bowel follow-through can identify hypomotility, strictures, diverticula, fistula, and partial obstruction. Small bowel biopsies are not diagnostic, but may be necessary to rule out other causes of malabsorption such as celiac sprue or giardiasis. The gold standard for the diagnosis of bacterial overgrowth is demonstrating greater than 10^5 organisms/mL in a jejunal aspirate, which can be obtained during endoscopy. Disadvantages include contamination by oropharyngeal flora at collection, sampling error, and missing the diagnosis of bacterial overgrowth by a single culture. Breath tests are viable alternatives to jejunal aspirate culture. The ^{14}C-xylose breath test measures the amount of radiolabeled $^{14}CO_2$ that is released in expired air after gram-negative aerobic bacteria catabolize ingested xylose. Patients with impaired gastric emptying may have false negative results, while rapid intestinal emptying may cause false positive results. This test also involves a minimal amount of radiation exposure and is not recommended in children or fertile women.

The hydrogen breath test is based on the principle that bacteria that ferment malabsorbed carbohydrates usually reside in the colon and fermentation releases hydrogen gas. An early rise in hydrogen concentration to 20 parts per million corresponds to small intestinal bacterial fermentation. No radiation is involved, so this test may be used in children and fertile women. However, up to 20% of patients with bacterial overgrowth are affected by bacteria that do not produce hydrogen. The bile acid breath test or ^{14}C-cholylglycine breath test is no longer used as it does not differentiate between bacterial overgrowth and ileal malabsorption.

Management

Fluid and nutrition support is critical for patients who have weight loss and evidence of micronutrient deficiency. Supplementation of vitamins A, D, and E and calcium may be necessary. Initial avoidance of lactose-containing food may improve symptoms associated with lactase deficiency. Reducing the proportion of carbohydrates ingested may decrease abdominal bloating and distention.

Correction of the underlying disorder forms the mainstay of management whenever possible. Antibiotic therapy is tailored to cover both aerobic and anaerobic enteric bacteria including *Bacteroides*, *Escherichia coli*, and *Klebsiella*. Initial therapy with one of the following drugs can be administered for 7 to 10 days: Amoxicillin-clavulanate 875 mg BID; metronidazole 250 mg TID plus trimethoprim-sulfamethoxazole double strength BID or a cephalosporin (cephalexin 250 mg QID); norfloxacin 800 mg QD; or gentamicin 80 mg QD orally and metronidazole 500 mg TID. For recurrent symptoms, patients may require a repeat course of antibiotics. Maintenance antibiotics administered on a regular schedule (for example, the first week of every month) sometimes are required, in which instance rotating the antibiotic regimen will help to decrease resistance. Some of the antibiotics used for patients requiring maintenance therapy are the following: tetracycline 250 mg QID or trimethoprim 200 mg BID, ciprofloxacin 250 mg BID, amoxicillin-clavulanate 500 mg TID, and metronidazole 250 mg TID. Metronidazole can be added to any of the other antibiotics used for maintenance.

Alternative therapies for patients who are unresponsive to antibiotics include intestinal lavage, administration of nonpathogenic strains of bacteria (probiotic therapy), and the use of corticosteroids and 5-ASA preparations. However, these measures offer marginal results and the benefits are seen mostly in the pediatric population. Prokinetic agents have not been proven to be beneficial in treating bacterial overgrowth syndrome.

Complications

The complications associated with bacterial overgrowth syndrome usually reflect the malabsorption of nutrients. Examples are neuropathy associated with vitamin B_{12} deficiency, night blindness from vitamin A deficiency, and tetany from hypocalcemia secondary to vitamin D deficiency.

DIVERTICULITIS

Diverticula are sac-like protrusions of the colonic wall, largely asymptomatic (diverticulosis) but rarely causing hemorrhage or inflammation resulting in diverticulitis. The prevalence of diverticulosis increases with age, ranging from 5% at 40 years of age to 65% at 85 years of age, and is more prevalent in Western nations. Diverticulosis is thought to result from the combination of increased intralumenal pressure and a weakened bowel wall, resulting in herniation of the mucosa at sites of penetrating blood vessels. Diverticulitus results when a microperforation of the diverticular sac results in peridiverticular inflammation and sometimes abscess formation. Approximately 15% to 25% of patients with diverticula develop diverticulitis.

Clinical features

The most common presenting symptom is left lower quadrant pain lasting more than 48 hours. Other symptoms include nausea, vomiting, diarrhea, or constipation. A few patients may have right lower quadrant pain indicating right-sided diverticulitis, which occurs in only 1.5% of patients. Physical exam may reveal a distended abdomen with tenderness in the left lower quadrant. A low-grade fever may be present. Laboratory values usually reflect leukocytosis.

Investigation

CT scanning is the test of choice for evaluation of suspected diverticulitis. CT scanning also may demonstrate complications of diverticulitis such as abscesses, fistulae, and obstruction. Contrast enema with water-soluble contrast is usually safe in uncomplicated disease and may identify a site of perforation. Unlike CT scanning, it provides examination of the colonic lumen and is less expensive. Colonoscopy is best performed after complete resolution of symptoms. This permits evaluation of the entire colon to determine the extent of diverticular disease and to exclude other lesions such as carcinoma.

Management

The choice of management modalities depends on the severity of the illness. Most patients with simple diverticulitis respond to conservative management with antibiotics (ciprofloxacin 500 mg orally BID, metronidazole 500 mg orally TID) and outpatient observation while on a clear liquid diet. Immunocompromised patients (diabetics, patients receiving chemotherapy or corticosteroid therapy) should be hospitalized. More complicated and recurrent cases may require surgical intervention.

Patients with moderate diverticulitis who typically cannot tolerate oral intake are hospitalized for IV antibiotics (eg, cefoxitin, piperacillin-tazobactam, a combination of gentamicin and clindamycin). Bowel rest and IV fluids are administered. Objective imaging studies are repeated, with consideration of surgery in those without improvement.

Patients with severe diverticulitis, typically with diffuse peritonitis, abscess formation, or obstruction usually require surgical intervention. Antibiotic regimens used include ampicillin 2 g IV every 4 to 6 hours, gentamicin 1.5 to 2 mg/kg IV every 8 hours, and metronidazole 500 mg IV every 8 hours; imipenem/cilastatin 500 mg IV every 6 hours; or piperacillin-tazobactam 3.375 to 4.5 g IV every 6 hours. Resection of the involved bowel with primary anastomosis is possible in elective situations (eg, a localized abscess). In emergency situations, in addition to resection of the affected colon, a colostomy may be necessary. Percutaneous drainage of abscesses may allow for elective surgery at a later date. Obstruction is usually partial and may allow for bowel preparation prior to surgical removal of the involved section of colon or stricture. Most cases of fistula formation can be managed with elective one stage surgery, resection, and primary anastomosis. Peritonitis requires immediate surgical exploration and usually results in a 2-stage procedure as described above. Elective surgery previously was recommended for those patients after a second episode of diverticulitis, based on the general belief that the prognosis was worse after a second bout of illness. This has not been substantiated in subsequent studies, so surgery is not for all patients who respond to medical therapy.

Complications

Major complications include fistula, abscess formation, or obstruction. The most common fistula is a colovesical fistula. Patients complain of pneumaturia, dysuria, or fecaluria. Others include colovaginal, coloenteric, and colouterine fistulae. Diagnosis is by flexible sigmoidoscopy and barium enema or, alternately, a CT scan. Direct visualization of the fistula is uncommon. Repair is surgical. Obstruction raises the concern of coexistent carcinoma and usually necessitates removal of the involved bowel segment or stricture, even if biopsy samples are negative for malignancy. Abscesses may be managed with percutaneous drains for up to 30 days, followed by elective surgery in most patients.

CLOSTRIDIUM DIFFICILE COLITIS

Clostridium difficile is a ubiquitous anaerobic, gram-positive, spore-forming rod. C. *difficile* has been cultured from hospital furniture, floors, bedpans, and mops and from the hands and clothing of health care workers. It is the leading cause of nosocomial diarrhea with up to 3 million new cases of diarrhea and colitis each year in the United States. The intestinal carriage rate, though not necessary for infection, is as high as 8% in healthy adults and up to 20% in hospitalized adult patients. The patients most at risk for infection are elderly, debilitated individuals in hospitals or nursing homes, especially those recently treated with antibiotics. Patients become infected when antibiotics alter the normal intestinal flora, permitting colonization with C. *difficile*. Transmission is patient-to-patient or through healthcare workers by the fecal-oral route. Any antibiotic can predispose to C. *difficile* colonization, including metronidazole and vancomycin, the 2 agents commonly used for treatment.

Clinical features

The clinical spectrum ranges from mild diarrhea to fulminant colitis. Symptoms may arise within a few days of initiating antibiotics and up to 30 days after discontinuation. In addition to watery bowel movements, there may be mild abdominal discomfort and fever with leukocytosis. More severe colitis results in moderate to severe lower abdominal pain, nausea and vomiting, tenesmus, and as many as 15 watery bowel movements daily, often with resulting dehydration. Low-grade fever and leukocytosis also may be present. A small number of patients are critically ill at presentation with fulminant colitis. In addition to severe abdominal pain, high fever, and significant leukocytosis, their course can be complicated by an ileus or toxic megacolon, in which case, diarrhea may be absent because of pooling of colonic contents. Rebound tenderness and a rigid abdomen with absent bowel sounds may signify intestinal perforation, a rare complication.

Investigation

The gold standard for detecting and diagnosing C. *difficile* infection is a cytotoxin assay. The test is 94% to 100% sensitive and up to 99% specific. However, the need for a tissue culture facility and the long incubation time makes this test cumbersome, so it is not available in many institutions. A number of enzyme-linked immunosorbent assays (ELISA) are available and are rapid and less expensive with comparable sensitivity and specificity. The disadvantage of the ELISA based assays is that they can miss up to 5% to 10% of cases that are eventually diagnosed by the cytotoxin assay.

Endoscopy generally is not necessary for the diagnosis of C. *difficile colitis*, and is reserved for situations where the diagnosis is in question or an immediate answer is necessary. If possible, colonoscopy is preferable to sigmoidoscopy, as some patients will have pseudomembranes in the proximal colon only. The characteristic appearance at endoscopy is that of white, raised plaques in a patchy distribution with normal-appearing mucosa in between. Some patients have a more confluent distribution of plaques covering the entire colon.

Management

In the mildest cases, cessation of the offending antibiotic may be all that is needed. For others with moderate disease, metronidazole or vancomycin is the drug of choice, both being equally effective. However, the cost and the concern of developing vancomycin-resistant organisms make metronidazole the agent of first choice. For initial therapy of moderate infection, metronidazole 500 mg orally TID or vancomycin 125 mg orally QID are recommended, each for a total of 10 to 14 days. For severe infections vancomycin may be started at 125 mg orally QID and can be advanced to 500 mg orally QID if no improvement. IV metronidazole 500 mg TID can be added if necessary. For fulminant colitis, vancomycin enemas can be considered if the patient is NPO. Some patients will require emergency colectomy because of the high risk of life-threatening complications such as colonic perforation.

Approximately 10% to 25% of patients will suffer relapsing infections that should not be mistaken for the development of antibiotic resistance. For the first relapse, the course of initial therapy can be repeated for 10 to 14 days. For recurrent relapses, longer courses of therapy or pulsed therapy are recommended after confirming the diagnosis. As an example, vancomycin can be given 125 mg orally QID for 7 to 14 days, then BID, QD, and QOD dosing each for 7 days, followed by vancomycin 125 mg orally every 3 days for 14 days. Alternate therapy for recurrent relapses includes cholestyramine 4 g BID in combination with a tapering vancomycin regimen or rifampin 600 mg orally BID with vancomycin 125 mg QID for 7 days. *Saccharomyces boulardii*, a nonpathogenic yeast, can be administered with metronidazole or vancomycin. Small studies have suggested that treatment with microorganism infusion orally or per rectum may be beneficial.

Complications

Patients with fulminant colitis are at the highest risk for developing complications, including a sepsis syndrome marked by fever, hypotension, and marked leukocytosis. Some patients develop a dilated colon or a "toxic megacolon" with increased risk for perforation.

INFECTIOUS COLITIS

The major bacterial pathogens that infect the colon include the *Shigella* species, *Campylobacter* species, and *Escherichia coli*. They produce a similar clinical picture of acute, bloody, low-volume (less than 1 L/day) diarrhea and abdominal cramps.

SHIGELLA INFECTION

Shigella species are aerobic, gram-negative bacilli that are transmitted via the fecal-oral route from person to person or in contaminated food. Children are particularly susceptible. *Shigella* is divided into 4 groups, A through D; *Shigella dysenteriae* type 1, a member of group A, is considered the most virulent. *Shigella sonnei* of group D is responsible for most of the cases of *Shigella* infection in the United States.

Clinical features

The clinical manifestations cover a wide spectrum, ranging from mild diarrhea and abdominal discomfort to toxic megacolon and bowel perforation. Most patients experience fever, moderate crampy abdominal pain, mucoid and bloody diarrhea, and vomiting. Tenesmus also can be a frequent complaint.

Investigation

The diagnosis should be suspected in patients with a compatible history. Stool culture is the test of choice for definitive diagnosis. Ideally the stool sample should be the mucoid portion of the diarrheal stool, immediately inoculated onto culture medium. Given the similarity in presentation, stool sample also should be examined for *Entamoeba histolytica*.

Management

Shigella infection usually is self-limited and antibiotic therapy may not be necessary for mild disease. However, antibiotic treatment has been shown to reduce the severity and duration of symptoms. For adults infected inside the United States, first line of therapy is ciprofloxacin 500 mg orally BID for 5 days (or the equivalent dosage of norfloxacin, ofloxacin, or levofloxacin for 5 days). Alternately, trimethoprim-sulfamethoxazole (TMP-SMX) 160/800 mg orally BID for 5 days can be used, but has been associated with a higher incidence of resistance. For adults infected outside the United States, first-line therapy is similar, with azithromycin as an alternative. For children inside the United States, TMP/SMX 10/50 mg/kg daily in 2 divided doses for 5 days is adequate, with ceftriaxone 50 mg/kg for 5 days as a viable alternative. Outside the United States, children are treated primarily with nalidixic acid 55 mg/kg/day in 4 divided doses.

Complications

Complications are rare and tend to occur with the virulent strains of *S. dysenteriae* type 1. They include bacteremia, toxic megacolon, and perforation with diffuse peritonitis. Reactive arthritis (Reiter syndrome) may occur and consists of a triad of arthritis, urethritis, and conjunctivitis. Another uncommon complication is the hemolytic uremic syndrome, characterized by hemolytic anemia, renal failure with uremia, and disseminated intravascular coagulopathy.

CAMPYLOBACTER COLITIS

Campylobacter species are the most common pathogens to cause acute infectious diarrhea in the United States. The organism is a gram-negative rod that has many subgroups, but *Campylobacter jejuni* and *Campylobacter coli* are the ones that typically cause gastroenteritis that is commonly acquired through the ingestion of poultry, eggs, and contaminated milk. Transmission is also possible by person-to-person contact via the fecal-oral route as well as through direct contact with animal hosts. Children and the elderly are most susceptible to infection. There is an increased incidence of *Campylobacter* infection in people with AIDS.

Clinical features

Clinical manifestations are similar to shigellosis. Patients may be asymptomatic or have a mild course of abdominal pain and diarrhea. Others experience a prodrome of fever, myalgia, and malaise for 24 to 72 hours. This is followed by severe lower abdominal pain and profuse, bloody diarrhea. Abdominal pain may radiate to the right lower quadrant and precede diarrhea, masquerading as acute appendicitis. The diarrhea may be watery and frequent and usually resolves in 5 to 7 days. A few patients report tenesmus. AIDS patients tend to have a more severe, protracted course requiring an extended course of antibiotics.

Investigation

A definitive diagnosis is made by demonstrating the organism in stool culture. Stool samples usually contain leukocytes and erythrocytes.

Management

Antibiotic therapy may not be necessary for patients with mild and resolving symptoms. For those with severe symptoms, antimicrobial therapy has been shown to decrease the duration of symptoms. Erythromycin 500 mg orally BID for 5 days is the first-line agent. An alternate agent is ciprofloxacin 500 mg orally BID for 5 days, which has the advantage of efficacy against *Salmonella, Shigella* and *E. coli* species. However, there are reports of increasing resistance to quinolones.

Complications

Acute complications include bacteremia, toxic megacolon and hemolytic uremic syndrome. An important post-infectious complication is the Guillain-Barre syndrome, thought to be due to cross-reacting antibodies to GM1 ganglioside present in peripheral nerve myelin.

ESCHERICHIA COLI INFECTION

Intestinal infection may be caused by any of the 5 strains of *E. coli*: Enterotoxigenic, enteropathogenic, enteroinvasive, enteroaggregative, and enterohemorrhagic *E. coli*. Enteroinvasive and enterohemorrhagic *E. coli* affect mainly the colon and result in a diarrheal illness similar to that caused by *Shigella* and *Campylobacter*. *E. coli* are normal inhabitants of the GI tract and become pathogenic by acquiring certain genetic material. Pathogenic strains are acquired through contaminated foods.

ENTEROINVASIVE *E. COLI*

Enteroinvasive *E. coli* produce an infectious illness much like shigellosis. Both invade enterocytes leading to cell death. Infection is acquired through contaminated food.

Clinical features

Patients have a watery diarrhea that is sometimes bloody, as well as abdominal pain, fever, and malaise.

Investigation

Stool examination for leukocytes and erythrocytes may be useful. To specifically identify EIEC, serotyping of the O and H antigens specifically identifies enteroinvasive *E. coli*. An ELISA for membrane protein also is available.

Management

Given the similarities shared with shigellosis, similar antibiotic regimens are used. Recommended regimens are TMP-SMX 160/800 mg orally BID or ciprofloxacin 500 mg orally QID.

Complications

Enteroinvasive *E. coli* infections typically are uncomplicated and do not result in chronic infection.

ENTEROHEMORRHAGIC *E. COLI*

Enterohemorrhagic *E. coli* is responsible for large outbreaks of diarrhea; the most notable occurred in 1982 in the United States after people ingested contaminated hamburgers. The strain was identified as O157:H7. Approximately 20,000 cases are reported annually in the United States.

Clinical features

Almost all patients have bloody diarrhea and severe abdominal pain. As with other causes of dysentery, the clinical course may be mild.

Investigation

Stool should be cultured for *E. coli* with special analysis for O157:H7 on sorbitol-MacConkey agar. Sorbitol-negative colonies can be diagnosed with serum antibody testing. Stool should be tested within the first few days of symptoms; testing 3 samples dramatically increases the yield.

Management

Antibiotic therapy generally is not recommended, as there is no definitive evidence that this shortens the duration of symptoms. In fact, antibiotics have been implicated in the subsequent development of the hemolytic uremic syndrome by increasing the production or release of toxins. Care is supportive and may include dialysis for patients who develop the hemolytic uremic syndrome.

Complications

The most dreaded complication is the hemolytic uremic syndrome, occuring mostly in children and elderly. Thrombotic thrombocytopenic purpura also occurs in a small number of cases, with fever and neurologic symptoms.

GASTROENTERITIS

Diarrheal illness is one of the leading causes of death worldwide. Fortunately, most cases are self-limited. This section will focus on the major pathogens that infect the small intestine. Some pathogens, such as *Giardia*, *Cryptosporidium*, and *E. coli*, have been covered elsewhere in this chapter.

STAPHYLOCOCCUS AUREUS

This gram-positive coccus is a normal inhabitant of the skin and mucous membranes of some healthy people. Infection results when these hosts contaminate food that is later ingested by susceptible individuals. *Staphylococcus aureus* exerts its pathogenic effects via enterotoxins, resulting in secretory diarrhea. Patients present with vomiting and, later, diarrhea within 6 to 8 hours after ingesting contaminated food. The illness usually resolves spontaneously and no specific antibiotic therapy is required. Treatment is supportive.

BACILLUS CEREUS

Bacillus cereus is an aerobic, gram-positive, spore-forming rod that is found in soil, water, and raw foods, and also colonizes healthy human beings. As in *S. aureus* infections, symptoms result within hours after ingesting contaminated food. Typical agents of transmission include rice, vegetables, and meats. The organism acts through release of a preformed toxin. Patients either have early onset of nausea and vomiting (within 5 to 6 hours) or abdominal cramping and watery diarrhea. Diagnosis is mostly by history. The disease is self-limited. Therapy is supportive and antibiotics are generally not recommended.

CLOSTRIDIUM BOTULINUM

Clostridium botulinum is an anaerobic, gram-positive, spore-forming organism that prefers anaerobic conditions where the pH is greater than 4. Home-canned foods and fish provide the ideal reservoir. After ingesting contaminated food, a neurotoxin is released that causes nausea, vomiting, diarrhea, and abdominal pain within 24 hours. Neurological symptoms such as lower extremity weakness, respiratory muscle weakness, dysphagia, and dysarthria can occur. The neurotoxin can be detected in stool or emesis as well as uncontaminated food. Treatment is with antitoxin; antibiotics are not indicated. Botulism may be fatal in as many as 15% of patients.

SALMONELLA

Salmonella are anaerobic, gram-negative, spore-forming rods classified as the species *Salmonella choleraesuis*, of which there are many subgroups. The serotypes of subgroup 1 are pathogenic to humans. Specifically, *S. typhi* and *S. paratyphi* reside in the human host, while the others are found in the environment and animal hosts. Clinical syndromes vary from asymptomatic carrier state to frank gastroenteritis, bacteremia, or enteric fever.

Nontyphoid salmonellosis

S. enteritidis and *S. typhimurium* are the most commonly isolated nontyphoid serotypes and are responsible for diarrheal outbreaks. Most cases can be attributed to contaminated milk and poultry products. Transmission also may be person-to-person through a fecal-oral route. Children, the elderly, and the immunosuppressed are most susceptible. The severity of the disease correlates with the size of the inoculum. Organisms invade enterocytes, causing inflammation and releasing toxins that lead to diarrhea.

Clinical features

The manifestations of *Salmonella* gastroenteritis are varied, ranging from a mild, self-limited, diarrheal illness to copious and occasionally bloody diarrhea. Patients experience fever, nausea, vomiting, and crampy abdominal pain.

Investigation

Organisms can be isolated in stool cultures within 48 to 72 hours.

Management

Most infections are asymptomatic or with mild symptoms and require only supportive care. For patients with severe symptoms, the elderly, or the immunocompromised, ciprofloxacin 500 mg orally BID for 3 to 7 days, TMP-SMX 160/800 mg orally BID, or a third generation cephalosporin is recommended. Patients with bacteremia or AIDS require IV antibiotics for 7 to 14 days. Some clinicians advocate an additional 4 weeks of oral therapy.

Complications

Complications include bacteremia, especially in children and immunocompromised individuals. Patients with sickle-cell disease are at increased risk of developing osteomyelitis.

Typhoid (enteric) fever

Although any of the *Salmonella* serotypes can cause typhoid fever, it occurs most commonly from S.*typhi* and S.*paratyphi* infection.

Clinical features

Symptoms appear 2 to 3 weeks after ingesting contaminated food. Patients may initially have transient enteritis, followed by a persisting fever, abdominal pain, and a characteristic salmon-colored rash on the trunk and abdomen. Still later, some patients develop intestinal bleeding and perforation. Other symptoms include mental status changes and anorexia. Hepatosplenomegaly and abdominal tenderness are commonly found on physical exam.

Investigation

Most patients have a positive blood culture. In addition, stool, urine, and duodenal aspirate cultures are helpful in making the diagnosis.

Management

Because of increased resistance to chloramphenicol and TMP/SMX, ciprofloxacin 500 mg orally BID or ofloxacin 400 mg orally BID for 7 to 10 days are currently the drugs of choice. Alternately, ceftriaxone 2 to 3 g QD for 7 to 14 days may be used.

Complications

Septic shock and intestinal perforation are two of the more common complications. Other complications include the formation of splenic or liver abscesses, orchitis, or carditis.

YERSINIA SPECIES

Yersiniae are gram-negative coccobacilli. Three species are known to cause disease in humans, *Yersinia enterocolitica*, *Yersinia pseudotuberuclosis*, and *Yersinia pestis*. While *Y. enterocolitica* and *Y. pseudotuberculosis* can both cause GI illness, *Y. enterocolitica* is the more commonly implicated in the United States. Children are affected most. Infection is transmitted through the ingestion of contaminated water and food, as well as through animals such as dogs and swine. Person-to-person transmission through the fecal-oral route is also possible.

Clinical features

Fever, diarrhea, abdominal pain, and, occasionally, nausea and vomiting highlight the course of gastroenteritis. Patients with right lower quadrant abdominal pain and less diarrhea may be misdiagnosed as acute appendicitis.

Investigation

Culture of stool remains the definitive diagnostic test. Culturing specimens from other involved sites such as blood, throat, and joint fluid also may be helpful. ELISAs and immunoblotting can be used to detect antibodies to *Yersinia*, but are not readily available in the United States.

Management

Antibiotic therapy is only indicated in severe, systemic illness in the form of ciprofloxacin 500 mg orally BID for 3 to 5 days or a third-generation cephalosporin (such as ceftriaxone) plus gentamicin for those in need of IV therapy. In patients with more complicated or extraintestinal infections, doxycycline or TMP-SMX is indicated.

Complications

Complications occur several weeks after onset of the infection and include suppurative appendicitis, intestinal perforation with peritonitis, bowel necrosis, and toxic megacolon. Extraintestinal complications are cholangitis, hepatic and splenic abscesses, osteomyelitis, septic arthritis, and mycotic aneurysms.

VIBRIO SPECIES

Cholera is a diarrheal disease caused by the gram-negative bacterium *Vibrio cholera*. There are 34 *Vibrio* species in all, of which one-third are pathogenic to humans. This section will focus on *V. cholera*, which is responsible for over 5.5 million cases of diarrheal illnesses worldwide annually. The reservoir is cold, salt water. Transmission of infection is by fecally contaminated water or undercooked seafood

Clinical features

Many infections are asymptomatic. Those with mild disease are indistinguishable from other causes of gastroenteritis. In patients with severe illness, the hallmark of cholera is profuse, watery diarrhea of up to 500 and 1000 mL/hour. This may be accompanied by crampy abdominal discomfort and nausea and vomiting.

Investigation

The history and clinical picture can suggest the diagnosis. Demonstrating the organism on stool dark field or phase contrast microscopy provides a definitive diagnosis. *V. cholerae* also can be detected by polymerase chain reaction.

Management

Rehydration and replacement of electrolytes are critical. The World Health Organization (WHO) has recommended an oral rehydration solution specially formulated to replace fluid and electrolytes, containing 3.5 g sodium chloride, 2.9 g trisodium citrate or 2.5 g sodium bicarbonate, 1.5 g potassium chloride, and 20 g glucose or 40 g sucrose in a liter of water. Caution should be used with sports drinks and carbonated beverages, as they do not provide the necessary fluid and electrolyte balance. Patients with severe dehydration will require hospitalization for IV rehydration. Antibiotic therapy with an oral quinolone or doxycycline has been shown to reduce the duration of symptoms and decrease the amount of diarrhea.

Complications

Complications are mostly caused by severe fluid and electrolyte imbalances, and include pre-renal azotemia, arrhythmia, and ileus from severe hypokalemia. Hypoglycemia can result in mental status changes and seizures.

ROTAVIRUS

Rotavirus is the most common cause of severe viral gastroenteritis in children worldwide. Approximately 1 million cases are reported in the United States annually. Although children are primarily affected, elderly adults also are susceptible. Infection generally is spread through the fecal-oral route or, less commonly, by contaminated water. The virus infects and destroys intestinal villous epithelial cells, which leads to brush border enzyme deficiency, malabsorption, and an osmotic diarrhea.

Clinical features

Symptoms are nonspecific and include fever, vomiting, and diarrhea. Up to 50% of children will have concurrent respiratory symptoms.

Investigation

Rotavirus can be detected in stool culture. However, the more rapid ELISA and polymerase chain reaction (PCR) techniques are routinely employed.

Management

Treatment is supportive with rehydration. No antiviral medication exists for the specific treatment of this disorder.

Complications

Many clinical illnesses may coexist with Rotavirus infection but a causal relationship is not always clear. These include necrotizing enterocolitis, intussusceptions, and biliary atresia.

NORWALK VIRUS

Norwalk virus is named for the 1968 epidemic outbreak of gastroenteritis in Norwalk, Ohio, and is associated with over one-third of nonbacterial gastroenteritis outbreaks in the United States. Ingesting contaminated food, especially raw shellfish, contaminated water, and stored, previously cooked food transmits disease.

Clinical features

Patients typically become symptomatic about 24 to 48 hours after infection. Symptoms include nausea, vomiting, headache, body aches, abdominal cramps, and fever. Diarrhea is watery and typically not bloody. Symptoms generally resolve spontaneously in 72 hours.

Investigation

Because of the usual mild, self-limiting nature of the disease, definitive diagnosis is not critical. Detection of the virus in cell culture or electron microscopy is difficult as it is shed in such small quantities. Detection by ELISA or PCR techniques is performed for epidemiologic and research purposes.

Management

Care is supportive with rehydration as necessary. No other specific therapy is recommended.

Complications

Infection is usually without complications or long-term sequelae

ENTERIC ADENOVIRUS

The enteric adenoviruses are a subgroup of the adenovirus family. Subgroup F adenoviruses types 40 and 41 have been designated the enteric adenovirus because of their association with gastroenteritis. They tend to infect children less than 2 years of age. Transmission is fecal-oral, especially in day care centers and hospitals.

Clinical features

The illness and natural course is indistinguishable from other viral gastroenteritis. Symptoms of watery diarrhea and vomiting present about 7 days after infection. It is usually self-limited, but protracted courses occasionally occur.

Investigation

Enteric adenoviruses do not grow well on routine culture. A virus specific enzyme immunoassay is the test of choice.

Management

Treatment is supportive.

Complications

There have been reports of lactose intolerance and malabsorption after resolution of acute infection with adenovirus.

PARASITES

GIARDIASIS

Giardia lamblia is a flagellated protozoan that is found in streams and surface reservoirs, uncooked food contaminated with cysts, and in the stool of infected persons. It is transmitted by ingesting contaminated food or water or through practices of poor hygiene or anal sex (direct fecal contact). Day care workers and attendees and male homosexuals are at increased risk. The organism exists as a cyst outside the body and is converted to its flagellated trophozoite form in the proximal small bowel. Approximately 2.5 million cases are reported annually in the United States.

Clinical features

Most patients have an asymptomatic course of infection. Others have an acute self-limited illness and present with foul-smelling diarrhea, abdominal cramps, bloating, flatulence, nausea, vomiting, and weight loss. Symptoms tend to last for a few weeks. A small number of patients will go on to have a chronic course of infection, when the stool is loose but not diarrheal and weight loss is more pronounced. Generalized malaise and depression also are common. Symptoms may last for months.

Investigation

Direct microscopic examination of stool for ova and parasites is the most common method of detecting infection, with a higher yield from examining 3 stool specimens. There is usually no fecal blood or leukocytes present. A number of *Giardia* antigen ELISA or immunoflorescence assays are readily available that are more sensitive and specific than the stool microscopic examination. Small bowel biopsy may be useful in ruling out other causes of diarrhea but there is usually no histopathologic abnormality specific for giardiasis.

Management

Metronidazole 250 mg orally TID for 5 days is first-line therapy. For resistant cases, metronidazole 750 mg orally TID for 10 days is effective. Tinidazole 2 gm orally one-time dosing is equally effective but not currently available in the United States. Albendazole 400 mg or 22.5 mg/kg orally for 5 days is also highly effective.

Complications

The most significant complications are severe malabsorption and weight loss.

CRYPTOSPORIDIOSIS

Cryptosporidium parvum exists as oocysts outside its human host. After ingestion, the sporozoite form is released and attaches to small bowel epithelial cell wall, which matures and releases merozoites intraluminally. *C. parvum*, like giardia, is one of the most common parasitic enteric pathogens in humans. It is commonly found in the feces of infected persons or contaminated food or water sources. High-risk populations include children and employees of day care centers and sexual partners of infected persons. *C. parvum* infection affects both immunocompetent and immunocompromised hosts, with a higher prevalence among patients with human immunodeficiency virus (HIV) infection.

Clinical features

Cryptosporidiosis can result in asymptomatic infection, especially in the immunocompetent host. Some patients have mild symptoms consisting of diarrhea, nausea, and crampy abdominal pain. Others have more severe enteritis with voluminous diarrhea and weight loss. The illness usually is self-limited and resolves in about 14 days. Immunocompromised patients tend to experience a more protracted course, especially AIDS patients with CD_4 lymphocyte count less than $100/mm^3$. Cryptosporidiosis can involve the hepatobiliary system as well, causing cholecystitis, cholangitis, hepatitis, or pancreatitis. These patients present with right upper quadrant pain and fever.

Investigation

The mainstay of diagnosis is stool microscopic analysis using modified acid-fast stains, hematoxylin and eosin and giemsa stains. Routine stool inspection for ova and parasites may miss the diagnosis. ELISA tests, though more expensive, have increased yield when compared to routine stool analysis. C. *parvum* also can be detected in small bowel aspirates and biliary secretions.

Management

There is no one treatment regimen that reliably results in a cure. Typically, immunocompetent patients recover spontaneously, while immunocompromised hosts recover once their immune status has been corrected. Results are disappointing with agents such as paromomycin, metronidazole, azithromycin, and clarithromycin. Currently, nitazoxanide 500 mg orally BID for 3 days is used but is not FDA approved. Supportive care with antidiarrheal agents is often indicated.

Complications

Prolonged diarrhea can result in nutrient deficiency and weight loss. Wasting is more severe in immunocompromised hosts.

AMEBIASIS

Entamoeba histolytica is the protozoan agent that causes intestinal and extraintestinal amebiasis. The organism exists as a cyst that, when ingested, releases an invasive trophozoite that penetrates the wall of the small intestine. As with the other parasites, it is acquired through contaminated food or water or contact with the feces of infected persons. Amebiasis is more prevalent in developing countries. The prevalence in the United States is about 4% and is usually seen in travelers with prolonged visits (greater than 1 month's duration) to endemic countries.

Clinical features

The vast majority of infections are asymptomatic with more severe symptoms seen in young patients and the immunosuppressed (especially with HIV infection). Patients present with abdominal pain and diarrhea with grossly bloody stools. Occasionally they are febrile. The most common extraintestinal manifestation is liver abscesses, presenting with fever and right upper quadrant pain for weeks to months. Rarely, jaundice or concomitant diarrhea also are seen.

Investigation

Stool microscopic examination may reveal cysts or trophozoites. Again, 3 stool samples increase the yield. Occasionally, distinguishing between *E. histolytica* and *E. dispar* (a nonpathogenic species) is difficult, and antigen detection tests using ELISA may be necessary. Amebic liver abscesses are best detected by ultrasound, CT, or magnetic resonance imaging (MRI), although none of these imaging modalities can differentiate between the various etiologies of liver cysts.

Management

Metronidazole 750 mg orally TID for 10 days is curative in 90% of cases. An alternate treatment regimen is tinidazole 2 g orally QD for 3 days, but this drug is not readily available in the United States. Dehydroemetine 1 to 1.5 mg/kg orally QD for 5 days is equally effective but its cardiotoxicity is prohibitive. Some clinicians advocate adding paromomycin 30 mg/kg orally QD for 5 to 10 days to metronidazole therapy in order to help eradicate luminal cysts. The treatment for amebic liver abscess is the same as that for intestinal amebiasis.

Complications

Invasion of the bowel wall with necrosis and perforation is a rare complication with a mortality approaching 40%. Granulation tissue can occasionally form masses known as amebomas, which may cause obstructive symptoms if large. Other complications include rectovaginal fistulae.

INTESTINAL HELMINTHS

Intestinal helminths tend to be more prevalent in areas of the world where sanitation is poor. Helminths typically have complex life cycles that involve multiplying or reproducing outside the host. Most have a lifespan of years and some can survive for decades.

ENTEROBIASIS

Enterobiasis is the most common helminthic infection in the United States, caused by the nematode *Enterobius vermicularis* (pinworm). Humans are the natural hosts, occurring most frequently in school-age children. Infection begins with ingestion of ova through the fecal-oral route. Once ingested, ova hatch and adult worms live in the cecum and appendix. Subsequently, the female migrates out the rectum to release her eggs onto the perianal skin. Eggs are transferred to the hands of the infected person through scratching. Later, the host can unknowingly ingest these eggs and the life cycle starts over again. Others who eat food prepared by the infected person can also become infected. The lifespan of an adult female is approximately 12 weeks.

Clinical features

Most infections are asymptomatic. The most common symptom is perianal itching. Excessive scratching with severe excoriations can lead to secondary bacterial skin infections. If the worm burden is sufficiently high, patients may complain of nausea, vomiting, and abdominal pain.

Investigation

The best test to detect eggs is the "tape test." A strip of transparent tape is attached to a tongue depressor. The tape is then pressed against the perianal skin, and the eggs stick to the tape. The tape is then transferred to a glass slide where the eggs can be visualized under the microscope. The test should be performed at night or first thing in the morning before bathing or showering. Worms and eggs are not typically passed in the stool, so stool examination generally is not required.

Management

Mebendazole or albendazole is the mainstay of therapy. Mebendazole is given in a 100 mg dose, and repeated in 1 to 2 weeks to prevent recurrence. Alternately, albendazole can be administered at a dose of 400 mg orally and repeated in 2 weeks. Pyrantel pamoate 11 mg/kg (maximum 1 g), is highly effective and the preferred therapy for pregnant patients. All household members are treated to prevent reinfection. All linen should be washed thoroughly.

Complications

Pinworms can migrate to the genital tract of females and cause vulvovaginits and, rarely, salpingitis, oophoritis, and cervical granulomas.

CHAPTER 9

NUTRITION AND VITAMIN DEFICIENCIES

MALNUTRITION IN GI DISEASE

Malnutrition contributes to increased morbidity and mortality in outpatients and hospitalized patients. Malnutrition is a common complication of many GI and liver conditions. Careful assessment allows the determination of which patients need nutritional support, as well as monitoring of the efficacy of nutritional support. The most common type of malnutrition encountered is protein-calorie malnutrition. This condition results in inadequate muscle and visceral protein stores and depleted adipose tissue calorie reserves. Protein-calorie malnutrition, especially if moderate or severe, increases morbidity and mortality. Consequently, early detection and management of protein-calorie malnutrition is essential. Specific vitamin and mineral deficiencies also may accompany many different disease states.

Clinical features

Many of the presenting features of malnutrition are nonspecific. Frequent symptoms include recent weight loss, poor intake, fatigue, muscle weakness, and peripheral edema. Common signs are temporal wasting, muscle wasting, thinning hair, abdominal distention, hepatomegaly, and decubitus ulcers. Because many of these findings are part of other chronic illnesses, a careful history will help determine if poor nutritional status or another disease state is contributing to the clinical manifestations.

If malnutrition is suspected based on any of the above presenting symptoms, questions should be directed at identifying a possible cause. A careful dietary history should be performed, including types and quantity of food, which may necessitate daily calorie counts by a dietician. Evidence of decreased oral intake should prompt further questions as to the reasons for inadequate intake. A change in appetite, poorly fitting dentures, difficulty chewing or swallowing, poor taste or smell, and inability to pay for food are common causes of decreased oral intake. The amount of weight loss should be calculated, with losses of more than 5% in 1 month or more than 10% in 6 months indicating significant weight loss. Symptoms of malaborption such as steatorrhea, bloating, or diarrhea may point to inadequate nutrient absorption. Ongoing alcohol use may limit the amount of nonalcohol calories consumed.

The most important part of the physical examination is a determination of the patient's body mass index (BMI). This is calculated according to the following formula: BMI = weight (kg)/(height)^2 (m^2). The BMI allows categorization of weight and determination of associated disease risk. Table 1 lists the BMI weight categories along with the associated disease risk.

Table 1. BMI and associated disease risk

Category	*BMI (kg/m^2)*	*Risk*
Extremely underweight	< 14.0	Extremely high
Underweight	14.1–18.4	Chronic illness
Normal	18.5–24.9	Normal
Overweight	25.0–29.9	Increased
Obesity Class I	30.0–34.9	High
Obesity Class II	35.0–39.9	Very high
Obesity Class III	> 40.0	Extremely high

Volume depletion may be apparent in patients with inadequate oral intake, manifested by confusion, orthostasis, and poor skin turgor. Muscle strength and endurance correlate well with malnutrition, and grip strength is a good indicator of nutritional status. Specific nutrient deficiencies may produce certain physical findings. These findings are described in the section of nutrient deficiencies. Finally, anthropomorphic measures, including triceps skinfold thickness and midarm muscle circumference, have been used to determine body fat and protein composition. However, these measures generally are not used in clinical practice.

Investigation

Various serum markers have been used as markers of nutritional status. Decreased levels of certain circulating proteins are often cited as evidence of malnutrition, but these are very nonspecific.

Albumin is synthesized by the liver and is the most abundant circulating protein. The half-life of albumin is approximately 20 days, making it a suitable candidate for long-term nutritional status. The levels correlate well with morbidity and mortality but correlate poorly with nutritional status. Albumin levels are a better marker of disease severity than of nutritional status. Serum albumin levels are decreased in liver disease, ascites, nephrotic syndrome, malignancy, inflammation, and any acute illness. Transferrin is a protein involved in iron transport and is synthesized mainly by the liver as well. The half-life is 8 to 9 days, but it is also a nonspecific marker of nutritional status. It is decreased in anemia of chronic disease, liver disease, burns, and nephrotic syndrome and is increased in hypoxia, pregnancy, and hormone therapy. Other serum proteins, such as retinol-binding protein and thyroxine-binding prealbumin, have been used as markers of nutritional status. These also are limited by poor specificity.

Many functions of the immune system are impaired in patients with malnutrition. Consequently, various measures of the immune system have been used as measures nutritional status. Total lymphocyte count and delayed-type hypersensitivity reactions, like many of the serum protein levels, are limited by poor specificity. Overall, laboratory data are not particularly helpful in the assessment of nutritional status.

Management

The combination of a careful history and physical examination allows most patients to be classified as normal/mildly malnourished, moderately malnourished, or severely malnourished. Once the nutritional assessment is complete, the need for nutritional support can be determined. Several important questions must be answered to determine whether nutritional support is needed, what type of support to utilize, and the duration of support.

Are nutritional requirements being met? The patient's daily protein and calorie requirements can be estimated based on the degree of metabolic stress: Normal/mild stress—25 kcal/kg and 0.75 g protein/kg; moderate/severe stress—35 kcal/kg and 1 to 1.5 g protein/kg. More complex calculations may be required for patients who are severely underweight or obese. The intake should be calculated based on history and daily calorie counts by a dietician. If the nutritional requirements are being attained based on measured intake, then no nutritional support is needed. If the nutritional needs are not being met, then additional questions must be answered to determine if nutritional support is needed.

What is the current nutritional status? This is generally assessed as described above. The degree of malnutrition will determine the urgency of initiating support.

What is the anticipated duration of inadequate intake? Often, it is difficult to predict the duration of negative balance. Most patients can tolerate a short duration of inadequate nutrition, but severely malnourished individuals will require earlier support. Therefore, an estimate of the time interval of inadequate intake allows planning of nutritional support. The duration of inadequate intake can be arbitrarily divided into short (less than 7 to 10 days) and long (greater than 7 to 10 days) intervals. The nutritional balance, current nutritional status, and anticipated duration of inadequate intake can be used to determine the need for nutritional support. No nutritional support is needed for patients with mild malnutrition with positive energy balance or negative energy balance but short duration of inadequate intake; patients with long duration of inadequate intake are encouraged to increase oral intake. On the other hand, patients with moderate or severe malnutrition generally need nutritional support unless they have positive nutritional balance. Patients with long duration of inadequate intake in this category need immediate nutritional support, while all others need to be given an initial trial of increased oral intake.

What type of support is needed? Once the decision has been made to initiate nutritional support, then the best method of delivery should be determined. Enteral feeding is the preferred option, but many patients will require parenteral feeding. In general, if the gut works, use it.

Enteral nutrition

Enteral nutrition is the administration of liquid-formula diets by mouth or tube into the GI tract. This is the preferred route for nutritional support. Relative contraindications to enteral feeding include ileus, intestinal obstruction, massive GI bleeding, high-output enteric fistulas, and severe inflammatory conditions that may worsen with enteral feeding. In the absence of any of these conditions, most individuals can be safely fed into the gut. For patients who can drink liquids, nutritional support may be given in the form of oral supplements. For individuals with inadequate oral intake, oropharyngeal dysphagia, or other contraindications to oral feeding, direct feeding via tube may be used. Options include placement of a nasogastric tube, nasoduodenal tube (Dobhoff), gastrostomy tube, or jejunostomy tube. Gastric feedings may be given as bolus feedings, whereas small bowel tube feedings generally must be given as continuous infusions. Gastric feedings generally are better tolerated than small bowel feedings but may increase aspiration risk in predisposed individuals.

Once the route of enteral feeding has been chosen, the appropriate formulation must be selected. Most liquid formula diets are either balanced or modified formulas. The balanced formulas contain carbohydrates, proteins, and fats in compositions similar to the typical American diet. Carbohydrates are supplied as oligosaccharides and polysaccharides, fat as medium and long chain triglycerides, and protein as intact or partially hydrolyzed natural proteins. The caloric density of these products ranges from 1 to 2 kcal/mL. The patient's fluid requirement helps determine which caloric density is most appropriate. Many commercially available formulas are available in flavored liquids. This type of nutritional support is appropriate for the majority of individuals who require enteral nutritional support.

Modified diets, or elemental diets, are composed of amino acids or short peptides, dextrose or oligosaccharides, and medium chain triglycerides or essential fatty acids. These are specially formulated for specific disease states. Patients with renal failure require low protein formulas with low electrolytes and only essential amino acids, while hepatic failure patients require low protein formulas with increased branched-chain amino acids. Formulas for pulmonary failure are low in carbohydrate but high in fat. Short peptides, medium chain triglycerides and glutamine are important components of formulas for patients with GI dysfunction.

Oral supplements generally are provided as drinks or shakes to increase calorie and protein intake to the desired level. For individuals starting gastric tube feedings, the rate should begin at 30 mL/hr in scheduled boluses. Small bowel feedings should begin at 30 mL/hr contInous infusion. If the patient tolerates the tube feedings, the rate is increased slowly until the target rate has been attained.

Parenteral nutrition

Many individuals who require nutritional support cannot be fed via the GI support. In these cases, nutrition must be given by IV infusion.

The 2 main types of parenteral nutrition are peripheral venous and central venous infusions. Peripheral vein infusions carry a lower risk of mechanical complications but are limited in usefulness by the large amount of fluid required to achieve adequate energy requirements. Therefore, peripheral vein infusions are used only as supplements in patients who require less intensive support or when central venous access cannot be obtained. The majority of patients who require parenteral support will receive central venous infusions. The remainder of this discussion will apply to central venous infusions.

The central venous solutions generally are formulated in the hospital pharmacy. The solutions are hypertonic (greater than 1900 mOsm/kg) and therefore must be given through a large central venous catheter, usually in the subclavian vein or internal jugular vein. Alternatively, a peripherally inserted central catheter (PICC) may be used. The solutions are combinations of hypertonic dextrose, amino acids, and fat emulsion, with electrolytes, vitamins, and minerals added as specified. The solution may be given as a 24-hour continuous infusion or cycled over 12-hour periods. Input from a nutrition support service can be invaluable in determining the optimal formulation for parenteral nutrition.

Complications

Individuals receiving enteral nutritional support require careful monitoring for adverse effects. The most frequent complication is diarrhea (approximately 75%). There are often many possible causes for diarrhea in a given patient. Decreasing the rate or osmolality or changing the type of formula often will decrease or eliminate the diarrhea. Antidiarrheals may be added if these measures fail. If none of these methods are effective, then other causes for the diarrhea should be sought. Other complications include clogging, leakage of feedings around the tube, and dislodgement of the tube. Clogging usually can be prevented with frequent flushes and effectively managed by instilling a carbonated beverage into the tube if clogging does occur. Leakage of feedings often results from a skin incision too large for the tube. Tube dislodgement often necessitates replacement of the tube. Prevention of these complications generally can be accomplished by careful attention to tube care. The refeeding syndrome may develop in enteral and parenteral nutrition. This condition is rare but may result in serious adverse effects, including CHF, hypokalemia, hypophosphatemia, hypomagnesemia, and edema. Patients with moderate or severe malnutrition should be monitored very closely for this complication when initiating nutritional support.

As with enteral nutrition, patients receiving parenteral nutrition need very close monitoring for complications. Catheter sepsis is the most serious problem related to central venous nutrition. If infection is suspected, the catheter site should be carefully examined. Other sources of infection should be excluded. If testing excludes other sources of infection, the catheter may need to be removed. This complication can be prevented or reduced by following strict protocols by a nurse specializing in the care of central venous catheters. Other complications associated with placement of the catheter include pneumothorax, bleeding, and deep venous thrombosis.

Metabolic complications are not uncommon with parenteral nutrition and are similar to those associated with enteral nutrition. Refeeding syndrome is a rare but potentially serious complication. Hyperglycemia is common, especially in patients with diabetes or impaired glucose intolerance, and usually requires addition of insulin to the solution. Elevated liver enzymes are common and may be due to a number of different conditions, including excessive total calories, excessive fat, choline deficiency, or passage of gallstones caused by gallbladder stasis. Once other causes of abnormal liver chemistries have been excluded, treatment of fatty infiltration caused by parenteral nutrition involves several measures. The total calorie infusion should be decreased if it exceeds requirements, and feeds may be cycled off for 4 to 6 hours a day.

MALABSORPTION

Absorption of nutrients from the intestinal lumen requires several important steps. The luminal phase begins with intraluminal processing by secreted pancreatic enzymes, bile salts, and specific proteins. The mucosal phase continues with brush border hydrolysis and epithelial transport and process. The transport phase moves nutrients into the portal system or the lymphatic system. Abnormalities at any step may result in malabsorption. Luminal abnormalities include pancreatic insufficiency, bile salt deficiency, bacterial overgrowth, and inactivation of intestinal enzymes in Zollinger-Ellison syndrome. Mucosal abnormalities can be seen in lactose intolerance, celiac and tropical sprue, Whipple disease, and Crohn disease. Transport abnormalities are seen in intestinal ischemia and infiltrative processes including lymphoma, amyloid, and scleroderma.

Clinical features

Diarrhea is the most common symptom of malabsorption. It occurs as a result of impaired water and sodium absorption or poorly absorbed carbohydrates or bile salts. Steatorrhea consists of bulky, oily stools that are foul-smelling and difficult to flush. Weight loss, fatigue, abdominal distention or cramps, and flatulence are other common complaints. Less common symptoms include amenorrhea, paresthesias, bone pain, or peripheral neuropathy. The physical examination often will reveal evidence of volume depletion, pallor caused by anemia, cachexia, temporal wasting, or peripheral edema. Certain clinical findings may provide a clue to the underlying cause of malabsorption. Patients with lactase deficiency develop abdominal cramps, flatulence, and diarrhea after consuming dairy products. Individuals with chronic pancreatitis and pancreatic insufficiency usually have a history of heavy alcohol use. Dermatitis herpetiformis is a blistering, pruritic rash on the extensor surfaces and back sometimes identified in patients with celiac sprue.

Investigation

There are a number of tests that can prove useful in the evaluation of malabsorption. Stool fat analysis is often the first test performed. Qualititative analysis is performed using the Sudan II stain to identify the presence of fat droplets in the stool. Quantitative stool fat analysis requires collection of stool samples while the patient is consuming at least 100 g fat/day. The intestine normally absorbs approximately 95% of ingested fat, so the normal value is 5 g/day or less. The d-xylose test helps distinguish between pancreatic insufficiency and small bowel disorders. Xylose is passively absorbed in the small intestine, so impaired absorption suggests a small bowel defect. The patient is given 25 g oral dose of d-xylose and either urinary xylose excretion or blood xylose level is measured. The test is limited somewhat by poor sensitivity and specificity.

If clinical features or initial studies suggest a small bowel disorder, then imaging of the small intestine may be helpful. An upper GI series with small bowel follow-through may identify mucosal thickening, evidence of prior surgery, or terminal ileum disease. Plain films or CT scans of the abdomen may identify pancreatic calcification in patients with chronic pancreatitis. If an abnormality of the small bowel is suspected, upper endoscopy with biopsy of the small bowel may identify the problem. Duodenal biopsies are generally sufficient, but occasionally jejunal or terminal ileal biopsies may be required.

The secretin stimulation test is the gold standard for the diagnosis of pancreatic function. A duodenal tube is used to collect pancreatic secretions in response to an IV secretin load. The test is limited by the invasive nature. The bentiromide test is less specific, but it may also be used to assess pancreatic function. In addition to identifying the cause of malabsorption, specific testing should be performed to identify specific nutrient, vitamin, and mineral deficiencies.

Management

The main management objectives are correction of nutritional deficiencies and specific treatment of the underlying disease, if possible. Careful assessment for protein-calorie assessment is performed as previously outlined and appropriate management initiated. Specific testing for vitamin and mineral deficiencies may be necessary. Specific management of the most common etiologies are described below.

Pancreatic insufficiency

One of the most common causes of malabsorption, pancreatic exocrine insufficiency usually results from chronic alcohol abuse and resultant pancreatitis. Other causes include cystic fibrosis, hereditary pancreatitis, surgical resection, and pancreatic cancer. Malabsorption does not usually occur until more than 90% of exocrine function has been lost. Enzyme replacement forms the cornerstone of therapy. Large doses of supplemental enzymes are required to control steatorrhea in most patients. The available enzyme preparations are composed of pancreatin or pancrelipase. At least 30,000 IU of lipase must be taken with each meal to control steatorrhea. As enzymes may be degraded in an acidic environment, administration of a proton-pump inhibitor or H_2-receptor antagonist may further decrease steatorrhea. Adequate control of steatorrhea generally results in significant improvement in nutritional status, and many of these patients will not require additional vitamin or mineral supplementation.

Bile salt deficiency

Inadequate luminal bile salt impairs micelle formation with resultant fat malabsorption. Bile salt deficiency may result from inadequate synthesis (cirrhosis), cholestasis with impaired secretion, bacterial overgrowth, terminal ileal disease, Zollinger-Ellison syndrome, or treatment with cholestyramine. Fat malabsorption may not be as severe as in untreated pancreatic insufficiency, but fat-soluble vitamin aborption may be significally decreased. In addition to symptoms of malabsorption, many patients have watery diarrhea from the secretory effect of fatty acids in the colon. Management is directed at correctly identifying and treating the underlying cause if possible. Individuals with bacterial overgrowth may benefit from antibiotics. Improved control of ileal Crohn disease may improve bile salt reabsorption in the terminal ileum. If no specific treatment is available, then treatment should focus on correction of nutritional deficits.

Disaccharidase deficiency

Lactase deficiency is by far the most common of the disaccharidase deficiencies. Many individuals begin to lose lactase around 5 years of age. Other individuals may develop transient lactase deficiency following an intestinal infection because of injury to the brush border enzymes. Patients usually complain of bloating, gas, and diarrhea after consuming lactose-containing foods (primarily dairy products). Weight loss or other signs of malnutrition are rare. Management involves avoiding lactose-containing products or adding lactase supplements to the diet to aid in digestion. This is a benign condition, but can be particularly bothersome to patients.

Celiac sprue

Celiac disease is an inflammatory disease of the small bowel caused by the ingestion of gluten-containing foods. In susceptible individuals, especially those of Irish descent, the ingestion of gluten (containing the toxic moiety, gliadin) induces an inflammatory response in the small bowel. The result is flattening of the villi with a resultant decrease in the surface area for nutrient absorption. The diagnosis of celiac disease is best on the finding of villous flattening that improves after instituting a gluten-free diet. Anti-endomysial IgA antibodies and anti-tissue transglutaminase (tTG) IgA antibodies are relatively sensitive and specific for the diagnosis of celiac sprue. Patients with celiac disease should institute a lifelong gluten-free diet. Because many foods, beers, and medications contain gluten, it is often helpful to enlist the assistance of a nutritionist to help formulate a diet. Most individuals have improvement in symptoms within a few weeks of starting a gluten-free diet. The most common reason for treatment failure is noncompliance with the gluten-free diet. Immunosuppressants may be considered for patients who continue to have problems despite strict adherence to a gluten-free diet.

SHORT BOWEL SYNDROME

Short bowel syndrome occurs after small bowel resection or intestinal bypass. Crohn disease is the most common reason for extensive bowel resection, but small bowel obstruction, trauma, mesenteric ischemia, and cancer also may necessitate resection. Management of patients with short bowel syndrome can be particularly challenging because of the significant changes in small bowel function that occur following extensive resection.

Clinical features

The clinical manifestations are determined not only by how much bowel has been resected, but also by which segments have been removed. Volume depletion is common in patients who have extensive small bowel resections. Patients with less than 100 cm remaining jejunum and an end-jejunostomy generally have high intestinal fluid outputs. If the ileum and colon are intact, then those segments may be able to compensate for the loss of absorptive area. Electrolyte losses, especially sodium, magnesium, and zinc are common. Malabsorption, with resulting protein-calorie malnutrition, is common and is more severe with more extensive resections. Renal stones may occur because of luminal calcium binding by unabsorbed fat with resulting increased absorption of oxalate and formation of oxalate stones. Bone disease, gallstones, and bacterial overgrowth also are common. D-lactic acidosis may occur because of overgrowth of bacteria in the intestine with conversion of carbohydrates to D-lactic acid. This condition may be life-threatening and must be identified and treated immediately.

Investigation

The most important aspect in the initial evaluation of a patient with suspected short bowel syndrome is a determination of how much and which part of the intestine remains. This will guide further testing and management. Surgical records, if available, are most useful, but barium studies also can provide this information. Careful attention must be paid to volume status and overall degree of malnutrition. Specific testing for individual nutrient deficiencies may be indicated depending on the clinical scenario. Serum electrolytes also should be measured. A thorough history and examination with specific testing, including radiologic studies if needed, will help determine whether continued enteral feeding is adequate, or whether parenteral nutrition or hydration is needed.

Management

All attempts should be made to manage the patient with oral nutrition and hydration, if possible. Oral rehydration solutions containing glucose, sodium, and other electrolytes improve jejunal absorption by utilizing the sodium cotransporters in the small intestine. The use of agents to slow intestinal transit increases the time available for fluid absorption and may prevent parenteral hydration. Antimotility agents that are useful include loperamide, deodorized tincture of opium (DTO), and belladonna. Loperamide can be given 2 mg TID in increased to a maximum of 40 mg/day. If this is not effective, then DTO (6 to 10 drops) and tincture of belladonna (6 to 15 drops) may be given before each meal. Frequent small meals also may slow diarrhea and improve hydration status. A proton-pump inhibitor may be added to decrease gastric output. Finally octreotide may be helpful to decrease pancreatic and intestinal secretion. Careful attention to electrolytes is essential. Many patients will require daily repletion of calcium, potassium, magnesium, or zinc. Most patients benefit from a multivitamin and need careful monitoring of fat- and water-soluble vitamin levels. Parenteral nutrition should be reserved for patients who cannot maintain adequate hydration or develop progressive protein-calorie malnutrition despite optimization of bowel function.

Complications

Complications include nutritional, electrolyte, and vitamin deficiencies. Oxalate renal stones, bone disease, and small bowel bacterial overgrowth are other complications. D-lactic acidosis is a rare complication that may result in life-threatening encephalitis.

VITAMIN DEFICIENCIES

Vitamin deficiencies are common in patients with protein-calorie malnutrition, but also may be seen in individuals with otherwise normal nutritional status. The manifestations of the various vitamin deficiencies are protean. Therefore, a high index of suspicion must be maintained for vitamin deficiencies, especially in susceptible individuals. Many cases are due to inadequate dietary intake, but several other factors may contribute to a specific deficiency. Early identification and treatment of vitamin deficiencies may prevent the development of more serious complications. The mechanisms of deficiency, clinical features, appropriate testing, and treatment are discussed for the most common vitamin deficiencies.

FAT SOLUBLE VITAMINS

Vitamin A

Inadequate dietary intake, especially in alcoholics, and malabsorption are the most frequent causes of vitamin A deficiency. The only known effects of deficiency are on the eye. The majority of patients have night blindness with impaired dark adaptation. In more severe cases, damage to the conjunctiva or cornea may result in serious visual problems. Serum levels of vitamin A and carotene can be used to identify deficiency, although the tests do not distinguish between poor intake and malabsorption. Deficient states will respond to daily oral doses of retinol (5000 to 30,000 IU). Higher doses generally are used in cases of malabsorption. Some caution must be used with higher doses of vitamin A (especially greater than 500,000 IU/day) as toxicity may develop. Vitamin A is also teratogenic at doses higher than 10,000 IU/day during the first trimester.

Vitamin D

The metabolism of vitamin D is relatively complex. Most of the vitamin D_3 is derived from ultraviolet light (sun exposure), converting 7-dehydrocholesterol to cholecalciferol (vitamin D_3). Normally, only about 10% is derived from dietary intake, so inadequate intake only becomes important in individuals without sun exposure. Vitamin D_3 is hydroxylated to 25-hydroxyvitamin D_3 in the liver, then an additional hydroxyl group is added in the kidney, producing 1,25-dihydroxyvitamin D_3. Deficiencies may arise with limited sun exposure, poor dietary intake, breast-fed infants, malabsorption, severe liver disease, or advanced renal disease. As vitamin D plays a critical role in calcium and phosphorus metabolism, the major clinical syndromes are related to decreased body stores of calcium or phosphorus. Rickets, or childhood osteomalacia, is a condition caused by poor bone mineralization. Affected children have bending of long bones (bow-legged), fractures, muscle weakness, inability to start walking, and seizures. Adult osteomalacia develops more slowly with skeletal pain and muscle weakness. Involutional osteoporosis, defined by low bone mass, with increased risk for fractures may occur. Serum 25-hydroxyvitamin D_3 and 1,25-dihydroxyvitamin D_3 are decreased in vitamin D deficiency. Occasionally, 24-hour urinary calcium (low in deficiency) and bone densitometry may be useful adjuncts to serum vitamin D levels. Vitamin D_2 (ergosterol, 600 to 1200 mcg/day) and vitamin D_3 (cholecalciferol, 10 to 25 mcg/day) are available for oral daily replacement. These are acceptable for patients without renal dysfunction. Patients with renal failure cannot form 1,25-dihydroxyvitamin D_3 (calcitriol) and should be treated with oral (0.25 to 0.5 mcg/day) or IV (0.01 to 0.05 mcg 3 times/week) calcitriol.

Vitamin E

Vitamin E (tocopherol) primarily acts as an antioxidant, and its actions have been studied in a number of clinical conditions, including cancer and cardiovascular disease. Newborns and patients with fat malabsorption or biliary obstruction are at risk for deficiency. Most of the clinical features are related to neurologic dysfunction. Patients may have unsteady gait, tremor, weakness, opthalmoplegia, cerebellar dysfunction, or myopathy. Newborns may develop a hemolytic anemia. Plasma α-tocopherol levels are low in vitamin E deficiency. Correction of vitamin E deficiency can be corrected with oral vitamin E and individuals with malabsorption may require large oral doses (up to 100 to 200 IU/kg/day).

Vitamin K

Vitamin K plays a critical role in the clotting cascade, activating factors II, VII, IX, and X. Deficiency states most commonly are due to warfarin therapy, which inhibits vitamin K. Other causes of vitamin K deficiency include malabsorption, liver disease, and antibiotic use with inadequate vitamin K intake. Most patients with vitamin K deficiency have abnormal coagulation, causing easy bruising or bleeding problems. The prothrombin time is prolonged in vitamin K deficiency. Vitamin K may be given via the oral, SC, or IM route (2 to 10 mg/day). If the prothrombin time does not correct with administration of vitamin K, then deficiencies of any of the clotting factors (II, VII, IX, X) should be suspected.

WATER-SOLUBLE VITAMINS

Thiamine (Vitamin B_1)

Thiamine, like the other B vitamins, acts as a coenzyme in various biochemical reactions. It is present in a broad variety of foods. Deficiency may result from poor intake (especially alcoholics), malabsorption, or increased tissue demand. The clinical spectrum in thiamine deficiency ranges from mild abnormalities such as fatigue, nausea, and irritability to a more severe syndrome with CHF (beriberi), polypneuritis, and edema. Neurologic problems may develop, including Wernicke encephalopathy or cerebellar signs. Signs of deficiency may worsen if glucose is given without thiamine. Serum levels of thiamine may be measured, but more commonly assessment is performed by measuring the ratio of transketolase with and without added thiamine. Treatment is with either oral or IM thiamine, up to 100 mg/day.

Riboflavin (Vitamin B_2)

Riboflavin also functions as a coenzyme in biologic oxidation reactions. Unlike other vitamins, it has no storage depot, so urinary excretion correlates with dietary intake. Deficiency results from inadequate dietary intake (alcoholism) or malabsorption. As many cases of riboflavin deficiency occur in patients with other B-vitamin deficiencies, it is difficult to identify exactly which symptoms are due to riboflavin deficiency. Clinical manifestations thought to be caused by riboflavin deficiency include angular stomatitis, cheilosis, glossitis, and seborrheic dermatitis. Urinary riboflavin excretion can be used to determine if a patient is deficient. Treatment is with oral or IV riboflavin (5 to 10 mg/day). Most multivitamins contain adequate riboflavin to prevent development of deficiency.

Niacin (Vitamin B_3)

Niacin, or nicotinic acid, is an essential component of the coenzyme NAD and NADP, which are involved in the mitochondrial electron transport system. Inadequate intake, alcoholism, malabsorption, and carcinoid syndrome may cause niacin deficiency. The classic deficiency syndrome is pellagra, a condition with skin, GI, and neurologic manifestations. Dermatitis, glossitis, and diarrhea caused by mucosal atrophy may occur. Early neurologic features include headache, anxiety, depression, and sleep disturbances, and may progess to psychomotor retardation, confusion, hallucinations, seizures, or catatonia. Urinary tests to measure the ratio of N'-methylnicotinamide to 2-pyridone-N'-methylnictoinamide can identify deficient intake. As isolated niacin deficiency, most patients are treated with a multivitamin. Replacement with niacin 100 to 500 mg/day will correct most cases of niacin deficiency. Caution must be used with niacin replacement as severe flushing, nausea, vomiting, diarrhea, or arrhythmias may occur with higher doses.

Pyridoxine (Vitamin B_6)

Pyridoxine is present in many foods and also is produced in intestinal bacteria, so dietary restriction rarely results in deficiency. Deficiency generally occurs in elderly patients, malabsorption, alcoholism, and use of vitamin B_6 antagonists (isoniazid, hydralazine, oral contraceptives, penicillamine). The clinical features of deficiency include seborrheic dermatitis, cheilosis, glossitis, microcytic anemia, and peripheral neuritis. Several tests are available for the assessment of vitamin B_6 status. Plasma pyridoxal-5'-phosphate and urinary 4-pyridoxic acid are low in deficiency. Erythrocyte AST and ALT activity coefficients are high in deficient states. Pyridoxine is available in oral and IV formulations. Individuals receiving isoniazid should take 25 mg/day to prevent neuropathy, and patients with established neuropathy require 50 to 300 mg/day. Most multivitamins contain approximately 2 mg each.

Folate

Folate coenzymes are involved in RNA, DNA, and protein synthesis. Deficiency may result from inadequate dietary intake, alcoholism, malabsorption, pregnancy, hemolysis, and anticonvulsant drugs. Normal individuals have 3 to 4 months of stored folate, so deficiency does not develop immediately with cessation of intake. Megaloblastic anemia, glossitis, and diarrhea are common manifestations of deficiency. Unlike vitamin B_{12} deficiency, patients do not develop a peripheral neuropathy. Neural tube defects are associated with inadequate folate intake in pregnancy. Patients with folate deficiency have low serum and red cell folate levels and peripheral blood smear shows macrocytosis and hypersegmented neutrophils. Serum homocysteine levels are elevated in folate deficiency, but methylmalonic acid levels are normal. Treatment is usually with oral folate (0.2 to 1.0 mg/day), but IV, IM, or SC folate may be used in severe deficiency.

Cobalamin (Vitamin B_{12})

Vitamin B_{12} is stored in the liver and cessation of intake will not result in deficiency for several years. The absorption of vitamin B_{12} is complex and abnormalities at any stage may result in deficiency. Vitamin B_{12} bound to ingested food is cleaved by gastric proteases and binds to haptocorrin. In the duodenum, pancreatic enzymes hydrolyze haptocorrin and free vitamin B_{12} then binds to intrinsic factor, which is produced by parietal cells. The intrinsic factor-vitamin B_{12} complex binds to specific receptors in the terminal ileum. Predisposing conditions include pernicious anemia with deficient intrinsic factor production, *Helicobacter pylori* gastritis, Crohn disease with ileal involvement, gastric surgery, bacterial overgrowth, and chronic pancreatitis. Clinical manifestations include megaloblastic anemia, dementia, and peripheral neuropathy. Serum cobalamin, homocysteine, and methylmalonic acid levels are low in advanced deficiency. The Schilling test may be used to identify the cause of the deficiency, but because of the high cost of this test, as well as the relatively ease of vitamin B_{12} replacement, this test rarely is performed. Dietary deficiency may be treated with daily oral doses of 1 to 3 mg/day, whereas patients with inadequate absorption are treated with monthly IM doses of 100 to 1000 mcg.

Ascorbic acid (Vitamin C)

The exact function of vitamin C is not known, but it is important in collagen formation, so deficiency causes connective tissue problems. Vitamin C deficiency is occurs with inadequate intake, usually in alcoholics. Scurvy is the clinical syndrome, with weakness, bleeding gums, and loose teeth. Patients also may have bleeding from the conjunctiva, nose, and GI or GU tracts. Anemia and hyperkeratosis also may occur. Infantile scurvy is characterized by cessation of long bone growth. Serum ascorbic acid and leukocyte ascorbate levels are low in deficiency. Scurvy is adequately treated with daily oral vitamin C (60 to 100 mg/day).

CHAPTER 10

MISCELLANEOUS TOPICS

DYSPHAGIA

Dysphagia is the term used to describe the sensation from impairment of passage of food upon swallowing. Oropharyngeal dysphagia refers to difficulty in transferring food from the mouth to the esophagus and is typically caused by neuromuscular or structural disorders involving the oropharynx and proximal esophagus. Acute stroke is an important cause of oropharyngeal dysphagia. Esophageal dysphagia results from disorders of the smooth muscle esophagus, including strictures, webs, mucosal inflammation (reflux and infectious esophagitis), motility disorders (achalasia, scleroderma), neoplasia and extrinsic compression. Odynophagia refers to painful swallowing, which can coexist particularly in infectious esophagitis and pill esophagitis. The elderly population is particularly prone to increased morbidity and mortality from dysphagia, especially from complications including aspiration pneumonia and malnutrition.

Clinical features

Patients describe dysphagia as food 'getting stuck' or 'hanging up' in the neck or chest area. This has to be distinguished from globus, which is a sensation of constant fullness or lump in the throat that may actually improve with swallowing. Patients with oropharyngeal dysphagia may have associated symptoms of drooling, nasal regurgitation, or coughing on attempted swallowing and the need to swallow repeatedly to clear food from the pharynx. Regurgitation of food and chest pain may coexist with esophageal dysphagia. Dysphagia caused by structural lesions starts with solids and progresses to liquids, while motility disorders may present as dysphagia with both solids and liquids. Achalasia, a motility disorder characterized by failure of relaxation of the lower esophageal sphincter and aperistalsis of the esophageal body, presents with dysphagia, regurgitation, chest pain, and weight loss. Benign esophageal disorders generally cause nonprogressive or slowly progressive dysphagia, while neoplastic disorders may present with rapidly progressive dysphagia with weight loss. Acute onset of dysphagia may suggest impaction of a food bolus at a site of a stricture or narrowing. Acute stroke also may result in acute dysphagia. Odynophagia generally suggests infectious esophagitis or pill esophagitis.

Investigation

A careful history can localize the level and sometimes the etiology of dysphagia. Physical examination can reveal features of the primary conditions responsible for dysphagia. Videofluoroscopic examination using a modified barium swallow assesses for abnormalities of the swallowing mechanism in oropharyngeal dysphagia. Nasal endoscopy provides complementary information. Additional tests include CT scans of the head and neck, laboratory tests (including acetyl choline receptor antibodies in myasthenia gravis, thyroid stimulating hormone levels in thyrotoxicosis, creatinine phosphokinase in inflammatory disorders of muscle), and electromyography. Motility studies have a low yield in oropharyngeal dysphagia but can be considered in the evaluation. Endoscopy is typically the preferred investigative procedure in esophageal dysphagia, especially because biopsies and dilation can be performed during the procedure. Barium studies may be superior to endoscopy when proximal esophageal lesions, subtle strictures, or motility disorders are suspected, and may provide a road map for the endoscopist in patients with tight or complex strictures. If initial studies fail to reveal the etiology, esophageal manometry is performed. Imaging studies are useful in patients with suspected extrinsic compression or esophageal neoplasia.

Management

Patients with oropharyngeal dysphagia benefit from modification of diet and swallowing therapy based on results of the modified barium swallow. Patients with frank tracheal aspiration on attempted swallowing despite these measures may need enteral feeding through nasoduodenal or gastrostomy tubes. Surgical or endoscopic therapy, preferably with cricopharyngeal myotomy, is recommended for Zenker's diverticulum. Certain tumors may be surgically resectable. Benign webs and strictures can be dilated endoscopically. Inflammatory myopathies and myasthenia can be treated medically. Patients with drooling of saliva may benefit from anticholinergic medication to decrease salivation, such as transdermal scopolamine.

Strictures and webs in the esophagus are amenable to endoscopic dilation. Reflux and infectious esophagitis can be treated medically as described elsewhere in this text. Urgent endoscopy is recommended for acute food bolus impaction, although IV glucagon administration can be attempted. Curative surgery and chemotherapy and radiotherapy are generally recommended for neoplastic disorders. Palliation can be provided by the placement of self-expanding endoluminal stents or by laser therapy to debulk tumors. Enteral nutrition through gastrostomy tubes is often necessary.

Therapies for achalasia attempt to decrease the lower esophageal sphincter pressure to facilitate esophageal emptying. Pharmacologic therapy using oral medications (nifedipine, isosorbide dinitrate) administered half an hour before meals may offer temporary relief in some patients, but are generally not very useful. Botulinum toxin can be injected to the lower esophageal sphincter for short-term relief of symptoms as a bridge to more definitive therapy or when more invasive therapies are contraindicated. Pneumatic dilation and surgical myotomy both offer lasting relief of symptoms. Pneumatic dilation is associated with a 3% to 5% likelihood of esophageal perforation requiring surgical correction. With the advent of laparoscopic techniques, surgical myotomy has replaced pneumatic dilation as the therapy of choice in patients who can tolerate the procedure.

Certain patients with diffuse esophageal spasm and nonspecific spastic disorders benefit from smooth muscle relaxants (nifedipine, isosorbide dinitrate, hyoscyamine), although conclusive data on their efficacy are lacking. Symptomatic patients also may benefit from low dose trazodone or tricyclic antidepressants. Botulinum toxin injection, pneumatic dilation, or surgical myotomy are reserved for refractory situations in patients with poor relaxation of the lower esophageal sphincter as a significant component of their disorder.

Complications

Oropharyngeal dysphagia may be complicated by tracheal aspiration and frequent pneumonias. Other complications include malnutrition, dehydration, and weight loss. Food bolus impaction can occur in patients with esophageal strictures or neoplasia. Patients with achalasia and esophageal strictures also are prone to aspiration pneumonia and weight loss. Long-standing achalasia can result in squamous cell carcinoma of the distal esophagus.

NAUSEA AND VOMITING

Nausea is the subjective feeling of an impending urge to vomit, occurring on its own or preceding vomiting. Vomiting consists of forceful ejection of gastric contents and may be accompanied by repetitive contraction of the abdominal wall musculature known as retching. These symptoms are associated with a significant impact on quality of life, especially in the setting of chemotherapy-associated or postoperative nausea and vomiting. Medications are among the most common causes of nausea and vomiting, and chemotherapeutic agents are an important cause. Ingestion of preformed bacterial toxins ('food poisoning'), other GI infections (gastroenteritis, colitis), or even systemic infections can cause nausea and vomiting. Obstruction of the luminal gut, motility disorders, and acute intraabdominal inflammatory conditions (appendicitis, cholecystitis, pancreatitis) can all lead to nausea and vomiting. Postoperative nausea and vomiting may be seen after general anesthesia. Psychiatric disorders such as eating disorders and bulimia are associated with nausea and vomiting. Other causes include raised intracranial pressure, metabolic disorders, pregnancy, motion sickness, and cyclic vomiting syndrome. When exhaustive investigation does not reveal a structural or metabolic cause, functional nausea and vomiting is sometimes diagnosed.

Clinical features

Nausea and vomiting are often accompanied by salivation, flushing, tachycardia, and retching. Regurgitation needs to be distinguished from vomiting, and consists of passive retrograde movement of esophageal contents without effort and typically without the associated symptoms of vomiting. Nausea and vomiting lasting longer than a month are considered chronic. Vomiting from raised intracranial pressure may be projectile, and may occur without preceding nausea. Gastroparesis or gastric outlet obstruction may result in vomiting of food eaten hours earlier, while eating disorders and bulimia are associated with vomiting soon after a meal. Vomiting of pregnancy typically occurs in the morning hours, although it can occur anytime during the day. Cyclic vomiting consists of stereotypic episodes of severe nausea and vomiting occurring at periodic intervals, and lasting hours to days, with asymptomatic intervals in between episodes. This disorder is thought to be linked to abdominal migraine. Physical examination may reveal features of the causative disorder.

Investigation

A careful history and physical examination, with particular attention to the patient's medication list, is an essential part of the initial evaluation. In the presence of dehydration or electrolyte imbalance, or if a mechanical or significant inflammatory or metabolic disorder is suspected, hospital admission and IV hydration may be necessary while further investigation is carried out. Measurement of serum electrolytes, pancreatic enzymes, liver chemistries, and a blood count may provide useful information. A pregnancy test is indicated in women of childbearing age. Plain abdominal X-rays or obstructive series help exclude bowel obstruction, ileus, and peforation. Imaging studies including CT and MRI may provide more detailed information when inflammatory or obstructive intra-abdominal pathology is suspected. Other imaging studies that can be performed include barium contrast studies that may help evaluate the upper GI tract and small bowel for obstructive lesions. Endoscopy may provide more information on mucosal pathology in the upper GI tract, especially in patients with undiagnosed or protracted nausea and vomiting. Gastric emptying scans may help quantify gastric emptying in patients with suspected gastroparesis. When a psychiatric or functional cause is suspected after negative evaluation, a formal psychiatric assessment may be useful.

Management

Supportive measures such as correction of fluid and electrolyte imbalances are important initial measures. When the etiology is found, specific management is recommended. Patients with acute nausea and vomiting generally avoid oral intake until symptoms subside. When symptoms are protracted or chronic, nutrition needs to be addressed. Patients with protracted vomiting from gastroparesis or gastric outlet obstruction can sometimes be fed in the jejunum using nasojejunal or percutaneously placed jejunal tubes. Rarely, in refractory nausea and vomiting, parenteral nutrition may be required.

Empiric therapy of nausea and vomiting often is initiated while investigation is in progress, or when the etiology is thought to be self-limited. Agents commonly used include phenothiazines (promethazine, prochlorperazine, chlorpromazine), dopamine receptor antagonists (metoclopramide), and antihistaminic agents (diphenhydramine, meclizine, cyclizine, cinnarizine). Prophylactic therapy is useful in patients undergoing general anesthesia or chemotherapy. In addition to the commonly used agents described above, serotonin receptor antagonists (5-HT_3 antagonists, eg, ondansetron, granisetron, tropisetron, dolasetron) and butyrophenones (haloperidol, droperidol) are useful in prophylaxis as well as therapy of postoperative and chemotherapy induced nausea and vomiting. Antihistaminics and anticholinergic agents (eg, scopolamine) are useful in motion sickness. Medications are avoided as far as possible in morning sickness of pregnancy, but when symptoms are severe, antihistaminics, phenothiazines, or dopamine receptor antagonists can be used. Low-dose tricyclic antidepressant agents are useful in functional nausea and vomiting and cyclic vomiting. Agents reserved for refractory symptoms include benzodiazepines, dronabinol, and steroids such as dexamethasone.

Complications

Dehydration and electrolyte imbalances can result from nausea and vomiting, with children and elderly patients being most susceptible. Repetitive retching can result in tears of the mucosa in the gastroesophageal junction (Mallory Weiss tears) that can present as GI bleeding. Full thickness tears are rare and can result in chemical mediastinitis and pleuritis (Boerhaave's syndrome). Abdominal wall muscle injury can sometimes result from violent retching. Reflux esophagitis can result from repeated vomiting of acidic stomach contents. In patients with protracted or chronic nausea and vomiting, nutrition may be affected, resulting in malnutrition and weight loss.

DIARRHEA

Diarrhea is defined as increased frequency or fluidity of stool. The main causes of acute diarrhea are infections, toxins, and medications, but inflammatory bowel disease also can present as acute diarrhea. Diarrhea is considered chronic when it lasts longer than 3 to 4 weeks. The pathophysiology responsible for chronic diarrhea includes secretory, osmotic, or inflammatory mechanisms. The differential diagnosis in chronic diarrhea is broad and includes inflammatory bowel disease, malabsorption or maldigestion, neoplastic disease, and irritable bowel syndrome.

Clinical features

A careful history can help determine the likely cause of acute diarrhea. Ingestion of poorly cooked food, recent travel, and antibiotic use are particularly relevant. Nausea, vomiting, abdominal cramps, and fever may coexist. Physical examination may demonstrate signs of volume depletion, including orthostatic hypotension, decreased skin turgor, and dry mucous membranes. These symptoms and signs may be less marked with chronic diarrhea. In general, diarrhea resulting from small bowel pathology is usually large in volume, while colonic pathology results in multiple smaller stools with distal colonic symptoms such as urgency. Greasy, foul-smelling stools that float in the toilet may indicate fat malabsorption. Patients with lactose intolerance may develop abdominal cramping and multiple loose bowel movements after ingestion of dairy products. Inflammatory etiologies can result in blood and mucus in the stool. As diarrhea becomes chronic, weight loss and vitamin deficiencies may result. Physical examination may reveal systemic manifestions of conditions like celiac sprue (dermatitis herpetiformis, vitamin deficiencies) and inflammatory bowel disease (pyoderma gangrenosum, arthritis).

Investigation

Acute self-limited diarrhea may require no investigation if symptoms rapidly resolve. In patients with severe symptoms and dehydration, serum electrolytes need to be checked and repleted if abnormal. Stool culture can identify infectious pathogens, and stool for ova and parasites can detect *Giardia* and other parasites. The presence of *Clostridium difficile* toxin in stool helps diagnose pseudomembranous colitis in patients taking antibiotics.

The diagnostic work-up of chronic diarrhea starts with a careful history. In addition to stool examination for organisms and toxins, sudan stain for fat can be performed when fat malabsorption is suspected. Quantitation of fat excretion over a 72-hour period also can be performed when indicated. Serum levels of fat-soluble vitamins are low in fat malabsorption. Endoscopic evaluation of the colon can help diagnose inflammatory bowel disease. Serum antigliadin, antiendomyseal and anti-tissue transglutaminase antibodies, and endoscopic small bowel biopsies are performed when celiac sprue is suspected. Secretory diarrhea persists during fasting and may have a hormonal etiology, identified from measurement of serum gastrin, glucagon, vasoactive intestinal peptide, or pancreatic polypeptide. Urine levels of 5-hydroxy indole acetic acid may be elevated in patients with carcinoid syndrome. Stool can be tested for laxatives when laxative abuse is suspected.

Management

Adequate hydration is essential in the management of diarrhea. In patients with moderate to severe volume depletion, IV hydration is necessary. Patients with mild volume depletion can be treated with oral rehydration and special rehydration solutions are available. Specific management is recommended whenever available, but it is often necessary to administer antidiarrheal agents for symptomatic benefit. Empiric antidiarrheal agents are recommended for symptomatic improvement while diagnostic testing is in progress, when specific management fails to improve symptoms, and when a specific etiology is not identified. Opiates (loperamide, diphenoxylate, tincture of opium) and anticholinergics are the commonest agents used. Kaolin and pectin preparations may bind toxins and bismuth subsalicylate has bactericidal properties; both agents may be useful in acute diarrhea. Cholestyramine binds bile acids and is useful in bile-acid induced diarrhea. Octreotide can be useful in hormone mediated secretory diarrhea.

Complications

Dehydration and electrolyte imbalance can result from severe acute diarrhea. Weight loss, malnutrition, and vitamin deficiencies are complications of chronic diarrhea, especially when the small bowel is involved. Protein loss from inflammatory diarrhea also can lead to malnutrition, sometimes necessitating parenteral nutrition, especially in inflammatory bowel disease.

CONSTIPATION

Constipation is defined by some as decreased frequency of bowel movements. Others use a broader definition, including features such as straining at defecation, hard stools, or a sensation of incomplete evacuation. Obstructive lesions including colorectal cancers are always a concern in new-onset constipation in older individuals. Other causes include medications (eg, opiates, anticholinergics, tricyclic antidepressants, calcium channel blockers), metabolic disorders (hypothyroidism, diabetes mellitus), pregnancy, neuropathic disorders (Hirschprung disease, spinal injury), and idiopathic disorders (irritable bowel syndrome, colonic inertia).

Clinical features

In addition to decreased frequency of bowel movements and straining at stool, other associated symptoms include abdominal discomfort, anal pain with defecation, rectal bleeding, and bloating. Frequency of bowel movements can vary widely among the general population, and a careful history will determine the patient's usual bowel habits. A recent change in frequency, especially in older individuals, is an alarm symptom that necessitates evaluation for an obstructive process or a growth in the colon. A history of constipation from birth may suggest a congenital condition, while a long history of constipation in adult life may suggest colonic inertia or functional bowel disease. A detailed neurologic examination may demonstrate evidence for a spinal cord or cauda equina lesion. A rectal examination may reveal pathology in the rectum and anal canal.

Investigation

Fecal occult blood may be positive and a complete blood count may demonstrate microcytic anemia in patients with occult bleeding from colonic neoplasms. These patients, as well as older patients with new-onset constipation, need further evaluation with colonoscopy or barium enema. Thyroid stimulating hormone levels and rheumatologic panels are useful in selected patients. Anorectal manometry is useful in the diagnosis of Hirschprung disease. Assessment of colonic transit using Sitz markers helps diagnose colonic inertia. Defecography defines the function of the perineal and anal musculature in defecation and helps exclude rectocele and pelvic floor dyssynergia.

Management

When an underlying cause is found, directed therapy is recommended. General measures including regular exercise, adequate fluid intake, and an increase in daily fiber intake to 20 to 30 g/day are useful initial steps in management. Fiber supplementation using products containing psyllium and methylcellulose are recommended after fecal impaction has been excluded. Osmotic laxatives (lactulose, milk of magnesia, magnesium citrate) act by retaining water in the bowel lumen and are useful agents for short-term use in patients needing immediate relief of constipation. Emollient laxatives (docusate, mineral oil) also are useful for intermittent use, as are stimulant laxatives (castor oil, cascara, senna, bisacodyl). For patients requiring long-term therapy, polyethylene glycol can be used in small daily doses *(Miralax, Golytely)*. Polyethylene glycol also is used for bowel cleansing prior to colonoscopy. Nonabsorbable phosphate (phosphosoda) also can be used intermittently in small doses, although phosphate retention and severe dehydration limit its use in the elderly and in patients with renal disease. Enemas (phosphate, tap water) and suppositories (glycerine, bisacodyl) also are useful for quick relief of symptoms. Oil-based enemas (hypaque, cottonseed colace, mineral oil) can soften hard, impacted stool and are reserved for refractory situations.

Complications

Rectal bleeding, hemorrhoids, rectal prolapse, and anal fissures can result from straining in patients with chronic constipation. Stercoral ulcers are induced by hard stool in the rectum or distal colon. Fecal impaction can result in colonic obstruction, necessitating manual disimpaction in some situations.

GI BLEEDING

GI bleeding can be overt, when fresh or altered blood is visible in emesis or stool, or occult, when the stool tests positive for occult blood or the patient presents with iron deficiency anemia. GI bleeding is designated obscure when routine endoscopy fails to determine a source and bleeding persists or recurs. Obscure bleeding can be either overt or occult depending on the presentation. Upper GI causes for overt bleeding include peptic ulcers, varices, angiodysplasia, Mallory Weiss tears, gastritis, esophagitis, and neoplasia. Colonic causes include diverticulosis, colitis, neoplasia, angiodysplasia and hemorrhoids. Angiodysplasia is the most common small bowel source for bleeding.

Clinical features

Emesis of fresh or altered blood is called hematemesis. When blood is altered by the action of gastric acid, it turns into a dark brown color resembling coffee grounds. Melena is the passage of dark, tarry stool, typically seen in patients with upper GI bleeding. Patients with bleeding further down the GI tract may have maroon, dark red, or bright red blood in the stool, termed hematochezia. Rapid blood loss from any site can result in volume depletion and tachycardia, low blood pressure, and orthostasis. Patients may have pallor, sweating, and cold, clammy extremities. Symptoms and signs of the causative lesion sometimes may be evident. Other patients may have systemic manifestations of anemia, including angina and heart failure. On the other hand, patients with occult GI bleeding may be completely asymptomatic, with the finding of fecal occult blood or microcytic anemia on routine physical or laboratory examination.

Investigation

Endoscopy is standard for the investigation of upper GI bleeding. Urgent colonoscopy after bowel cleansing has been reported to increase the likelihood of finding a source for acute lower GI bleeding. However, in patients with rapid bleeding, radionuclide scans and angiograms may be useful in localizing the bleeding source. Push enteroscopy and capsule endoscopy are utilized for further investigation when a bleeding source is not identified on routine endoscopy. Barium studies including small bowel follow-through x-rays and enteroclysis, do not have a high yield but can be employed to exclude gross small bowel lesions prior to capsule endoscopy. Investigation of occult bleeding starts with routine endoscopy, usually bi-directional in older age groups. This can be followed by barium studies, push enteroscopy, and capsule endoscopy to evaluate the small bowel when indicated. Intraoperative enteroscopy is indicated in refractory situations and can be associated with significant complications and morbidity.

Management

IV fluids and blood transfusions may be urgently indicated to replete lost intravascular volume. Anticoagulants are discontinued and prolonged coagulation parameters are corrected with vitamin K, fresh frozen plasma or protamine as indicated. Platelet infusions are necessary when the platelet count is less than 50,000/cu mm. Octreotide bolus and infusion is indicated when variceal bleeding is suspected. Endoscopic therapy can be performed during endoscopy to potential bleeding lesions, including endoscopic variceal ligation for esophageal varices. Selective vasopressin infusion or embolization can be performed during angiography, especially in acute lower GI bleeding. Surgery is sometimes indicated when endoscopic or radiologic techniques are unsuccessful in controlling acute bleeding. Specific management of the etiologic lesion is recommended whenever available.

Medical therapy of angiodysplasia presents a vexing problem in certain patients. Presentation can be in the form of acute or obscure bleeding. Whenever identified, endoscopic ablation is performed. However, angiodysplasia may be present beyond the reach of conventional endoscopy and, hence, not amenable to ablation. Iron supplementation usually is the first step in the medical management of iron deficiency anemia from angiodysplasia. A proportion of patients may maintain their blood counts with just iron supplementation. Others need intermittent blood transfusions to keep their blood counts within acceptable range. In patients who do not maintain their blood counts despite iron supplementation and intermittent transfusions, options include intraoperative enteroscopy to ablate lesions beyond reach of conventional endoscopy and combination hormone (estrogen and progesterone) therapy. The latter option is a final resource available to patients with refractory anemia from angiodysplasia. The potential side effects of estrogen and progesterone have to be given due consideration, especially in older women and men. When indicated, birth-control pills containing estrogen and progesterone (ethinyl estradiol, 0.035 to 0.05 mg; norethisterone, 1 mg) administered twice a day may be effective in decreasing GI blood loss from angiodysplasia. Treatment courses of 4 to 6 months followed by treatment holidays lasting several weeks to months may be beneficial in patients with side effects.

Complications

Exsanguination and death can result from uncontrolled bleeding. Intravascular volume depletion can lead to hemorrhagic shock and ischemic complications including MI, stroke, and ischemic colitis. In patients with chronic anemia, angina, shortness of breath, fatigue, and heart failure can limit activities.

ACETAMINOPHEN (N-Acetyl-P-Aminophenol, APAP)

ACETAMINOPHEN	
Suppositories: 80, 120, 125, 300, 325, and 650 mg (*otc*)	Various, *Acetaminophen Uniserts* (Upsher-Smith), *Acephen* (G & W Labs), *Neopap* (PolyMedica)
Tablets, chewable: 80 mg (*otc*)	Various, *St. Joseph Aspirin-Free for Children* (Schering-Plough), *Tylenol, Children's*, *Tylenol, Junior Strength* (McNeil-CPC)
Capsules: 80, 160, and 500 mg (*otc*)	Various, *Feverall Sprinkle Caps* (Upsher-Smith), *Dapa Extra Strength* (Ferndale)
Granules: 80 mg (*otc*)	*Snaplets-FR Granules* (Baker Cummins)
Caplets: 160 mg (*otc*)	*Junior Strength Panadol* (Sterling Health)
Caplets, extended release: 650 mg (*otc*)	*Tylenol Extended Relief* (McNeil-CPC)
Tablets: 160, 325, 500, and 650 mg (*otc*)	Various, *Tylenol Regular Strength Tablets* (McNeil-CPC), *Aspirin Free Anacin Maximum Strength* (Whitehall)
Elixir: 80, 120, 130, 160, and 325 mg/5 mL (*otc*)	Various, *Ridenol* (RID), *Dolanex* (Lannett), *Oraphen-PD* (Great Southern), *Tylenol Children's* (McNeil-CPC)
Liquid: 160 mg/5 mL and 500 mg/15 mL (*otc*)	Various, *St. Joseph Aspirin-Free Fever Reducer for Children* (Schering-Plough), *Tylenol Extra Strength* (McNeil-CPC)
Solution: 100 mg/mL and 120 mg/2.5 mL (*otc*)	Various, *Tempra Drops* (Mead Johnson Nutritional), *Liquiprin Infants' Drops* (Menley & James)
Suspension: 80 mg/0.8 mL and 160 mg/5 mL (*otc*)	*Tylenol Infants' Drops* (McNeil-CPC), *Tylenol, Children's* (McNeil-CPC)
ACETAMINOPHEN, BUFFERED	
Effervescent granules: 325 mg w/2.781 g sodium bicarbonate & 2.224 g citric acid/dose measure (*otc*)	*Bromo Seltzer* (Warner-Lambert)

Indications

An analgesic-antipyretic in the presence of aspirin allergy, hemostatic disturbances (including anticoagulant therapy), bleeding diatheses (eg, hemophilia), upper GI disease (eg, ulcer, gastritis, hiatus hernia), and gouty arthritis; variety of arthritic and rheumatic conditions involving musculoskeletal pain, as well as in other painful disorders; diseases accompanied by discomfort and fever such as the common cold, "flu" and other bacterial or viral infections.

Unlabeled uses: Prophylactic APAP use in children receiving DTP vaccination appears to decrease incidence of fever and injection site pain. A dose immediately following vaccination and every 4 to 6 hrs thereafter for 48 to 72 hrs is suggested.

Administration and Dosage

Oral:

Adults – 325 to 650 mg every 4 to 6 hours, or 1 g 3 to 4 times/day. Do not exceed 4 g/day.

Children – May repeat doses 4 or 5 times/day; do not exceed 5 doses in 24 hours.

Acetaminophen Dosage for Children

Age	Dosage (mg)	Age (years)	Dosage (mg)
0-3 months	40	4-5	240
4-11 months	80	6-8	320
1-2 years	120	9-10	400
2-3 years	160	11	480

A 10 mg/kg/dose schedule has also been recommended.

Suppositories:

Adults – 650 mg every 4 to 6 hrs. Give no more than 6 in 24 hours.

Children –

(3 to 11 months of age): 80 mg every 6 hours.

(1 to 3 years of age): 80 mg every 4 hours.

(3 to 6 years of age): 120 to 125 mg every 4 to 6 hours. Give no more than 720 mg/24 hours.

(6 to 12 years of age): 325 mg every 4 to 6 hours. Give no more than 2.6 g/24 hours.

Actions

Pharmacology: The site and mechanism of the analgesic effect is unclear. APAP reduces fever by a direct action on the hypothalamic heat-regulating centers, which increases dissipation of body heat (via vasodilatation and sweating). APAP is almost as potent as aspirin in inhibiting prostaglandin synthetase in the CNS, but its peripheral inhibition of prostaglandin synthesis is minimal.

APAP does not inhibit platelet aggregation, affect prothrombin response, or produce GI ulceration.

Pharmacokinetics:

Absorption – Absorption of acetaminophen is rapid and almost complete from the GI tract.

Distribution – Usual analgesic doses produce total serum concentrations of 5 to 20 mcg/mL.

Metabolism/Excretion – Average elimination half-life is 1 to 3 hours; half-life is slightly prolonged in neonates (2.2 to 5 hours) and in cirrhotics.

Contraindications

Hypersensitivity to acetaminophen.

Warnings

Do not exceed recommended dosage. Consult physician for use in children < 3 years of age, or for oral use longer than 5 days (children), 10 days (adults) or 3 days for fever. Chronic excessive use (> 4 g/day) eventually may lead to transient hepatotoxicity. The kidneys may undergo tubular necrosis; the myocardium may be damaged.

Hepatic function impairment: Hepatotoxicity and severe hepatic failure occurred in chronic alcoholics following therapeutic doses. Caution chronic alcoholics to limit acetaminophen intake to ≤ 2 g /day.

Pregnancy: Acetaminophen crosses the placenta. It is routinely used during all stages of pregnancy; when used in therapeutic doses, it appears safe for short-term use.

Lactation: Acetaminophen is excreted in breast milk. No adverse effects in nursing infants were reported.

Precautions

If a sensitivity reaction occurs, discontinue use.

Severe or recurrent pain or high or continued fever may indicate serious illness. If pain persists for more than 5 days, if redness is present or in arthritic and rheumatic conditions affecting children < 12 years of age, consult physician immediately.

Drug Interactions

Drugs that may affect APAP include barbiturates, carbamazepine, hydantoins, isoniazid, rifampin, sulfinpyrazone, ethyl alcohol, and activated charcoal.

Drug/Lab test interactions: Acetaminophen may interfere with *Chemstrip bG*, *Dextrostix*, and *Visidex II* home blood glucose measurement systems; decreases of > 20% in mean glucose values may be noted. This effect appears to be drug-, concentration-, and system-dependent.

Adverse Reactions

Used as directed, acetaminophen rarely causes severe toxicity or side effects.

ANTACIDS

MAGNESIA (Magnesium Hydroxide)	
Tablets, chewable: 311 mg (*otc*)	*Phillips' Chewable* (Sterling Health)
Liquid: 400 mg/5 mL, 800 mg/5 mL (*otc*)	Various, *Phillips' Milk of Magnesia* (Sterling Health), *Phillips' Concentrated Milk of Magnesia* (Sterling Health)
ALUMINUM HYDROXIDE GEL	
Tablets: 300, 500, 600 mg (*otc*)	*Amphojel* (Wyeth-Ayerst), *Alu-Tab* (3M Pharm)
Capsules: 400, 500 mg (*otc*)	*Alu-Cap* (3M Pharm), *Dialume* (Aventis)
Suspension: 320 mg/5 mL, 450 mg/5 mL, 675 mg/5 mL (*otc*)	Various, *Amphojel* (Wyeth-Ayerst)
Liquid: 600 mg/5 mL (*otc*)	Various, *AlternaGEL* (J & J-Merck)
ALUMINUM CARBONATE GEL, BASIC	
Tablets: Equiv. to 608 mg dried aluminum hydroxide gel or 500 mg aluminum hydroxide (*otc*)	*Basaljel* (Wyeth-Ayerst)
Capsules: Equiv. to 608 mg dried aluminum hydroxide gel or 500 mg aluminum hydroxide (*otc*)	*Basaljel* (Wyeth-Ayerst)
Suspension: Equiv. to 400 mg aluminum hydroxide/5 mL (*otc*)	*Basaljel* (Wyeth-Ayerst)
CALCIUM CARBONATE	
Tablets, chewable: 350, 420, 750, 850, 1000 mg (*otc*)	*Amitone* (Menley & James), *Mallamint* (Roberts), *Extra Strength Tums E-X* (GlaxoSmithKline), *Alka-Mints* (Bayer), *Tums Ultra* (GlaxoSmith-Kline), *Extra Strength Alkets Antacid* (Roberts Pharm), *Dicarbosil* (BIRA)
Tablets: 500, 600, 650, 1000, 1250 mg (*otc*)	Various, *Maalox Antacid Caplets* (Aventis)
Gum tablets: 500 mg (*otc*)	*Chooz* (Schering-Plough)
Suspension: 1250 mg/5 mL (*otc*)	Various
Lozenges: 600 mg (*otc*)	*Mylanta* (J & J-Merck)
MAGNESIUM OXIDE	
Tablets: 400, 420, 500 mg (*otc*)	Various, *Mag-Ox 400* (Blaine), *Maox 420* (Kenneth A. Manne)
Capsules: 140 mg (*otc*)	*Uro-Mag* (Blaine)
MAGALDRATE	
Suspension: 540 mg/5 mL (*otc*)	*Riopan* (Whitehall)
Liquid: 540 mg/5 mL (*otc*)	Various, *Iosopan* (Goldline)
SODIUM BICARBONATE	
Tablets: 325, 520, 650 mg (*otc*)	Various, *Bell/ans* (C.S. Dent)
SODIUM CITRATE	
Solution: 450 mg (*otc*)	*Citra pH* (ValMed)

Indications

Hyperacidity: Symptomatic relief of upset stomach associated with hyperacidity (heartburn, gastroesophageal reflux, acid indigestion, and sour stomach); hyperacidity associated with peptic ulcer and gastric hyperacidity.

Aluminum carbonate: Treatment, control, or management of hyperphosphatemia, or for use with a low phosphate diet.

Calcium carbonate: Treating calcium deficiency states.

Magnesium oxide: Treatment of magnesium deficiencies or magnesium depletion.

Unlabeled uses: Antacids with aluminum and magnesium hydroxides or aluminum hydroxide alone effectively prevent significant stress ulcer bleeding. Antacids also are effective in treatment and maintenance of duodenal ulcer, and may be effective in treating gastric ulcer. Antacids also are recommended, initially, for gastroesophageal reflux disease (GERD).

Aluminum hydroxide has been used to reduce phosphate absorption in hyperphosphatemia in patients with chronic renal failure.

Calcium carbonate also may be used to bind phosphate.

Administration and Dosage

MAGNESIA (*Magnesium Hydroxide*):

Antacid dose, adults, and children > 12 years of age –

Liquid: 5 to 15 mL up to 4 times daily with water.

Liquid, concentrated: 2.5 to 7.5 mL up to 4 times daily with water.

Tablets: 622 mg to 1244 mg up to 4 times daily.

ALUMINUM HYDROXIDE GEL:

Tablets/Capsules – 500 to 1500 mg 3 to 6 times daily, between meals and at bedtime.

Suspension – 5 to 30 mL as needed between meals and at bedtime or as directed.

ALUMINUM CARBONATE GEL, BASIC:

Antacid – 2 capsules or tablets or 10 mL of regular suspension (in water or fruit juice) as often as every 2 hours, up to 12 times daily.

CALCIUM CARBONATE: 0.5 to 1.5 g, as needed.

MAGNESIUM OXIDE:

Capsules – 140 mg 3 to 4 times daily.

Tablets – 400 to 800 mg/day.

MAGALDRATE (*Aluminum Magnesium Hydroxide Sulfate*):

Suspension/Liquid – 5 to 10 mL between meals and at bedtime.

SODIUM BICARBONATE: 0.3 to 2 g 1 to 4 times daily.

SODIUM CITRATE: 30 mL daily.

Actions

Pharmacology: Antacids neutralize gastric acidity, resulting in an increase in the pH of the stomach and duodenal bulb. Additionally, by increasing the gastric pH above 4, they inhibit the proteolytic activity of pepsin. Antacids do not "coat" the mucosal lining, but may have a local astringent effect. Antacids also increase the lower esophageal sphincter tone. Aluminum ions inhibit smooth muscle contraction, thus inhibiting gastric emptying.

Acid neutralizing capacity (ANC) – ANC is a consideration in selecting an antacid. It varies for commercial antacid preparations and is expressed as mEq/mL. Milliequivalents of ANC is defined by the mEq of HCl required to keep an antacid suspension at pH 3.5 for 10 minutes in vitro. An antacid must neutralize at least 5 mEq/dose. Also, any ingredient must contribute at least 25% of the total ANC of a given product to be considered an antacid.

Aluminum hydroxide and calcium-containing antacids may reduce LDL cholesterol and increase the HDL/LDL ratio.

Warnings

Sodium content: Sodium content of antacids may be significant. Patients with hypertension, CHF, marked renal failure, or those on restricted or low-sodium diets should use a low sodium preparation.

"Acid rebound": Antacids may cause dose-related rebound hyperacidity because they may increase gastric secretion or serum gastrin levels.

Milk-alkali syndrome: Milk-alkali syndrome, an acute illness with symptoms of headache, nausea, irritability, and weakness, or a chronic illness with alkalosis, hypercalcemia and, possibly, renal impairment, has occurred following the concurrent use of high-dose calcium carbonate and sodium bicarbonate.

Hypophosphatemia: Prolonged use of aluminum-containing antacids may result in hypophosphatemia in normophosphatemic patients if phosphate intake is not adequate.

Renal function impairment: Use magnesium-containing products with caution, particularly when > 50 mEq magnesium is given daily. Hypermagnesemia and toxicity may occur because of decreased clearance of the magnesium ion.

Prolonged use of aluminum-containing antacids in patients with renal failure may result in or worsen dialysis osteomalacia.

Pregnancy: If pregnant, consult a physician before using.

Precautions

GI hemorrhage: Use aluminum hydroxide with care in patients who have recently suffered massive upper GI hemorrhage.

Drug Interactions

Drugs that may be affected by antacids include allopurinol, amphetamines, benzodiazepines, captopril, chloroquine, corticosteroids, dicumarol, diflunisal, digoxin, ethambutol, flecainide, fluoroquinolones, histamine H_2 antagonists, hydantoins, iron salts, isoniazid, ketoconazole, levodopa, lithium, methenamine, methotrexate, nitrofurantoin, penicillamine, phenothiazines, quinidine, salicylates, sodium polystyrene sulfonate, sulfonylureas, sympathomimetics, tetracyclines, thyroid hormones, ticlopidine, and valproic acid.

Adverse Reactions

Magnesium-containing antacids – Laxative effect as saline cathartic, may cause diarrhea; hypermagnesemia in renal failure patients.

Aluminum-containing antacids – Constipation (may lead to intestinal obstruction); aluminum-intoxication; osteomalacia and hypophosphatemia; accumulation of aluminum in serum, bone, and the CNS (aluminum accumulation may be neurotoxic); encephalopathy.

Antacids – Dose-dependent rebound hyperacidity and milk-alkali syndrome.

ANTHELMINTIC INTRODUCTION

Indications

	Major Parasite Infections		
	Infection (common name)	Organism	Drug(s) of Choice
Intestinal Nematodes	Ascariasis[1] (Roundworm)	*Ascaris lumbricoides*	Mebendazole, Pyrantel pamoate or Diethylcarbamazine
	Uncinariasis (Hookworm)	*Ancylostoma duodenale* *Necator americanus*	Mebendazole or Pyrantel pamoate[2]
	Strongyloidiasis (Threadworm)	*Strongyloides stercoralis*	Thiabendazole
	Trichuriasis (Whipworm)	*Trichuris trichiura*	Mebendazole
	Enterobiasis[3] (Pinworm)	*Enterobius vermicularis*	Mebendazole, Pyrantel pamoate or Albendazole
	Capillariasis	*Capillaria philippinensis*	Mebendazole, Thiabendazole or Albendazole
Tissue Nematodes	Trichinosis	*Trichinella spiralis*	Steroids for severe symptoms plus Thiabendazole, Albendazole, Flubendazole[6] or Mebendazole[2]
	Cutaneous larva migrans (Creeping eruption)	*Ancylostoma braziliense* and others	Thiabendazole, Albendazole or Ivermectin[4]
	Onchocerciasis (River blindness)	*Onchocerca volvulus*	Suramin[5], Diethylcarbamazine or Ivermectin[4]
	Dracontiasis (Guinea worm)	*Dracunculus medinensis*	Thiabendazole or Mebendazole
	Angiostrongyliasis (Rat lungworm)	*Angiostrongylus cantonensis*	Thiabendazole or Mebendazole
	Loiasis	*Loa loa*	Diethylcarbamazine
Cestodes	Taeniasis (Beef tapeworm)	*Taenia saginata*	Praziquantel[2] or Niclosamide[6]
	(Pork tapeworm)	*Taenia solium*	Praziquantel[2], Niclosamide[6] or Albendazole
	Diphyllobothriasis (Fish tapeworm)	*Diphyllobothrium latum*	Praziquantel[2] or Niclosamide[6]
	Dog tapeworm	*Dipylidium caninum*	Praziquantel[2]
	Hymenolepiasis (Dwarf tapeworm)	*Hymenolepis nana*	Praziquantel[2] or Niclosamide[6]
	Hydatid cysts	*Echinococcus granulosus*	Albendazole or Praziquantel
Trematodes	Schistosomiasis	*Schistosoma mansoni*	Praziquantel or Oxamniquine
		Schistosoma japonicum	Praziquantel
		Schistosoma haematobium	Praziquantel
		Schistosoma mekongi	Praziquantel
	Hermaphroditic Flukes Fasciolopsiasis (Intestinal fluke)	*Fasciolopsis buski*	Praziquantel
		Heterophyes heterophyes *Metagonimus yokogawai*	Praziquantel
	Clonorchiasis (Chinese liver fluke)	*Clonorchis sinensis*	Praziquantel
	Fascioliasis (Sheep liver fluke)	*Fasciola hepatica*	Praziquantel or Bithionol[4]
	Opisthorchiasis (Liver fluke)	*Opisthorchis viverrini*	Praziquantel
	Paragonimiasis (Lung fluke)	*Paragonimus westermani*	Praziquantel or Bithionol[4] (alternate)

[1] Thiabendazole is also indicated in Ascariasis.
[2] Unlabeled use.
[3] Thiabendazole is also indicated in Enterobiasis.
[4] Available from the CDC.
[5] Available from the CDC, although generally not recommended.
[6] Not available in the US.

MEBENDAZOLE

Tablets, chewable: 100 mg	Various, *Vermox* (Janssen)

Indications

Helminths: Treatment of *Trichuris trichiura* (whipworm), *Enterobius vermicularis* (pinworm), *Ascaris lumbricoides* (roundworm), *Ancylostoma duodenale* (common hookworm), or *Necator americanus* (American hookworm), in single or mixed infections.

Administration and Dosage

The same dosage schedule applies to children and adults.

Tablets may be chewed, swallowed, or crushed and mixed with food. No special procedures, such as fasting or purging, are required.

If the patient is not cured 3 weeks after treatment, a second treatment course is advised.

Trichuriasis, ascariasis, and hookworm infection: One tablet morning and evening on 3 consecutive days. In one study, treatment with a single 500 mg dose was effective against *A. lumbricoides*.

Enterobiasis: A single tablet given once.

Actions

Pharmacology: Mebendazole inhibits the formation of the worms' microtubules and irreversibly blocks glucose uptake by the susceptible helminths, thereby depleting endogenous glycogen stored within the parasite that is required for survival and reproduction of the helminth. Mebendazole does not affect blood glucose concentrations in the host.

Pharmacokinetics: Mebendazole is poorly absorbed (5% to 10%) after oral administration. Peak plasma levels are reached in 2 to 4 hours. Approximately 2% of the drug is excreted in the urine during the first 24 to 48 hours. Most of the dose is excreted in the feces as unchanged drug or primary metabolites.

Contraindications

Hypersensitivity to mebendazole.

Warnings

Hydatid disease: There is no evidence that mebendazole is effective for hydatid disease.

Pregnancy: Category C. Mebendazole was embryotoxic and teratogenic in pregnant rats. This drug is not recommended for use in pregnant women. During pregnancy, especially during the first trimester, use mebendazole only if the potential benefit justifies the potential risk to the fetus.

Lactation: Exercise caution when mebendazole is administered to a nursing woman.

Children: Safety and efficacy for use in children < 2 years of age have not been established; consider the relative benefit vs risk.

Drug Interactions

Carbamazepine and hydantoins: May reduce the plasma levels of concomitant mebendazole, possibly decreasing its therapeutic effect.

Adverse Reactions

Transient abdominal pain, diarrhea, neutropenia, fever.

ALBENDAZOLE

Tablets: 200 mg *Albenza* (GlaxoSmithKline)

Indications

Neurocysticercosis: For the treatment of parenchymal neurocysticercosis due to active lesions caused by larval forms of the pork tapeworm, *Taenia solium.*

Hydatid disease: For the treatment of cystic hydatid disease of the liver, lung, and peritoneum caused by the larval form of the dog tapeworm, *Echinococcus granulosus.*

When medically feasible, surgery is considered the treatment of choice for hydatid disease. When administering albendazole in the pre- or post-surgical setting, optimal killing of cyst contents is achieved when 3 courses of therapy have been given.

Administration and Dosage

Dosing of Albendazole According to the Parasitic Infection

Indication	Weight	Dose	Duration
Hydatid disease	≥ 60 kg	400 mg twice a day with meals	28-day cycle followed by a 14-day albendazole-free interval, for a total of three cycles
	< 60 kg	15 mg/kg/day given in divided doses twice a day with meals (maximum total daily dose 800 mg)	
Neurocysticercosis	≥ 60 kg	400 mg twice a day with meals	8 to 30 days
	< 60 kg	15 mg/kg/day given in divided doses twice a day with meals (maximum total daily dose 800 mg)	

Patients being treated for neurocysticercosis should receive appropriate steroid and anticonvulsant therapy as required. Consider oral or IV corticosteroids to prevent cerebral hypertensive episodes during the first week of treatment.

Actions

Pharmacology: Albendazole's principal mode of action is its inhibitory effect on tubulin polymerization, which results in the loss of cytoplasmic microtubules.

Pharmacokinetics:

Absorption – Albendazole is poorly absorbed from the GI tract because of its low aqueous solubility. Albendazole concentrations are negligible or undetectable in plasma as it is rapidly converted to the sulfoxide metabolite prior to reaching the systemic circulation. Oral bioavailability appears to be enhanced when albendazole is coadministered with a fatty meal.

The mean apparent terminal elimination half-life of albendazole sulfoxide typically ranged from 8 to 12 hours.

Distribution – Albendazole sulfoxide is 70% bound to plasma protein and is widely distributed throughout the body; it has been detected in urine, bile, liver, cyst wall, cyst fluid and cerebral spinal fluid (CSF). Concentrations in plasma were 3- to 10-fold and 2- to 4-fold higher than those simultaneously determined in cyst fluid and CSF, respectively. Limited in vitro and clinical data suggest that albendazole sulfoxide may be eliminated from cysts at a slower rate than observed in plasma.

Metabolism/Excretion – Albendazole is rapidly converted in the liver to the primary metabolite, albendazole sulfoxide, which is further metabolized to albendazole sulfone and other primary oxidative metabolites that have been identified in human urine.

Special populations –

Renal function impairment: It is unlikely that clearance of these compounds would be altered in these patients.

Hepatic function impairment: In patients with evidence of extrahepatic obstruction, the systemic availability of albendazole sulfoxide is increased. The rate of absorption/conversion and elimination of albendazole sulfoxide appeared to be prolonged with mean T_{max} and serum elimination half-life values of 10 hours and 31.7 hours, respectively.

Children: Albendazole sulfoxide pharmacokinetics were similar to those observed in fed adults.

Elderly: Pharmacokinetics are similar to those in young healthy subjects.

Contraindications

Hypersensitivity to the benzimidazole class of compound or any components of albendazole.

Warnings

Hepatic function impairment: Mild to moderate elevations of hepatic enzymes in ≈ 16% of patients. These have returned to normal upon discontinuation of therapy. Perform liver function tests (transaminases) before the start of each treatment. If enzymes are significantly increased, discontinue albendazole therapy. Therapy can be reinstituted when liver enzymes have returned to pretreatment levels, but perform laboratory tests frequently during repeated therapy.

Fertility impairment: Patients should not become pregnant for at least 1 month following cessation of albendazole therapy.

Elderly: No problems associated with an older population have been observed.

Pregnancy: Category C. Albendazole is teratogenic in animals. Do not use albendazole in pregnant women except in clinical circumstances where no alternative management is appropriate. If a patient becomes pregnant while taking this drug, discontinue albendazole immediately.

Lactation: Use caution when administering to a nursing woman.

Children: Experience in children < 6 years of age is limited. In hydatid disease, infection in infants and young children is uncommon, but no problems have been encountered in those who have been treated.

Precautions

Monitoring: Albendazole has been shown to cause occasional (< 1% of treated patients) reversible reductions in total white blood cell count.

Cysticercosis: It may, in rare cases, involve the retina. Before initiating therapy for neurocysticercosis, examine the patient for the presence of retinal lesions.

Drug Interactions

Albendazole may be affected by dexamethasone, praziquantel, and cimetidine.

Adverse Reactions

Adverse reactions affecting at least 3% of patients include the following: Abnormal liver function tests, abdominal pain, nausea, vomiting, headache, raised intracranial pressure.

PYRANTEL

Capsules, soft gel: 180 mg pyrantel pamoate (equiv. to 62.5 mg pyrantel base)	*Pin-Rid* (Apothecary), *Reese's Pinworm* (Reese)
Oral suspension: 50 mg pyrantel (as pamoate) per mL	*Antiminth* (Pfizer Labs)
Liquid: 50 mg pyrantel (as pamoate) per mL	*Pin-X* (Effcon), *Reese's Pinworm* (Reese)

Indications

Helminths: Treatment of ascariasis (roundworm infection) and enterobiasis (pinworm infection).

Administration and Dosage

A single dose of 11 mg/kg (5 mg/lb). Maximum total dose is 1 g.

May be administered without regard to ingestion of food or time of day. Purging is not necessary. May be taken with milk or fruit juices.

Actions

Pharmacology: Pyrantel is a depolarizing neuromuscular blocking agent, resulting in spastic paralysis of the worm. It also inhibits cholinesterases. It is active against *Enterobius vermicularis* (pinworm) and *Ascaris lumbricoides* (roundworm); it is also effective against *Ancylostoma duodenale* (hookworm).

Pharmacokinetics: Pyrantel is poorly absorbed from the GI tract. Plasma levels of unchanged drug are low. Greater than 50% is excreted in feces as unchanged drug; ≤ 7% of the dose is found in the urine as parent drug and metabolites.

Contraindications

Hepatic disease; pregnancy (see Warnings); hypersensitivity to pyrantel.

Warnings

Pregnancy: Do not use during pregnancy unless otherwise directed by a physician.

Children: Safety and efficacy for use in children < 2 years have not been established.

Drug Interactions

Pyrantel may interact with piperazine and theophylline.

Adverse Reactions

CNS: Headache; dizziness; drowsiness; insomnia.

Dermatologic: Rash.

GI: Anorexia; nausea; vomiting; abdominal cramps; diarrhea.

DIFENOXIN HCl WITH ATROPINE SULFATE

Tablets: 1 mg difenoxin (as HCl) and 0.025 mg atropine sulfate (*c-iv*)	*Motofen* (Carnrick)

Indications

Adjunctive therapy in management of acute nonspecific diarrhea and acute exacerbations of chronic functional diarrhea.

Administration and Dosage

Adults: Recommended starting dose: 2 tablets, then 1 tablet after each loose stool; 1 tablet every 3 to 4 hours as needed. The total dosage during any 24-hour treatment period should not exceed 8 tablets. For diarrhea in which clinical improvement is not observed in 48 hours, continued administration is not recommended. For acute diarrhea and acute exacerbations of functional diarrhea, treatment beyond 48 hours is usually not necessary.

Actions

Pharmacology: Difenoxin is an antidiarrheal agent chemically related to meperidine. Atropine sulfate is present to discourage deliberate overdosage.

Difenoxin manifests its antidiarrheal effect by slowing intestinal motility. The mechanism of action is by a local effect on the GI wall.

Difenoxin is the principal active metabolite of diphenoxylate and is effective at one-fifth the dosage of diphenoxylate.

Pharmacokinetics: Difenoxin is rapidly and extensively absorbed orally. Mean peak plasma levels occur within 40 to 60 minutes. Plasma levels decline to < 10% of their peak values within 24 hours and to < 1% of their peak values within 72 hours. This decline parallels the appearance of difenoxin and its metabolites in the urine. Difenoxin is metabolized to an inactive hydroxylated metabolite. The drug and its metabolites are excreted, mainly as conjugates, in urine and feces.

Contraindications

Diarrhea associated with organisms that penetrate the intestinal mucosa (eg, toxigenic *E. coli*, *Salmonella* sp., *Shigella;*) and pseudomembranous colitis associated with broad-spectrum antibiotics. Antiperistaltic agents may prolong or worsen diarrhea.

Children: Children < 2 years of age because of the decreased margin of safety of drugs in this class in younger age groups.

Hypersensitivity to difenoxin, atropine, or any of the inactive ingredients; jaundice.

Warnings

Difenoxin HCl with atropine sulfate is not innocuous; strictly adhere to dosage recommendations. Overdosage may result in severe respiratory depression and coma, possibly leading to permanent brain damage or death.

Fluid and electrolyte balance: The use of this drug does not preclude the administration of appropriate fluid and electrolyte therapy. Dehydration, particularly in children, may further influence the variability of response and may predispose to delayed difenoxin intoxication. Drug-induced inhibition of peristalsis may result in fluid retention in the colon, and this may further aggravate dehydration and electrolyte imbalance.

Ulcerative colitis: Agents that inhibit intestinal motility or delay intestinal transit time have induced toxic megacolon. Consequently, carefully observe patients with acute ulcerative colitis.

Liver and kidney disease: Use with extreme caution in patients with advanced hepatorenal disease and in all patients with abnormal liver function tests because hepatic coma may be precipitated.

Atropine: A subtherapeutic dose of atropine has been added to difenoxin to discourage deliberate overdosage. A recommended dose is not likely to cause prominent anticholinergic side effects, but avoid in patients in whom anticholinergic drugs are contraindicated. In children, signs of atropinism may occur even with recommended doses, particularly in patients with Down's Syndrome.

Pregnancy: Category C.

Lactation: Decide whether to discontinue nursing or to discontinue the drug, taking into account the importance of the drug to the mother.

Children: Contraindicated in children under 2 years of age. Safety and efficacy in children below the age of 12 have not been established.

Precautions

Drug abuse and dependence: Addiction to (dependence on) difenoxin is theoretically possible at high dosage. Therefore, do not exceed recommended dosage.

Drug Interactions

Drugs that may interact include MAO inhibitors, barbiturates, tranquilizers, narcotics, and alcohol.

Adverse Reactions

Adverse reactions may include nausea, dry mouth, dizziness, lightheadedness, and drowsiness.

DIPHENOXYLATE HCl WITH ATROPINE SULFATE

Tablets: 2.5 mg diphenoxylate HCl and 0.025 mg atropine sulfate (*c-v*)	Various, *Logen* (Goldline), *Lomotil* (Searle), *Lonox* (Geneva)
Liquid: 2.5 mg diphenoxylate HCl and 0.025 mg atropine sulfate per 5 mL (*c-v*)	Various, *Lomotil* (Searle)

Indications

Adjunctive therapy in the management of diarrhea.

Administration and Dosage

Adults: Individualize dosage. Initial dose is 5 mg 4 times/day.

Children: In children 2 to 12 years of age, use liquid form only. The recommended initial dosage is 0.3 to 0.4 mg/kg daily, in 4 divided doses.

Diphenoxylate w/Atropine Pediatric Dosage

Age (years)	Approximate weight kg	Approximate weight lb	Dosage (mL) (4 times daily)
2	11-14	24-31	1.5-3
3	12-16	26-35	2-3
4	14-20	31-44	2-4
5	16-23	35-51	2.5-4.5
6-8	17-32	38-71	2.5-5
9-12	23-55	51-121	3.5-5

Reduce dosage: Reduce dosage as soon as initial control of symptoms is achieved. Maintenance dosage may be as low as ¼ of the initial daily dosage. Do not exceed recommended dosage. Clinical improvement of acute diarrhea is usually observed within 48 hours. If clinical improvement of chronic diarrhea is not seen within 10 days after a maximum daily dose of 20 mg, symptoms are unlikely to be controlled by further use.

Actions

Pharmacology: Diphenoxylate, a constipating meperidine congener, lacks analgesic activity. High doses cause opioid activity.

Pharmacokinetics: Bioavailability of tablet vs liquid is ≈ 90%. Diphenoxylate is rapidly, extensively metabolized to diphenoxylic acid (difenoxine), the active major metabolite. Elimination half-life is ≈ 12 to 14 hours. An average of 14% of drug and metabolites are excreted over 4 days in urine, 49% in feces. Urinary excretion of unmetabolized drug is < 1%; difenoxine plus its glucuronide conjugate constitutes ≈ 6%.

Contraindications

Children < 2 years of age because of greater variability of response; hypersensitivity to diphenoxylate or atropine; obstructive jaundice; diarrhea associated with pseudomembranous enterocolitis or enterotoxin-producing bacteria.

Warnings

Diarrhea: Diphenoxylate may prolong or aggravate diarrhea associated with organisms that penetrate intestinal mucosa (ie, toxigenic *Escherichia coli, Salmonella, Shigella*) or in pseudomembranous enterocolitis associated with broad-spectrum antibiotics. Do not use diphenoxylate in these conditions. In some patients with acute ulcerative colitis, diphenoxylate may induce toxic megacolon.

Fluid/Electrolyte balance: Dehydration, particularly in younger children, may influence variability of response and may predispose to delayed diphenoxylate intoxication. Inhibition of peristalsis may result in fluid retention in the intestine, which may further aggravate dehydration and electrolyte imbalance.

Hepatic function impairment: Use with extreme caution in patients with advanced hepatorenal disease or abnormal liver function; hepatic coma may be precipitated.

Pregnancy: Category C.

Lactation: Diphenoxylic acid may be excreted in breast milk and atropine is excreted in breast milk.

Children: Use with caution; signs of atropinism may occur with recommended doses, particularly in Down's syndrome patients. Use with caution in young children because of variable response. Not recommended in children < 2 years of age.

Precautions

Drug abuse and dependence: In recommended doses, diphenoxylate has not produced addiction and is devoid of morphine-like subjective effects. At high doses, it exhibits codeine-like subjective effects; therefore, addiction to diphenoxylate is possible. A subtherapeutic dose of atropine may discourage deliberate abuse.

Drug Interactions

Drugs that may interact include MAO inhibitors, barbiturates, tranquilizers, and alcohol.

Adverse Reactions

Adverse reactions may include dry skin and mucous membranes, flushing, hyperthermia, tachycardia, urinary retention (especially in children), pruritus, gum swelling, angioneurotic edema, urticaria, anaphylaxis, dizziness, drowsiness, sedation, headache, malaise, lethargy, restlessness, euphoria, depression, numbness of extremities, confusion, anorexia, nausea, vomiting, abdominal discomfort, toxic megacolon, and pancreatitis.

LOPERAMIDE HCl

Tablets: 2 mg (*otc*)	*Imodium A-D Caplets* (McNeil-CPC), *Kaopectate II Caplets* (Upjohn), *Maalox Anti-Diarrheal Caplets* (Aventis)
Capsules: 2 mg (*Rx*)	Various, *Imodium* (Janssen)
Liquid: 1 mg/5 mL (*otc*)	Various, *Imodium A-D* (McNeil-CPC)
Liquid: 1 mg/mL (*otc*)	*Pepto Diarrhea Control* (Procter & Gamble)

Indications

Rx: Control and symptomatic relief of acute nonspecific diarrhea and of chronic diarrhea associated with inflammatory bowel disease.

For reducing the volume of discharge from ileostomies.

OTC: Control of symptoms of diarrhea, including traveler's diarrhea.

Administration and Dosage

Rx:

Acute diarrhea –

Adults: 4 mg followed by 2 mg after each unformed stool. Do not exceed 16 mg/day. Clinical improvement is usually observed within 48 hours.

Children:

Loperamide Pediatric Dosage (First Day Schedule)			
Age (years)	Weight (kg)	Doseform	Amount
2-5	13-20	liquid	1 mg tid
6-8	20-30	liquid or capsule	2 mg bid
8-12	> 30	liquid or capsule	2 mg tid

Subsequent doses: Administer 1 mg/10 kg only after a loose stool. Total daily dosage should not exceed recommended dosages for the first day.

Chronic diarrhea –

Adults: 4 mg followed by 2 mg after each unformed stool until diarrhea is controlled. When optimal daily dosage (average, 4 to 8 mg) has been established, administer as a single dose or in divided doses.

If clinical improvement is not observed after treatment with 16 mg/day for at least 10 days, symptoms are unlikely to be controlled by further use.

Children – Dose has not been established.

OTC:

Acute diarrhea, including traveler's diarrhea –

Adults: 4 mg after first loose bowel movement followed by 2 mg after each subsequent loose bowel movement but no more than 8 mg/day for no more than 2 days.

Children:

9 to 11 years of age (60 to 95 lbs) – 2 mg after first loose bowel movement followed by 1 mg after each subsequent loose bowel movement but no more than 6 mg/day for no more than 2 days.

6 to 8 years of age (48 to 59 lbs) – 1 mg after first loose bowel movement followed by 1 mg after each subsequent loose bowel movement but no more than 4 mg/day for no more than 2 days.

< 6 years of age (up to 47 lbs) – Consult physician (not for use in children < 6).

Actions

Pharmacology: Loperamide slows intestinal motility and affects water and electrolyte movement through the bowel. It inhibits peristalsis by a direct effect on the circular and longitudinal muscles of the intestinal wall. It reduces daily fecal volume, increases viscosity and bulk density and diminishes the loss of fluid and electrolytes.

Pharmacokinetics:

Absorption/Distribution – Loperamide is 40% absorbed after oral administration and does not penetrate well into the brain. Peak plasma levels occur ≈ 5 hours after capsule administration, 2.5 hours after liquid administration and are similar for both formulations.

Metabolism/Excretion – The apparent elimination half-life is 10.8 hours (range, 9.1 to 14.4 hrs). Of a 4 mg oral dose, 25% is excreted unchanged in the feces, and 1.3% is excreted in the urine as free drug and glucuronic acid conjugate within 3 days.

Contraindications

Hypersensitivity to the drug and in patients who must avoid constipation.

OTC use: Bloody diarrhea; body temperature > 101°F.

Warnings

Diarrhea: Do not use loperamide in acute diarrhea associated with organisms that penetrate the intestinal mucosa (enteroinvasive *Escherichia coli*, *Salmonella*, and *Shigella*) or in pseudomembranous colitis associated with broad-spectrum antibiotics.

Acute ulcerative colitis: In some patients with acute ulcerative colitis, agents that inhibit intestinal motility or delay intestinal transit time may induce toxic megacolon.

Fluid/electrolyte depletion: Fluid/electrolyte depletion may occur in patients who have diarrhea. Loperamide use does not preclude administration of appropriate fluid and electrolyte therapy.

Pregnancy: *Category B.*

Lactation: It is not known whether loperamide is excreted in breast milk.

Children: Not recommended for use in children < 2 years of age. Use special caution in young children because of the greater variability of response in this age group. Dehydration may further influence variability of response. Dosage has not been established for children in treatment of chronic diarrhea.

Precautions

Acute diarrhea: If clinical improvement is not observed in 48 hours, discontinue use.

Hepatic dysfunction: Monitor patients with hepatic dysfunction closely for signs of CNS toxicity because of the apparent large first-pass biotransformation.

Adverse Reactions

Adverse reactions may include abdominal pain, distention, or discomfort; constipation; dry mouth; nausea; vomiting; tiredness, drowsiness, or dizziness; hypersensitivity reactions (including skin rash).

BISMUTH SUBSALICYLATE (BSS)

Tablets, chewable: 262 mg (*otc*)	Various, *Pepto-Bismol* (Procter & Gamble)
Caplets: 262 mg (*otc*)	*Pepto-Bismol* (Procter & Gamble)
Liquid: 130 mg/15 mL (*otc*), 262 mg/15 mL (*otc*), 524 mg/15 mL (*otc*)	Various, *Pepto-Bismol* (Procter & Gamble)

Indications

For indigestion without causing constipation; nausea; control of diarrhea, including traveler's diarrhea, within 24 hours. Also relieves abdominal cramps.

Administration and Dosage

Adults: 2 tablets or 30 mL.

Children: 9 to 12 years of age – 1 tablet or 15 mL.
6 to 9 years of age – ⅔ tablet or 10 mL.
3 to 6 years of age – ⅓ tablet or 5 mL.
< 3 years of age – Consult physician.

Repeat dosage every 30 minutes to 1 hour, as needed, up to 8 doses in 24 hours.

Actions

Pharmacology: BSS appears to have antisecretory and antimicrobial effects in vitro and may have some anti-inflammatory effects. The salicylate moiety provides the antisecretory effect, while the bismuth moiety may exert direct antimicrobial effects against bacterial and viral enteropathogens.

Pharmacokinetics: BSS undergoes chemical dissociation in the GI tract. Two BSS tablets yield 204 mg salicylate. Following ingestion, salicylate is absorbed, with > 90% recovered in the urine; plasma levels are similar to levels achieved after a comparable dose of aspirin. Absorption of bismuth is negligible.

Precautions

Impaction: Impaction may occur in infants and debilitated patients.

Radiologic examinations: May interfere with radiologic examinations of GI tract. Bismuth is radiopaque.

Drug Interactions

Drugs that may be affected by bismuth include aspirin and tetracyclines.

ANTIEMETIC/ANTIVERTIGO AGENTS

Product	Manufacturer
CHLORPROMAZINE	
Tablets: 10, 25, 50, 100, and 200 mg (*Rx*)	Various, *Thorazine* (GlaxoSmithKline)
Capsules, sustained release: 30, 75, 150, 200, and 300 mg (*Rx*)	*Thorazine Spansules* (GlaxoSmithKline)
Syrup: 10 mg/5 mL (*Rx*)	*Chlorpromazine HCl* (Geneva), *Thorazine* (GlaxoSmithKline)
Concentrate: 30 and 100 mg/mL (*Rx*)	Various, *Thorazine* (GlaxoSmithKline)
Suppositories (as base): 25 and 100 mg (*Rx*)	*Thorazine* (GlaxoSmithKline)
Injection: 25 mg/mL (*Rx*)	Various, *Ormazine* (Hauck), *Thorazine* (GlaxoSmithKline)
PERPHENAZINE	
Tablets: 2, 4, 8, and 16 mg (*Rx*)	Various, *Trilafon* (Schering)
Concentrate: 16 mg/5 mL (*Rx*)	*Trilafon* (Schering)
Injection: 5 mg/mL (*Rx*)	*Trilafon* (Schering)
TRIFLUPROMAZINE	
Injection: 10 and 20 mg/mL (*Rx*)	*Vesprin* (Princeton)
PROCHLORPERAZINE	
Tablets (as maleate): 5, 10, and 25 mg (*Rx*)	Various, *Compazine* (GlaxoSmithKline)
Capsules, sustained release: 10, 15, and 30 mg (*Rx*)	*Compazine Spansules* (GlaxoSmithKline)
Suppositories: 2.5, 5, and 25 mg (*Rx*)	Various, *Compazine* (GlaxoSmithKline)
Syrup: 5 mg/5 mL (*Rx*)	*Compazine* (GlaxoSmithKline)
Injection (as edisylate): 5 mg/mL (*Rx*)	Various, *Prochlorperazine* (Wyeth-Ayerst), *Compazine* (GlaxoSmithKline)
THIETHYLPERAZINE	
Tablets: 10 mg (*Rx*)	*Norzine* (Purdue Frederick), *Torecan* (Roxane)
Suppositories: 10 mg (*Rx*)	
Injection: 5 mg/mL (*Rx*)	
METOCLOPRAMIDE	
Tablets: 5 mg (*Rx*)	Various, *Reglan* (Robins)
Tablets: 10 mg (*Rx*)	Various, *Clopra* (Quantum), *Maxolon* (GlaxoSmithKline), *Octamide* (Adria), *Reclomide* (Major), *Reglan* (Robins)
Syrup: 5 mg/5 mL (*Rx*)	Various, *Reglan* (Robins), *Maxolon* (GlaxoSmithKline)
Concentrated solution: 10 mg/mL (*Rx*)	*Metoclopramide Intensol* (Roxane)
Injection: 5 mg/mL (*Rx*)	Various, *Octamide PFS* (Adria), *Reglan* (Robins)

Administration and Dosage

CHLORPROMAZINE HCl:

Adults –

Nausea and vomiting:

Oral – 10 to 25 mg every 4 to 6 hours, as needed; increase if necessary.

Rectal – 50 to 100 mg every 6 to 8 hours, as needed.

IM – 25 mg. If no hypotension occurs, give 25 to 50 mg every 3 to 4 hours, as needed, until vomiting stops. Then switch to oral dosage.

Intractable hiccoughs: Orally, 25 to 50 mg 3 or 4 times/day. If symptoms persist 2 to 3 days, give 25 to 50 mg IM. If still persistent, use slow IV infusion with patient flat in bed. Give 25 to 50 mg in 500 to 1000 mL saline. Monitor blood pressure.

Children –

Nausea and vomiting: Do not use in children < 6 months of age except where potentially lifesaving. Do not use in conditions for which specific children's dosages have not been established. The activity following IM use may last 12 hours.

Oral – 0.25 mg/lb (0.55 mg/kg) every 4 to 6 hours.

Rectal – 0.5 mg/lb (1.1 mg/kg) every 6 to 8 hours, as needed.

IM – 0.25 mg/lb (0.55 mg/kg) every 6 to 8 hours, as needed.

Maximum IM dosage –

Children up to 5 years of age: 40 mg/day.

Children 5 to 12 years of age: 75 mg/day, except in severe cases.

PERPHENAZINE:

Oral – 8 to 16 mg/day in divided doses; occasionally, 24 mg may be necessary. Early dosage reduction is desirable.

IM – Give to seated or recumbent patient; observe patient for a short period afterward.

Adults: 5 mg repeated every 6 hours as necessary. Do not exceed 15 mg in ambulatory or 30 mg in hospitalized patients. For severe conditions, an initial dose of 10 mg may be given. Place patients on oral therapy as soon as possible, usually within 24 hours. In general, reserve higher dosages for hospitalized patients.

Children (> 12 years of age): The lowest adult dose (5 mg). Pediatric dose not established.

IV – Use only when necessary to control severe vomiting, intractable hiccoughs or acute conditions such as violent retching during surgery. Limit use to recumbent hospitalized adults in doses not exceeding 5 mg. Give as a diluted solution by either fractional injection or slow drip infusion. In the surgical patient, slow infusion is preferred. When administered in divided doses, dilute to 0.5 mg/mL (1 mL mixed with 9 mL saline solution) and give not more than 1 mg per injection at not less than 1 to 2 minute intervals. Discontinue as soon as symptoms are controlled. Do not exceed 5 mg.

TRIFLUPROMAZINE HCl:

Adults –

IM (range): 5 to 15 mg repeated every 4 hours, up to 60 mg maximum daily dose.

Elderly or debilitated – 2.5 mg; maximum daily dose, 15 mg.

IV (range): 1 mg, up to 3 mg total daily dose.

Children (over 2½ years of age) –

IM: 0.2 to 0.25 mg/kg; maximum 10 mg/day. The duration of activity following IM administration may last up to 12 hours. Do not administer IV.

PROCHLORPERAZINE: Do not crush or chew sustained release preparations.

Adults: Control of severe nausea and vomiting –

Oral: Usually, 5 or 10 mg, 3 or 4 times/day; *sustained release* -15 mg on arising or 10 mg every 12 hours.

Rectal: 25 mg twice/day.

IM: Initially, 5 to 10 mg. If necessary, repeat every 3 or 4 hours. Do not exceed 40 mg/day.

SC: Do not administer SC because of local irritation.

Adult surgery: Control of severe nausea and vomiting – Total parenteral dosage should not exceed 40 mg/day. Hypotension may occur if the drug is given IV or by infusion.

IM: 5 to 10 mg, 1 to 2 hours before induction of anesthesia (may repeat once in 30 minutes), or to control acute symptoms during and after surgery (may repeat once).

IV injection: 5 to 10 mg, 15 to 30 minutes before induction of anesthesia, or to control acute symptoms during or after surgery. Repeat once if necessary. Prochlorperazine may be administered either undiluted or diluted in isotonic solution, but do not exceed 10 mg in a single dose of the drug. Do not exceed 5 mg/mL/min. Do not use bolus injection.

IV infusion: 20 mg/L of isotonic solution. Do not dilute in less than 1 L of isotonic solution. Add to IV infusion 15 to 30 minutes before induction.

Children (over 20 pounds or 2 years of age): Control of severe nausea and vomiting –

Oral or rectal: More than one day of therapy is seldom necessary.

9.1 to 13.2 kg – 2.5 mg 1 or 2 times/day (not to exceed 7.5 mg/day).

13.6 to 17.7 kg – 2.5 mg 2 or 3 times/day (not to exceed 10 mg/day).

18.2 to 38.6 kg – 2.5 mg 3 times/day or 5 mg twice/day (not to exceed 15 mg/day).

IM: 0.06 mg/lb (0.132 mg/kg). Give by deep IM injection. Control is usually obtained with one dose. Duration of action may be 12 hours. Subsequent doses may be given if necessary.

PROMETHAZINE:

Oral and rectal –

Motion sickness: The average adult dose is 25 mg twice/day. Take the initial dose 1 hour before travel, and repeat 8 to 12 hours later, if necessary. On succeeding days, administer 25 mg on arising and again before the evening meal. For children, administer 12.5 to 25 mg twice/day.

Nausea and vomiting: The average dose for active therapy in children or adults is 25 mg. Repeat as necessary in doses of 12.5 to 25 mg at 4 to 6 hour intervals.

Children – 0.25 to 0.5 mg/kg every 4 to 6 hours rectally, as needed. Do not use in children < 2 years of age. Adjust dose based on age, weight, and severity of condition.

Parenteral – Administer preferably by deep IM injection. Proper IV administration is well tolerated, but hazardous. When used IV, give in a concentration no greater than 25 mg/mL, and at a rate not to exceed 25 mg/min; it is preferable to inject through an appropriate site in tubing of an IV infusion set.

Motion sickness: 12.5 to 25 mg; may repeat as necessary 3 or 4 times a day.

Nausea and vomiting: 12.5 to 25 mg; do not repeat more frequently than every 4 hours. For postoperative nausea and vomiting, administer IM or IV.

In children < 12 years of age, do not exceed half the adult dose. As an adjunct to premedication, use 0.5 mg/lb (1.1 mg/kg) with an equal dose of narcotic or barbiturate and the appropriate dose of an atropine-like drug. Do not use in premature infants or neonates or in vomiting of unknown etiology in children.

THIETHYLPERAZINE MALEATE: Do not use IV (may cause severe hypotension).

When used for nausea or vomiting associated with anesthesia and surgery, administer by deep IM injection at, or shortly before, termination of anesthesia.

Adults –

Oral and rectal: 10 to 30 mg/day in divided doses.

IM: 2 mL, 1 to 3 times/day.

Children – Dosage not determined. Not recommended in children < 12 years of age.

THIETHYLPERAZINE: Do not use IV (may cause severe hypotension). Use of this drug has not been studied following intracardiac or intracranial surgery.

When used for nausea or vomiting associated with anesthesia and surgery, administer by deep IM injection at, or shortly before, termination of anesthesia.

Adults –

Oral and Rectal: 10 to 30 mg/day in divided doses.

IM: 2 mL, 1 to 3 times/day.

Children – Dosage not determined. Not recommended in children < 12 years of age.

METOCLOPRAMIDE:

Prevention of chemotherapy-induced emesis – For doses in excess of 10 mg, dilute injection in 50 mL of a parenteral solution (Dextrose 5% in Water, Sodium Chloride Injection, Dextrose 5% in 0.45% Sodium Chloride, Ringer's or Lactated Ringer's Injection). Infuse slowly IV over not less than 15 minutes, 30 minutes before beginning cancer chemotherapy; repeat every 2 hours for 2 doses, then every 3 hours for 3 doses.

The initial 2 doses should be 2 mg/kg if highly emetogenic drugs such as cisplatin or dacarbazine are used alone or in combination. For less emetogenic regimens, 1 mg/kg/dose may be adequate.

Metoclopramide may have some potential value (10 mg orally or IV 30 minutes before each meal and at bedtime) in nausea and vomiting of a variety of etiologies (uncontrolled studies report 80% to 90% efficacy), including emesis during pregnancy and labor (5 to 10 mg orally or 5 to 20 mg IV or IM, 3 times a day).

Actions

Pharmacology: Drug-induced vomiting (eg, drugs, radiation, metabolic disorders) is generally stimulated through the chemoreceptor trigger zone (CTZ), which in turn stimulates the vomiting center (VC) in the brain. Nausea of motion sickness is initiated by stimulation of labyrinthine mechanism of the ear, which sends impulses to CTZ. VC may also be stimulated directly by GI irritation, motion sickness, vestibular neuritis.

The following table indicates manufacturers' recommended uses for agents in this group. Several of these are indicated for uses other than as antiemetic/antivertigo agents.

Recommended Uses for Antiemetic/Antivertigo Agents

	Drug	Indications		
		Nausea and Vomiting	Motion Sickness	Vertigo
ANTIDOPAMINERGICS				
Phenothiazines	Chlorpromazine [1]	✓		
Phenothiazines	Triflupromazine	✓		
Phenothiazines	Perphenazine [1]	✓		
Phenothiazines	Prochlorperazine	✓		
Phenothiazines	Promethazine[2]	✓	✓	
Phenothiazines	Thiethylperazine	✓		
Other	Metoclopramide	✓		
ANTICHOLINERGICS				
Antihistamines	Cyclizine	✓	✓	
Antihistamines	Meclizine	✓	✓	✓[3]
Antihistamines	Buclizine	✓	✓	
Antihistamines	Diphenhydramine		✓	
Antihistamines	Dimenhydrinate	✓	✓	✓
Other	Trimethobenzamide	✓		
Other	Scopolamine		✓	
MISCELLANEOUS				
Miscellaneous	Diphenidol	✓		✓
Miscellaneous	Benzquinamide	✓		
Miscellaneous	Phosphorated Carbohydrate Solution	✓		
Miscellaneous	Hydroxyzine HCl	✓[4]		
Miscellaneous	Corticosteroids	✓[4]		
Miscellaneous	Cannabinoids	✓		

[1] Also indicated for relief of intractable hicoughs.
[2] For complete listing of promethazine products refer to Antihistamine Product Pages.
[3] Classified "possibly effective" by the FDA.
[4] This is an *unlabeled* use.

Warnings

Children: Not recommended for uncomplicated vomiting in children; limit use to prolonged vomiting of known etiology.

Children with acute illnesses (eg, chickenpox, CNS infections, measles, gastroenteritis) or dehydration seem to be much more susceptible to neuromuscular reactions, particularly dystonias, than are adults. Do not use dimenhydrinate in children under 2 years of age unless directed by a doctor.

Severe emesis – Severe emesis should not be treated with an antiemetic drug alone; where possible, establish cause of vomiting. Direct primary emphasis toward restoration of body fluids and electrolyte balance, and relief of fever and causative disease process. Avoid overhydration which may result in cerebral edema.

CYCLIZINE AND MECLIZINE

CYCLIZINE	
Tablets: 50 mg (as HCl) (*otc*)	*Marezine* (Himmel)
MECLIZINE	
Tablets: 12.5, 25, and 50 mg (*Rx*)	Various, *Antivert* (Roerig), *Ru-Vert-M* (Solvay), *Dramamine II* (Pharmacia)
Tablets, chewable: 25 mg (*Rx*)	Various
Tablets, chewable: 25 mg (*otc*)	Various, *Bonine* (Leeming)
Capsules: 25 mg (*Rx*)	Various, *Meni-D* (Seatrace)
Capsules: 30 mg (*otc*)	*Vergon* (Marnel)

Indications

Motion sickness, vestibular system disease: Prevention and treatment of nausea, vomiting, and dizziness of motion sickness.

Meclizine is "possibly effective" for the management of vertigo associated with diseases affecting the vestibular system.

Administration and Dosage

CYCLIZINE:

Oral –

Adults: 50 mg taken ½ hour before departure; repeat every 4 to 6 hours. Do not exceed 200 mg/day.

Children (6 to 12 years of age): 25 mg, up to 3 times/day.

Parenteral – For IM use only. Not recommended for use in children.

Adults: 50 mg every 4 to 6 hours, as necessary.

MECLIZINE:

Motion sickness – Take an initial dose of 25 to 50 mg, 1 hour prior to travel. May repeat dose every 24 hours for the duration of the journey.

Vertigo – 25 to 100 mg/day in divided doses.

Actions

Pharmacology: Cyclizine and meclizine have antiemetic, anticholinergic, and antihistaminic properties.

Cyclizine and meclizine have an onset of action of 30 to 60 minutes, depending on dosage; their duration of action is 4 to 6 hours and 12 to 24 hours, respectively.

Contraindications

Hypersensitivity to cyclizine or meclizine.

Warnings

Pregnancy: Category B. Meclizine presents the lowest risk of teratogenicity and is the drug of first choice in treating nausea and vomiting during pregnancy.

Lactation: Safety for use in the nursing mother has not been established.

Children: Safety and efficacy for use in children have not been established. Not recommended for use in children < 12 years of age.

Precautions

Hazardous tasks: May produce drowsiness; patients should observe caution while driving or performing other tasks requiring alertness.

Because of the anticholinergic action of these agents, use with caution and with appropriate monitoring in patients with glaucoma, obstructive disease of the GI or GU tract, and in elderly males with possible prostatic hypertrophy. These drugs may have a hypotensive action, which may be confusing or dangerous in postoperative patients.

May have additive effects with alcohol and other CNS depressants (eg, hypnotics, sedatives, tranquilizers, antianxiety agents); use with caution.

Adverse Reactions

Adverse reactions include the following: Hypotension; palpitations; tachycardia; drowsiness; restlessness; excitation; nervousness; insomnia; euphoria; blurred vision; diplopia; vertigo; tinnitus; auditory and visual hallucinations (particularly when dosage recommendations are exceeded); urticaria; rash; dry mouth; anorexia; nausea; vomiting; diarrhea; constipation; cholestatic jaundice (cyclizine); urinary frequency; difficult urination; urinary retention; dry nose and throat.

BUCLIZINE HCl

Tablets: 50 mg (*Rx*)	*Bucladin-S Softabs* (Stuart)

Indications

For the control of nausea, vomiting, and dizziness of motion sickness.

Administration and Dosage

Tablets can be taken without swallowing water. Place tablet in mouth and allow to dissolve, or chew or swallow whole.

Adults: A 50 mg dose usually alleviates nausea. In severe cases, 150 mg/day may be taken. Usual maintenance dose is 50 mg, 2 times/day. In prevention of motion sickness, take 50 mg at least hour before beginning travel. For extended travel, a second 50 mg dose may be taken after 4 to 6 hours.

Actions

Pharmacology: Acts centrally to suppress nausea and vomiting.

Contraindications

Hypersensitivity to buclizine HCl; pregnancy (see Warnings).

Warnings

Pregnancy: Clinical data are not adequate to establish safety in early pregnancy.

Children: Safety and efficacy for use in children have not been established.

Adverse Reactions

Drowsiness, dry mouth, headache, and jitteriness.

DIPHENHYDRAMINE

Indications

Treatment and prophylaxis (oral only) of motion sickness.

Administration and Dosage

Oral: Adults – 25 to 50 mg 3 or 4 times/day.

Children > 20 lbs (9.1 kg) – 12.5 to 25 mg 3 or 4 times/day (5 mg/kg/24 hr, or 150 mg/m^2/24 hr. Do not exceed 300 mg.

Give first dose 30 minutes before exposure to motion and repeat before meals and upon retiring for the duration of journey.

Parenteral: For use only when the oral form is impractical.

Adults – 10 to 50 mg IV or deep IM; 100 mg if required. Maximum daily dosage is 400 mg.

Children – 5 mg/kg/24 hrs or 150 mg/m^2/24 hr, in 4 divided doses, IV or deep IM. Maximum daily dosage is 300 mg.

DIMENHYDRINATE

Tablets: 50 mg (*Rx*)	*Dimetabs* (Jones Medical)
Tablets: 50 mg (*otc*)	Various, *Calm-X* (Republic Drug), *Dramamine* (Pharmacia), *Triptone Caplets* (Commerce)
Tablets, chewable: 50 mg (*otc*)	*Dramamine* (Pharmacia)
Capsules: 50 mg (*otc*)	*Vertab* (UAD)
Injection: 50 mg/mL (*Rx*)	Various, *Dinate* (Seatrace), *Dramamine* (Pasadena), *Dymenate* (Keene), *Hydrate* (Hyrex)
Liquid: 12.5 mg/4 mL (*otc*)	Various, *Dramamine* (Pharmacia),
Liquid: 12.5 mg/5 mL (*otc*)	*Children's Dramamine* (Pharmacia)
Liquid: 15.62 mg/5 mL (*Rx*)	*Dramamine* (Pharmacia)

Indications

For the prevention and treatment of nausea, vomiting, dizziness, or vertigo of motion sickness.

Administration and Dosage

Adults:

Oral – 50 to 100 mg every 4 to 6 hours. Do not exceed 400 mg in 24 hours.

IM – 50 mg, as needed.

IV – 50 mg in 10 mL Sodium Chloride Injection given over 2 minutes. Do not inject intra-arterially.

Children:

Oral (6 to 12 years of age) – 25 to 50 mg every 6 to 8 hours; do not exceed 150 mg in 24 hours.

Oral (2 to 6 years of age) – Up to 12.5 to 25 mg every 6 to 8 hours; do not exceed 75 mg in 24 hours.

IM – 1.25 mg/kg or 37.5 mg/m^2 4 times/day; do not exceed 300 mg/day.

Children (under 2 years of age): Only on advice of a physician.

Actions

Pharmacology: Dimenhydrinate consists of equimolar proportions of diphenhydramine and chlorotheophylline.

Pharmacokinetics: Dimenhydrinate has a depressant action on hyperstimulated labyrinthine function. The precise mode of action is not known. The antiemetic effects are believed to be caused by the diphenhydramine, an antihistamine also used as an antiemetic agent.

Contraindications

Neonates; patients hypersensitive to dimenhydrinate or its components.

Note: Most IV products contain Benzyl Alcohol, which has been associated with a fatal "gasping syndrome" in premature infants and low birth weight infants.

Warnings

Pregnancy: Category B.

Lactation: Small amounts of dimenhydrinate are excreted in breast milk.

Children: For infants and children especially, an overdose of antihistamines may cause hallucinations, convulsions, or death. Mental alertness may be diminished. In the young child, dimenhydrinate may produce excitation. Do not give to children under 2 years of age unless directed by a physician.

Precautions

Use with caution in conditions which might be aggravated by anticholinergic therapy (eg, prostatic hypertrophy, stenosing peptic ulcer, pyloroduodenal obstruction, bladder neck obstruction, narrow angle glaucoma, bronchial asthma, cardiac arrhythmias).

Drug Interactions

Drugs that may interact with dimenhydrinate may include CNS depressants and antibiotics.

Adverse Reactions

Adverse reactions may include drowsiness; confusion; nervousness; restlessness; headache; insomnia (especially in children); tingling, heaviness and weakness of hands; vertigo; dizziness; lassitude; excitation; nausea; vomiting; diarrhea; epigastric distress; constipation; anorexia; blurring of vision; diplopia; palpitations; hypotension; tachycardia; anaphylaxis; photosensitivity; urticaria; drug rash; hemolytic anemia; difficult or painful urination; nasal stuffiness; tightness of chest; wheezing; thickening of bronchial secretions; dryness of mouth, nose, and throat.

TRIMETHOBENZAMIDE HCl

Capsules: 100 mg (*Rx*)	*Tigan* (Roberts), *Trimazide* (Major)
Capsules: 250 mg (*Rx*)	Various, *Tigan* (Roberts)
Pediatric suppositories: 100 mg (*Rx*)	Various, *Pediatric Triban* (Great Southern), *Tebamide* (G&W Labs), *T-Gen* (Goldline), *Tigan* (Roberts), *Trimazide* (Major)
Suppositories: 200 mg (*Rx*)	Various, *Tebamide* (G&W), *T-Gen* (Goldline), *Tigan* (Roberts), *Triban* (Great Southern), *Trimazide* (Major)
Injection: 100 mg/mL (*Rx*)	Various, *Pediatric Triban* (Great Southern), *Ticon* (Hauck), *Tigan* (Roberts)

Indications

Control of nausea and vomiting.

Administration and Dosage

Oral:

Adults – 250 mg, 3 or 4 times/day.

Children (30 to 90 lbs; 13.6 to 40.9 kg) – 100 to 200 mg, 3 or 4 times/day.

Rectal:

Adults – 200 mg, 3 or 4 times/day.

Children (30 to 90 lbs; 13.6 to 40.9 kg) – 100 to 200 mg, 3 or 4 times/day.

(< 30 lbs) – 100 mg, 3 or 4 times/day. Do not use in premature or newborn infants.

Injection: For IM use only.

Adults – 200 mg 3 or 4 times/day. Pain, stinging, burning, redness, and swelling may develop at injection site.

Actions

Pharmacokinetics: Mechanism is obscure, but may be mediated through the chemoreceptor trigger zone; direct impulses to vomiting center are not inhibited.

Contraindications

Hypersensitivity to trimethobenzamide, benzocaine or similar local anesthetics; parenteral use in children; suppositories in premature infants or neonates.

Warnings

Pregnancy: Safety for use has not been established.

Lactation: Safety for use in the nursing mother has not been established.

Precautions

Encephalitides, gastroenteritis, dehydration, electrolyte imbalance (especially in children and the elderly or debilitated), and CNS reactions have occurred when used during acute febrile illness.

Exercise caution when giving the drug with alcohol and other CNS-acting agents such as phenothiazines, barbiturates, and belladonna derivatives.

Adverse Reactions

Adverse reactions may include: Hypersensitivity reactions; parkinson-like symptoms; hypotension or pain following IM injection; blood dyscrasias; blurred vision; coma; convulsions; depression; diarrhea; disorientation; dizziness; drowsiness; headache; jaundice; muscle cramps; opisthotonos; allergic-type skin reactions.

DRONABINOL

Gelatin capsules: 2.5, 5, and 10 mg *(c-iii)*	*Marinol* (Roxane)

Indications

Antiemetic: Treatment of nausea and vomiting associated with cancer chemotherapy in patients not responding adequately to conventional antiemetic treatment.

Appetite stimulation: Treating anorexia associated with weight loss in AIDS patients.

Administration and Dosage

Antiemetic: Initially, give 5 mg/m^2 1 to 3 hours prior to the administration of chemotherapy, then every 2 to 4 hours after chemotherapy is given, for a total of 4 to 6 doses/day. If the 5 mg/m^2 dose is ineffective, and there are no significant side effects, increase the dose by 2.5 mg/m^2 increments to a maximum of 15 mg/m^2 per dose. Use caution, however, as the incidence of disturbing psychiatric symptoms increases significantly at this maximum dose. Administration with phenothiazines may improve efficacy (vs either drug alone) without additional toxicity.

Appetite stimulation: Initially, give 2.5 mg twice/day before lunch and supper. For patients who cannot tolerate 5 mg/day, reduce dosage to 2.5 mg/day as a single evening or bedtime dose. When adverse reactions are absent or minimal and further therapeutic effect is desired, increase to 2.5 mg before lunch and 5 mg before supper (or 5 mg at lunch and 5 mg after supper). Although most patients respond to 2.5 mg twice/day, 10 mg twice/day has been tolerated in about 50% of patients. The dosage may be increased to a maximum of 20 mg/day in divided doses. Use caution in escalating the dosage because of the increased frequency of dose-related adverse reactions at higher dosages.

Actions

Pharmacology: Dronabinol is the principal psychoactive substance present in *Cannabis sativa* L (marijuana). The mechanism of action is unknown.

Cannabinoids have complex CNS effects, including central sympathomimetic activity.

Pharmacokinetics:

Absorption/Distribution – Following oral administration, dronabinol is almost completely absorbed (90% to 95%). It has an onset of action of ≈ 0.5 to 1 hour and peak effect at 2 to 4 hours. Duration for psychoactive effects is 4 to 6 hours, but the appetite stimulant effect may continue for ≥ 24 hours after administration.

Metabolism/Excretion – Dronabinol undergoes extensive first-pass hepatic metabolism.

Biliary excretion is the major route of elimination. Extended use at the recommended doses may cause accumulation of toxic amounts of dronabinol and its metabolites.

Contraindications

Hypersensitivity to dronabinol, marijuana, or sesame oil.

Warnings

Tolerance: Following 12 days of dronabinol, tolerance to the cardiovascular and subjective effects developed at doses ≤ 210 mg/day. An initial tachycardia induced by dronabinol was replaced successively by normal sinus rhythm and then bradycardia. A fall in supine blood pressure, made worse by standing, was also observed initially. Within days, these effects disappeared, indicating development of tolerance. Tachyphylaxis and tolerance did not, however, appear to develop to the appetite stimulant effect.

Patient supervision: Because of individual variation, determine clinically the period of patient supervision required.

Elderly: Use caution because the elderly are generally more sensitive to the psychoactive effects. In antiemetic studies, no difference in tolerance or efficacy was apparent in patients > 55 years of age.

Pregnancy: Category B.

Lactation: Dronabinol is concentrated and excreted in breast milk; nursing mothers should not use dronabinol.

Children: Not recommended for AIDS-related anorexia in children because it has not been studied in this population. Dosage for chemotherapy-induced emesis is the same as in adults. Use caution in children because of the psychoactive effects.

Precautions

Hypertension or heart disease: Use with caution since dronabinol may cause a general increase in central sympathomimetic activity.

Psychiatric patients: In manic, depressive, or schizophrenic patients, symptoms of these disease states may be exacerbated by the use of cannabinoids.

Drug abuse and dependence: Dronabinol is highly abusable. Limit prescriptions to the amount necessary for a single cycle of chemotherapy.

A withdrawal syndrome consisting of irritability, insomnia, and restlessness was observed in some subjects within 12 hours following abrupt withdrawal of dronabinol. The syndrome reached its peak intensity at 24 hours when subjects exhibited hot flashes, sweating, rhinorrhea, loose stools, hiccoughs, and anorexia. The syndrome was essentially complete within 96 hours. EEG changes following discontinuation were consistent with a withdrawal syndrome. Several subjects reported impressions of disturbed sleep for several weeks after discontinuing high doses.

Hazardous tasks: Because of its profound effects on mental status, warn patients not to drive, operate complex machinery, or engage in any activity requiring sound judgment and unimpaired coordination while receiving treatment. Effects may persist for a variable and unpredictable period of time.

Drug Interactions

Drugs that may be affected by dronabinol include amphetamines, cocaine, sympathomimetics, anticholinergics, antihistamines, tricyclic antidepressants, alcohol, sedatives, hypnotics, psychomimetics, disulfiram, fluoxetine, and theophylline.

Adverse Reactions

Adverse reactions occurring in ≥ 3% of patients include euphoria, nausea, vomiting, dizziness, paranoid reaction, and somnolence.

KETOCONAZOLE

Tablets: 200 mg (*Rx*)	Various, *Nizoral* (Janssen)

Warning:

Ketoconazole has been associated with hepatic toxicity, including some fatalities. Closely monitor patients and inform them of the risk.

Indications

Treatment of the following systemic fungal infections: Candidiasis, chronic mucocutaneous candidiasis, oral thrush, candiduria, blastomycosis, coccidioidomycosis, histoplasmosis, chromomycosis, and paracoccidioidomycosis.

Treatment of severe recalcitrant cutaneous dermatophyte infections not responding to topical therapy or oral griseofulvin or in patients unable to take griseofulvin.

Do not use ketoconazole for fungal meningitis because it penetrates poorly into the CSF.

Administration and Dosage

If antacids, anticholinergics, or H_2 blockers are needed, give at least 2 hours after administration. Take with food to alleviate GI disturbance.

Adults: Initially, 200 mg once daily. In very serious infections, or if clinical response is insufficient, increase dose to 400 mg once daily.

Children:

(> 2 years of age) – 3.3 to 6.6 mg/kg/day as a single daily dose.

(< 2 years of age) – Daily dosage has not been established.

Minimum treatment is 1 or 2 weeks for candidiasis and 6 months for the other indicated systemic mycoses. Chronic mucocutaneous candidiasis usually requires maintenance therapy.

Minimum treatment of recalcitrant dermatophyte infections is 4 weeks in cases involving glabrous skin. Palmar and plantar infections may respond more slowly.

Actions

Pharmacology: Ketoconazole, an imidazole broad-spectrum antifungal agent, impairs the synthesis of ergosterol, the main sterol of fungal cell membranes, allowing increased permeability and leakage of cellular components.

Pharmacokinetics:

Absorption/Distribution – Bioavailability depends on an acidic pH for dissolution and absorption. In vitro, plasma protein binding is ≈ 95% to 99%, mainly to albumin.

Metabolism/Excretion – The drug undergoes extensive hepatic metabolism to inactive metabolites. Plasma elimination is biphasic; half-life is 2 hours during the first 10 hours, 8 hours thereafter. The major excretory route is enterohepatic. From 85% to 90% is excreted in bile and feces, 13% in urine.

Contraindications

Hypersensitivity to ketoconazole. Do not use ketoconazole for the treatment of fungal meningitis because it penetrates poorly into the CSF. Concomitant administration of ketoconazole with oral triazolam is contraindicated.

Warnings

Hepatotoxicity: Hepatotoxicity, primarily of the hepatocellular type, has been associated with ketoconazole, including rare fatalities. Measure liver function before starting treatment and frequently during treatment. Monitor patients receiving ketoconazole concurrently with other potentially hepatotoxic drugs, particularly those patients requiring prolonged therapy or those with a history of liver disease. Transient minor elevations in liver enzymes have occurred.

Prostatic cancer: In clinical trials involving 350 patients with metastatic prostatic cancer, 11 deaths were reported within 2 weeks of starting high-dose ketoconazole (1200 mg/day). It is not known whether death was related to therapy. High ketoconazole doses are known to suppress adrenal corticosteroid secretion.

Hypersensitivity reactions: Anaphylaxis occurs rarely after the first dose. Hypersensitivity reactions, including urticaria, have been reported.

Pregnancy: Category C.

Lactation: Ketoconazole is excreted in breast milk. Administer to nursing mothers only if the potential benefits outweigh the potential risks to the infant.

Children: Safety for use in children < 2 years of age has not been established.

Precautions

Hormone levels: Testosterone levels are impaired with doses of 800 mg/day and abolished by 1600 mg/day. It also decreases ACTH-induced corticosteroid serum levels at similar high doses.

Gastric acidity: Ketoconazole requires acidity for dissolution and absorption. In achlorhydria, dissolve each tablet in 4 mL aqueous solution of 0.2 N HCl. Use a glass or plastic straw to avoid contact with teeth. Follow with a glass of water.

Drug Interactions

Ketoconazole is a potent inhibitor of the cytochrome P450 3A4 enzyme system. Coadministration of ketoconazole with other drugs metabolized by the same enzyme system may result in increased plasma concentrations of the drugs that could increase or prolong both therapeutic and adverse effects. Unless otherwise specified, dosage adjustment may be necessary.

Drugs that may affect ketoconazole include antacids, didanosine, histamine H_2 antagonists, isoniazid, sucralfate, proton pump inhibitors, and rifampin. Drugs that may be affected by ketoconazole include oral anticoagulants, corticosteroids, cyclosporine, protease inhibitors, tricyclic antidepressants, carbamazepine, quinidine, sulfonylureas, benzodiazepines, buspirone, oral contraceptives, donepezil, nisoldipine, tacrolimus, vinca alkaloids, zolpidem, and theophylline.

Adverse Reactions

Adverse reactions occurring in ≥ 3% of patients include nausea and vomiting.

AMPHOTERICIN B

Powder for injection: 50 mg (as deoxycholate) (*Rx*)	*Amphotericin B* (PharmaTek), *Fungizone Intravenous* (Apothecon), *Amphocin* (Pharmacia)
Suspension for injection: 100 mg/20 mL (as lipid complex) (*Rx*)	*Abelcet* (Liposome Co.)
Powder for injection: 50 mg and 100 mg (as cholesteryl) (*Rx*)	*Amphotec* (Sequus Pharmaceuticals)
Powder for injection: 50 mg (as liposomal) (*Rx*)	*AmBisome* (Fujisawa)

Warning:

Use primarily for treatment of patients with progressive and potentially fatal fungal infections. Do not use to treat noninvasive forms of fungal disease such as oral thrush, vaginal candidiasis, and esophageal candidiasis in patients with normal neutrophil counts.

Indications

Fungal infections, systemic:

Amphotericin B deoxycholate – Intended to treat the following potentially life-threatening invasive fungal infections: Aspergillosis; cryptococcosis (torulosis); North American blastomycosis; candidiasis; coccidioidomycosis; histoplasmosis; zygomycosis including mucormycosis caused by *Mucor*, *Rhizopus*, and *Absidia* sp.; infections caused by related susceptible species of *Conidiobolus* and *Basidiobolus*; sporotrichosis.

Lipid-based formulations – For use in patients refractory to conventional amphotericin B deoxycholate therapy or where renal impairment or unacceptable toxicity precludes the use of the deoxycholate formulation for the treatment of invasive fungal infections (lipid complex); for the treatment of invasive aspergillosis (cholesteryl); for the treatment of infections caused by *Aspergillus*, *Candida*, or *Cryptococcus* sp. (liposomal).

Fungal infections, empirical: For empirical treatment in febrile, neutropenic patients with presumed fungal infection (liposomal only).

Cryptococcal meningitis in HIV: Treatment of cryptococcal meningitis in HIV-infected patients (*AmBisome* only).

Leishmaniasis: For treatment of visceral leishmaniasis (liposomal only); treatment of American mucocutaneous leishmaniasis but not as primary therapy (deoxycholate).

Unlabeled uses: Prophylaxis for fungal infection in patients with bone marrow transplantation (0.1 mg/kg/day).

Administration and Dosage

Fungal infection, empirical: Administer 3 mg/kg/day of liposomal amphotericin B using a controlled infusion device over ≈ 120 minutes; infusion time may be reduced to 60 minutes if well tolerated or increased if patient experiences discomfort.

Fungal infection, systemic:

Amphotericin B deoxycholate (eg, Fungizone) –

Suggested Indication-Specific Dosage Regimens for Amphotericin B Deoxycholate

Fungal infection, systemic	Treatment regimen	Dose[1] (mg/kg/day)
Aspergillosis	up to 3.6 g total dose	1 to 1.5
Blastomyces	4 to 12 weeks	0.5 to 0.6
Candidiasis	4 to 12 weeks	0.5 to 1
Coccidioidomycosis	4 to 12 weeks	0.5 to 1
Cryptococcus	4 to 12 weeks	0.5 to 0.7
Histoplasmosis	4 to 12 weeks	0.5 to 0.6
Mucormycosis	4 to 12 weeks	1 to 1.5
Rhinocerebral phycomycosis	3 to 4 g total dose	0.25 to 0.3 up to 1 to 1.5
Sporotrichosis	up to 2.5 g total dose	0.5

[1] Some of these dosages are not FDA-approved.

Because patient tolerance varies greatly, a test dose may be preferred; 1 mg in 20 mL of 5% Dextrose delivered IV over 20 to 30 minutes. Record patient's temperature, pulse, respiration, and blood pressure every 30 minutes for 2 to 4 hours.

The recommended initial dose is 0.25 to 0.3 mg/kg/day prepared as 0.1 mg/mL infusion and delivered slowly over 2 to 6 hours. Depending on the patient's cardiorenal status, dosage may be gradually increased by 5 to 10 mg/day up to a total dose of 0.5 to 0.7 mg/kg/day. Some mycoses may require total doses up to 1 to 1.5 mg/kg/day. Do not exceed a total daily dose of 1.5 mg/kg; overdoses can result in cardiorespiratory arrest. Alternate daily dosing is recommended for total daily doses of 1.5 mg/kg.

In patients with impaired cardio-renal function or a severe reaction to the test dose, initiate therapy with smaller daily doses (eg, 5 to 10 mg).

An in-line membrane filter of ≥ 1 micron mean pore diameter may be used.

Amphotericin B cholesteryl (Amphotec) – A test dose is advisable (eg, 10 mL of final preparation containing between 1.6 to 8.3 mg infused over 15 to 30 min). The recommended dose is 3 to 4 mg/kg/day prepared as a 0.6 mg/mL (range, 0.16 to 0.83 mg/mL) infusion delivered at a rate of 1 mg/kg/hr. Do not use an in-line filter.

Amphotericin B lipid complex (Abelcet) – The recommended dose is 5 mg/kg/day prepared as a 1 mg/mL infusion and delivered at a rate of 2.5 mg/kg/hr. For pediatric patients and patients with cardiovascular disease, the drug may be diluted to a final concentration of 2 mg/mL. If the infusion exceeds 2 hours, mix the contents by shaking the infusion bag every 2 hours. Do not use an in-line filter.

Liposomal amphotericin B (AmBisome) – The recommended dose is 3 to 5 mg/kg/day prepared as a 1 to 2 mg/mL infusion delivered initially over 120 minutes; infusion time may be reduced to 60 minutes if well tolerated or increased if patient experiences discomfort. Lower infusion concentrations of 0.2 to 0.5 mg/mL may be appropriate for infants and small children to provide sufficient volume for infusion. An in-line membrane filter of ≥ 1 micron mean pore diameter may be used.

Cryptococcal meningitis in HIV:

AmBisome – Administer 6 mg/kg/day using a controlled infusion device over ≈ 120 minutes; infusion time may be reduced to 60 minutes if well tolerated or increased if patient experiences discomfort.

Leishmaniasis:

Liposomal amphotericin B (AmBisome) – Administer 3 mg/kg/day on days 1 through 5, 14 and 21 to immunocompetent patients; a repeat course of therapy may be useful if parasitic clearance is not achieved. Administer 4 mg/kg/day on days 1 through 5, 10, 17, 24, 31, and 38 to immunosuppressed patients; seek expert advice regarding further therapy if parasitic clearance is not achieved.

Amphotericin B deoxycholate (eg, Fungizone) – 0.5 mg/kg/day administered on alternate days for 14 doses has been effective but is not recommended as primary therapy.

Rhinocerebral phycomycosis: A cumulative dose of ≥ 3 g amphotericin B is recommended. Although a total dose of 3 to 4 g will infrequently cause lasting renal impairment, it is a reasonable minimum where there is clinical evidence of deep tissue invasion. Rhinocerebral phycomycosis usually follows a rapidly fatal course; therapy must be more aggressive than that for more indolent mycoses.

Unlabeled:

Cystitis, candidal – Irrigate bladder with a 50 mcg/mL solution, instilled periodically or continuously for 5 to 10 days.

Meningitis, coccidioidal or cryptococcal – Adminsiter amphotericin B deoxycholate intrathecally at initial doses of 0.025 mg, gradually increased to the maximum tolerable dose. The usual dose is 0.25 to 1 mg every 48 to 72 hours. A maximum total dose of 15 mg has been suggested.

Paracoccidioidomycosis – Administer 0.4 to 0.5 mg/kg/day slow IV infusion, treat for 4 to 12 weeks.

Actions

Pharmacology: Amphotericin B is fungistatic or fungicidal, depending on the concentration obtained in body fluids and on the susceptibility of the fungus. It acts by binding to sterols in the fungal cell membrane with a resultant change in membrane permeability, allowing leakage of a variety of intracellular components.

Liposomal encapsulation or incorporation in a lipid complex can substantially affect a drug's functional properties relative to those of the unencapsulated or nonlipid-associated drug. Lipid-based formulations increase the circulation time and alter the biodistribution of associated amphotericin. Increasing drug levels at site of action and reducing levels in normal tissues offers 2 distinct clinical advantages: An increased therapeutic index and altered toxicity profile relative to free drug.

Different lipid-based formulations with a common active ingredient may vary from one another in the chemical composition (eg, phospholipid and cholesterol content) and physical form of the lipid component (eg, sphere, disc, or ribbon). Such differences may affect functional properties of these drug products.

Pharmacokinetics:

Absorption/Distribution – Amphotericin B is highly protein bound (> 90%) and is poorly dialyzable.

Metabolism/Excretion – Amphotericin B has a relatively short initial serum half-life of 24 hours, followed by a second elimination phase with a half-life of ≈ 15 days. The drug is slowly excreted by the kidneys with 2% to 5% as the biologically active form. The following table presents pharmacokinetic parameters at steady-state for lipid-based formulations of amphotericin B; the assay used to measure serum levels did not distinguish between free and complex amphotericin B.

Pharmacokinetic Parameters of Lipid-Based Amphotericin B Formulations[1]						
Parameter	*AmBisome* 1 mg/kg/day (n = 7)	*AmBisome* 2.5 mg/kg/day (n = 7)	*AmBisome* 5 mg/kg/day (n = 9)	*Amphotec* 3 mg/kg/day (predicted)[2]	*Amphotec* 4 mg/kg/day (predicted)[2]	*Abelcet* 5 mg/kg/day (n = varied)[3]
Cmax (mcg/mL)	≈ 12.2	≈ 31.4	≈ 83	2.6	2.9	≈ 1.7
AUC (mcg/mL•hr)	≈ 60	≈ 197	≈ 555	29	36	≈ 14
t½ (hrs)	≈ 7	≈ 6.3	≈ 6.8	27.5 (100 to 153)[4]	28.2 (100 to 153)[4]	≈ 173.4
Vss (L/kg)	≈ 0.14	≈ 0.16	≈ 0.1	3.8	4.1	≈ 131
CL (mL/hr/kg)	≈ 17	≈ 22	≈ 11	105	112	≈ 436

[1] Data are pooled from separate studies and are not necessarily comparable.
[2] Values based on the population model developed from 51 bone marrow transplant patients with systemic fungal infections given *Amphotec* 0.5 to 8 mg/kg/day.
[3] Data obtained from various studies in patients with mucocutaneous leishmaniasis or cancer with presumed or proven fungal infections.
[4] Based on total amphotericin B levels measured within a 24-hour dosing interval (or up to 49 days after dosing).

Contraindications

Hypersensitivity to amphotericin B, unless the condition requiring treatment is life-threatening and amenable only to amphotericin B therapy.

Warnings

Fatal fungal diseases: Amphotericin B is frequently the only effective treatment for potentially fatal fungal diseases. Balance its possible lifesaving effect against its dangerous side effects.

Nephrotoxicity: Renal damage is a limiting factor for the use of amphotericin B. Renal dysfunction usually improves upon interruption of therapy, dose reduction or increased dosing interval; however, some permanent impairment often occurs, especially in patients receiving large doses (> 5 g) or receiving other nephrotoxic agents. Decreased glomerular filtration rate and renal blood flow, increased serum creatinine and renal tubular dysfunction are prominent. In some patients, hydration and sodium repletion prior to amphotericin B administration may reduce the risk of developing nephrotoxicity.

Lipid formulations of amphotericin B have been shown to reduce the severe kidney toxicity of amphotericin B and are indicated in patients with renal impairment or when unacceptable toxicity precludes the use of amphotericin B deoxycholate in effective doses.

Infusion reactions: Acute reactions including fever, shaking chills, hypotension, anorexia, vomiting, nausea, headache, and tachypnea are common 1 to 3 hours after starting an IV infusion. These reactions usually are more severe with the first few doses of amphotericin B and usually diminish with subsequent doses. Avoid rapid IV infusion because it has been associated with hypotension, hypokalemia, arrhythmias, bronchospasm, and shock.

Leukoencephalopathy: This has been reported following use of amphotericin B. The literature has suggested that total body irradiation may be a predisposition.

Rhinocerebral phycomycosis: A fulminating disease, this generally occurs in association with diabetic ketoacidosis. Diabetic control must be instituted before successful treatment with amphotericin B can be accomplished. Pulmonary phycomycosis, which is more common in association with hematologic malignancies, is often an incidental finding at autopsy.

Hypersensitivity reactions: Anaphylaxis has been reported with amphotericin B. If severe respiratory distress occurs, discontinue the infusion immediately. Do not give further infusions. Have cardiopulmonary resuscitation facilities available during administration.

Renal function impairment: Use amphotericin B desoxycholate with care in patients with reduced renal function; frequent monitoring is recommended (see Precautions). Lipid formulations have been reported to overcome most problems of chronic nephrotoxicity, even in patients with impaired renal function following previous treatment with amphotericin B desoxycholate.

Pregnancy: Category B.

Lactation: It is not known whether amphotericin B is excreted in breast milk; however, consider discontinuing nursing.

Children: Safety and efficacy of amphotericin B desoxycholate in children have not been established. Systemic fungal infections have been successfully treated in children without reports of unusual side effects. Limit administration to the least amount compatible with an effective therapeutic regimen.

Pediatric patients < 16 years of age (n = 97) with systemic fungal infections have been treated with amphotericin B cholesteryl at daily mg/kg doses similar to those given in adults and had significantly less renal toxicity than the desoxycholate formulation (12% vs 52%); 273 pediatric patients age 1 month to 16 years with presumed fungal infections, confirmed systemic fungal infections or with visceral leishmaniasis have been successfully treated with liposomal amphotericin B (*AmBisome*); 111 children < 16 years of age, including 11 patients < 1 year of age, have been treated with amphotericin B lipid complex (*Abelcet*) at 5 mg/kg/day and 5 children with hepatosplenic candidiasis were effectively treated with 2.5 mg/kg/day. Safety and efficacy in patients < 1 month of age have not been established.

Precautions

Monitoring: Monitor renal function frequently during amphotericin B therapy. It is also advisable to monitor liver function, serum electrolytes (particularly magnesium and potassium), blood counts, and hemoglobin concentrations on a regular basis. Use laboratory test results as a guide to subsequent dose adjustments. Monitor complete blood count and prothrombin time as medically indicated.

Record the patient's temperature, pulse, respiration, and blood pressure every 30 minutes for 2 to 4 hours after administration.

Resistance: Variants with reduced susceptibility to amphotericin B have been isolated from several fungal species after serial passage in cell culture media containing the drug and from some patients receiving prolonged therapy with amphotericin B desoxycholate. The relevance of drug resistance to clinical outcome has not been established.

Therapy interruption: Whenever medication is interrupted for > 7 days, resume therapy with the lowest dosage level; increase gradually.

Pulmonary reactions: Pulmonary reactions characterized by acute dyspnea, hypoxemia, and interstitial infiltrates have been observed in neutropenic patients receiving amphotericin B and leukocyte transfusions. Separate the infusion as far as possible from the time of a leukocyte transfusion.

Lab test abnormalities:

Serum electrolyte abnormalities – Hypomagnesemia, hyperkalemia, hypokalemia, hypercalcemia, hypocalcemia, hypophosphatemia.

Liver function test abnormalities – Increased AST, ALT, GGT, bilirubin, alkaline phosphatase, and LDH.

Renal function impairment – Increased BUN and serum creatinine.

Other test abnormalities – Acidosis, hyperamylasemia, hypoglycemia, hyperglycemia, hyperuricemia.

Drug Interactions

Drugs that may interact with amphotericin B include antineoplastic agents, corticosteroids, zidovudine, other nephrotoxic agents, digitalis glycosides, flucytocine, skeletal muscle relaxants, cyclosporine, azole antifungal agents, and thiazides.

Adverse Reactions

Prevention of adverse reactions – Most patients will exhibit some intolerance, often at less than full therapeutic dosage. Severe reactions may be lessened by giving aspirin, antipyretics (eg, acetaminophen), antihistamines, and antiemetics before the infusion and by maintaining sodium balance. Administration on alternate days may decrease anorexia and phlebitis. Small doses of IV adrenal corticosteroids given prior to or during the infusion may decrease febrile reactions. Meperidine (25 to 50 mg IV) has been shown in some patients to decrease the duration of shaking chills and fever that may accompany infusion of amphotericin B.

Adverse reactions may include abdominal pain; acidosis; anemia; anorexia; anxiety; apnea; asthenia; asthma; arrhthmias; azotemia; bilirubinemia; blood product transfusion reaction; chest/back pain; coagulation disorder; confusion; cough increased; cramping; decreased prothrombin time; depression; diarrhea; dizziness; dry mouth; dyspepsia; dyspnea; edema; epigastric pain; epistaxis; eye hemorrhage; face edema; fever (sometimes with shaking chills); generalized pain, including muscle and joint pains; GI hemorrhage; headache; heart arrest; hematemesis; hematuria; hemoptysis; hemorrhage; hypernatremia; hypertension; hyperventilation; hypokalemia; hypovolemia; hyposthenuria; hypotension; hypoxia; increased serum creatinine; infection; insomnia; jaundice; leukopenia; lung disorder; maculopapular rash; malaise; mucous membrane disorder; multiple organ failure; nausea; normochromic, normycytic anemia; pain; peripheral edema; pleural effusion; pneumonia; pruritus; rash; renal tubular acidosis and nephrocalcinosis; respiratory disorder; respiratory failure; rhinitis; sepsis; somnolence; stomatitis; sweating; tachycardia; tachypnea; thinking abnormal; thrombocytopenia; tremor; vomiting; venous pain at the injection site with phlebitis and thrombophlebitis; weight loss/gain.

FLUCONAZOLE

Tablets: 50, 100, 150, and 200 mg (*Rx*)	*Diflucan* (Roerig)
Powder for oral suspension: 10 and 40 mg/mL when reconstituted (*Rx*)	
Injection: 2 mg/mL (*Rx*)	

Indications

Candidiasis:

Treatment – Oropharyngeal and esophageal candidiasis.

Candidal urinary tract infections, peritonitis, and systemic candidal infections including candidemia, disseminated candidiasis and pneumonia.

Vaginal candidiasis (vaginal yeast infections caused by *Candida*).

Prophylaxis – To decrease the incidence of candidiasis in patients undergoing bone marrow transplantation who receive cytotoxic chemotherapy or radiation therapy.

Cryptococcal meningitis: Treatment of cryptococcal meningitis.

Administration and Dosage

Single dose:

Vaginal candidiasis – 150 mg as a single oral dose.

Multiple dose: The daily dose of fluconazole is the same for oral and IV administration. In general, a loading dose of twice the daily dose is recommended on the first day of therapy to result in plasma levels close to steady state by the second day of therapy.

Patients with AIDS and cryptococcal meningitis or recurrent oropharyngeal candidiasis usually require maintenance therapy to prevent relapse.

Adults –

Oropharyngeal candidiasis: 200 mg on the first day, followed by 100 mg once daily. Continue treatment for at least 2 weeks to decrease the likelihood of relapse.

Esophageal candidiasis: 200 mg on the first day, followed by 100 mg once daily. Doses up to 400 mg/day may be used, based on the patient's response. Treat patients with esophageal candidiasis for a minimum of 3 weeks and for at least 2 weeks following resolution of symptoms.

Candidiasis, other: For candidal UTIs and peritonitis, 50 to 200 mg/day has been used. For systemic candidal infections (including candidemia, disseminated candidiasis, and pneumonia), optimal dosage and duration have not been determined, although doses up to 400 mg/day have been used.

Prevention of candidiasis in bone marrow transplant: 400 mg once daily. In patients who are anticipated to have severe granulocytopenia (< 500 neutrophils/mm^3), start fluconazole prophylaxis several days before the anticipated onset of neutropenia, and continue for 7 days after the neutrophil count rises above 1000 cells/mm^3.

Cryptococcal meningitis: 400 mg on the first day, followed by 200 mg once daily. A dosage of 400 mg once daily may be used, based on the patient's response to therapy. The duration of treatment for initial therapy of cryptococcal meningitis is 10 to 12 weeks after the cerebrospinal fluid becomes culture negative. The dosage of fluconazole for suppression of relapse of cryptococcal meningitis in patients with AIDS is 200 mg once daily.

Children –

Fluconazole Dosage in Children	
Pediatric Patients	Adults
3 mg/kg	100 mg
6 mg/kg	200 mg
12 mg/kg[1]	400 mg

[1] Some older children may have clearances similar to that of adults. Absolute doses > 600 mg/day are not recommended.

Based on the prolonged half-life seen in premature newborns (gestational age 26 to 29 weeks), these children, in the first 2 weeks of life, should receive the same dosage (mg/kg) as older children, but administered every 72 hours. After the first 2 weeks, dose these children once daily.

Oropharyngeal candidiasis: The recommended dosage is 6 mg/kg on the first day, followed by 3 mg/kg once daily. Administer treatment for at least 2 weeks.

Esophageal candidiasis: The recommended dosage is 6 mg/kg on the first day followed by 3 mg/kg once daily. Doses up to 12 mg/kg/day may be used based on medical judgment of the patient's response to therapy. Treat patients with esophageal candidiasis for a minimum of 3 weeks and for at least 2 weeks following the resolution of symptoms.

Systemic Candida infections: For the treatment of candidemia and disseminated *Candida* infections, daily doses of 6 to 12 mg/kg/day have been used.

Cryptococcal meningitis: The recommended dosage is 12 mg/kg on the first day, followed by 6 mg/kg once daily. A dosage of 12 mg/kg once daily may be used. The recommended duration of treatment for initial therapy of cryptococcal meningitis is 10 to 12 weeks after the CSF becomes culture negative. For suppression of relapse of cryptococcal meningitis in children with AIDS, the recommended dose is 6 mg/kg once daily.

Renal function impairment: There is no need to adjust single dose therapy for vaginal candidiasis in patients with impaired renal function. In patients with impaired renal function who will receive multiple doses, give an initial loading dose of 50 to 400 mg. After the loading dose, base the daily dose on the following table:

Fluconazole Dose in Impaired Renal Function	
Ccr (mL/min)	Percent of recommended dose
> 50	100%
≤ 50	50%
Patients receiving regular hemodialysis	One recommended dose after each dialysis

Injection: Fluconazole injection has been used safely for up to 14 days of IV therapy. Administer the IV infusion of fluconazole at a maximum rate of ≈ 200 mg/hr, given as a continuous infusion. Fluconazole injections are intended only for IV administration.

Actions

Pharmacology: Fluconazole, a synthetic broad spectrum bis-triazole antifungal agent, is a highly selective inhibitor of fungal cytochrome P450 and sterol C-14 alpha-demethylation.

Pharmacokinetics:

Absorption/Distribution – The pharmacokinetic properties of fluconazole are similar following administration by the IV or oral routes. In healthy volunteers, the bioavailability of oral fluconazole is > 90% compared with IV administration.

Peak plasma concentrations (C_{max}) in fasted healthy volunteers occur between 1 and 2 hours with a terminal plasma elimination half-life of ≈ 30 hours (range, 20 to 50 hours) after oral administration.

Steady-state concentrations are reached within 5 to 10 days following oral doses of 50 to 400 mg given once daily. The apparent volume of distribution approximates that of total body water. Plasma protein binding is low (11% to 12%).

Metabolism/Excretion – Fluconazole is cleared primarily by renal excretion, with ≈ 80% of the dose appearing in the urine unchanged, ≈ 11% as metabolites. The dose may need to be reduced in patients with impaired renal function. A 3-hour hemodialysis session decreases plasma concentrations by ≈ 50%.

Contraindications

Hypersensitivity to fluconazole or to any excipients in the product. There is no information regarding cross-hypersensitivity between fluconazole and other azole antifungal agents; use with caution in patients with hypersensitivity to other azoles.

Warnings

Hepatic injury: Fluconazole has been associated with rare cases of serious hepatic toxicity. Instances of fatal hepatic reactions occurred primarily in patients with serious underlying medical conditions (predominantly AIDS or malignancy) and often while taking multiple concomitant medications.

Anaphylaxis: In rare cases, anaphylaxis has occurred.

Dermatologic changes: Patients have rarely developed exfoliative skin disorders during treatment with fluconazole.

Pregnancy: Category C.

Lactation: The use of fluconazole in nursing mothers is not recommended.

Children: Efficacy has not been established in children < 6 months of age.

Precautions

Single-dose use: Weigh the convenience and efficacy of the single dose regimen for treatment of vaginal yeast infections against the acceptability of a higher incidence of adverse reactions with fluconazole (26%) vs intravaginal agents (16%).

Drug Interactions

Fluconazole is a potent inhibitor of the cytochrome P450 3A4 enzyme system. Coadministration of fluconazole with other drugs metabolized by the same enzyme system may result in increased plasma concentrations of the drugs, which could increase or prolong therapeutic and adverse effects. Unless otherwise specified, dosage adjustment may be necessary.

Drugs that may affect fluconazole include cimetidine, hydrochlorothiazide, and rifampin. Drugs that may be affected by fluconazole include oral contraceptives, cyclosporine, phenytoin, theophylline, sulfonylureas, warfarin, alfentanil, zolpidem, vinca alkaloids, tacrolimus, nisoldipine, benzodiazepines, corticosteroids, buspirone, tricyclic antidepressants, losartan, and zidovudine.

Adverse Reactions

Adverse reactions occurring in ≥ 3% of patients include headache, nausea, abdominal pain, and diarrhea.

ITRACONAZOLE

Capsules: 100 mg (*Rx*)	*Sporanox* (Janssen-Ortho)
Oral solution: 10 mg/mL (*Rx*)	*Sporanox* (Janssen-Ortho)
Injection: 10 mg/mL (*Rx*)	*Sporanox* (Ortho Biotech)

Warning:

CHF: Do not administer itraconazole for the treatment of onychomycosis or dermatomycoses in patients with evidence of cardiac dysfunction, such as CHF or a history of CHF. Discontinue if signs and symptoms of CHF occur during treatment of onychomycosis or dermatomycoses. If signs and symptoms of CHF occur during treatment for more serious fungal infections involving other parts of the body, reassess continued use of itraconazole.

Drug interactions: Coadministration of pimozide, dofetilide, or quinidine with itraconazole is contraindicated. Itraconazole is a potent inhibitor of the cytochrome P450 3A4 isoenzyme system and may raise plasma concentrations of drugs metabolized by this pathway. Serious cardiovascular events, including QT prolongation, torsades de pointes, ventricular tachycardia, cardiac arrest, or sudden death have occurred in patients taking itraconazole concomitantly with cisapride, pimozide, or quinidine, which are inhibitors of the cytochrome P450 3A4 system.

Indications

Capsules: For treatment of the following fungal infections in normal, predisposed, or immunocompromised patients:

- Dermatomycoses caused by tinea corporis, tinea cruris, tinea pedis, and pityriasis versicolor when oral therapy is considered appropriate
- Onychomycosis
- Invasive and noninvasive pulmonary aspergillosis
- Oral and oral/esophageal candidiasis
- Chronic pulmonary histoplasmosis
- Cutaneous and lymphatic sporotrichosis
- Paracoccidioidomycosis
- Chromomycosis
- Blastomycosis

Oral solution:

Candidiasis – Treatment of oral or esophageal candidiasis in adult HIV-positive or other immunocompromised patients.

Injection: For empiric therapy of febrile neutropenic patients with suspected fungal infections.

For treatment of the following fungal infections in immunocompromised and nonimmunocompromised patients:

- Blastomycosis, pulmonary and extrapulmonary
- Histoplasmosis, including chronic cavitary pulmonary disease and disseminated, nonmeningeal histoplasmosis
- Aspergillosis, pulmonary and extrapulmonary, in patients who are intolerant of or refractory to amphotericin B therapy.

Unlabeled uses: Itraconazole appears to be beneficial in the treatment of the following conditions. Dosage is generally 50 to 400 mg/day; duration of therapy varies from 1 day to ≥ 6 months depending on the condition and mycological response.

Itraconazole Unlabeled Uses

Superficial mycoses	Systemic mycoses	Miscellaneous
Dermatophytoses Tinea capitis Tinea manuum Tinea pedis Sebopsoriasis	Cryptococcal infections Disseminated Meningitis Dimorphic infections Coccidioidomycosis	Alternariosis Fungal keratitis Leishmaniasis, cutaneous Zygomycosis

Administration and Dosage

Do not use capsules and oral solution interchangeably.

Capsules: Taking immediately after a full meal is essential to ensure maximal absorption. Capsules must be swallowed whole.

Blastomycosis/Chronic pulmonary histoplasmosis – The recommended dose is 200 mg once daily. If there is no obvious improvement or there is evidence of progressive fungal disease, increase the dose in 100 mg increments to a maximum of 400 mg daily. Give doses > 200 mg/day in 2 divided doses.

Continue treatment for a minimum of 3 months and until clinical parameters and laboratory tests indicate that the active fungal infection has subsided. An inadequate period of treatment may lead to recurrence of active infection.

Oral and oral/esophageal candidiasis – The recommended dose is 100 mg daily for 2 weeks. Increase the dose to 200 mg/day in patients with AIDS and neutropenic patients. In patients with oral/esophageal candidiasis, treatment should last 4 weeks.

Other systemic mycoses –

Other Systemic Mycoses Dose and Duration of Therapy

Indication	Dose	Median duration (months)
Aspergillosis		
Pulmonary	200 mg QD	3 to 4
Invasive pulmonary	200 mg BID	3 to 4
Sporotrichosis	100 mg QD	3
Paracoccidioidomycosis	100 mg QD	6
Chromomycosis		
Caused by *Fonsecaea pedrosoi*	200 mg QD	6
Caused by *Cladosporium carrioni*	100 mg QD	3

Dermatomycoses –

Standard dosages:

Tinea corporis/tinea cruris – Recommended dose is 100 mg once daily for 14 consecutive days.

Tinea pedis – Recommended dose is 100 mg once daily for 28 consecutive days.

Pityriasis versicolor – Recommended dose is 200 mg once daily for 7 consecutive days.

Alternative dosages: Shorter dosing schedules have also been found to be effective in the treatment of tinea corporis/tinea cruris and tinea pedis. The shorter dosages are:

Tinea corporis/tinea cruris – 200 mg once daily for 7 consecutive days.

Tinea pedis – 200 mg BID for 7 consecutive days.

Equivalency between standard and alternative dosages was not established. Patients with chronic recalcitrant tinea pedis may benefit from the standard dosage of a lower daily dose (100 mg) for a longer period of time (4 weeks).

Onychomycosis – A 1-week treatment course consists of 200 mg twice daily for 7 days. Treatment with 2 one-week courses is recommended for fingernail infections and 3 one-week courses for toenail infections. The one-week courses are always separated by a 3-week drug-free interval. Clinical response will become evident as the nail regrows, following discontinuation of the treatment.

Itraconazole Onychomycosis Dosing Schedule

	Pulse 1[1]				Pulse 2[1]				Pulse 3[1]
Site of onychomycosis	Week 1	Week 2	Week 3	Week 4	Week 5	Week 6	Week 7	Week 8	Week 9
Toenails with/without fingernail involvement	200 mg BID for 7 days	Itraconazole-free weeks			200 mg BID for 7 days	Itraconazole-free weeks			200 mg BID for 7 days
Fingernails only	200 mg BID for 7 days	Itraconazole-free weeks			200 mg BID for 7 days				

[1] A pulse = 1 week course of treatment.

Oral solution: For optimal absorption, do not take with food. Swish in oral cavity and swallow. Do not rinse after swallowing. Discard unused product 3 months after opening.

Oropharyngeal candidiasis – The recommended dosage for oropharyngeal candidiasis is 200 mg (20 mL) daily in single or divided doses for 1 to 2 weeks to decrease likelihood of relapse.

Esophageal candidiasis – The recommended dosage for esophageal candidiasis is 100 mg (10 mL) daily for a minimum of 3 weeks. Continue treatment for 2 weeks following resolution of symptoms. Doses ≤ 200 mg (20 mL) per day may be used based on medical judgement of the patient's response to therapy.

Injection: Use only the components provided in the kit. Do not substitute.

Admixture incompatibility – The compatibility of itraconazole injection with diluents other than 0.9% Sodium Chloride Injection (Normal Saline) is not known. Do not dilute with 5% Dextrose Injection or with Lactated Ringer's Injection alone or in combination with any other diluent. Not for IV bolus injection.

Preparation/Administration – Use only a dedicated infusion line for administration of itraconazole injection. Do not introduce concomitant medication in the same bag or through the same line used for itraconazole injection. Other medications may be administered after flushing the line/catheter with 0.9% Sodium Chloride Injection.

Empiric therapy in febrile, neutropenic patients with suspected fungal infections (ETFN) – The recommended dose of itraconazole injection is 200 mg twice daily for 4 doses, followed by 200 mg once daily for up to 14 days. Infuse each IV dose over 1 hour. Continue treatment with itraconazole oral solution 200 mg (20 mL) twice daily until resolution of clinically significant neutropenia. The safety and efficacy of itraconazole use exceeding 28 days in ETFN is not known.

Blastomycosis, histoplasmosis, and aspergillosis – 200 mg IV twice daily for 4 doses, followed by 200 mg/day. Infuse each IV dose over 1 hour.

For the treatment of blastomycosis, histoplasmosis, and aspergillosis, itraconazole can be given as oral capsules or IV. The safety and efficacy of the injection administered for > 14 days are not known.

Continue total itraconazole therapy (injection followed by capsules) for a minimum of 3 months and until clinical parameters and laboratory tests indicate that the active fungal infection has subsided. An inadequate period of treatment may lead to recurrence of active infection.

Renal function impairment: Do not use in patients with Ccr < 30 mL/min.

Actions

Pharmacology: Itraconazole is a synthetic triazole antifungal agent. In vitro, itraconazole inhibits the cytochrome P450-dependent synthesis of ergosterol, which is a vital component of fungal cell membranes.

Pharmacokinetics:

Absorption/Distribution –

Oral solution/injection: The oral bioavailability is maximal when itraconazole oral solution is taken without food. Steady state is reached after 1 to 2 weeks during chronic administration. Peak plasma levels are observed 2 hours (fasting) to 5 hours (with food) following oral administration. Steady-state plasma concentrations are

≈ 25% lower when the oral solution is taken with food.

Plasma protein binding is 99.8%. It is extensively distributed into tissues that are prone to fungal invasion. Concentrations in the lung, kidney, liver, bone, stomach, spleen, and muscle were found to be 2 to 3 times higher than the corresponding plasma concentration. Following IV administration, the volume of distribution averaged 796 ± 185 L.

Metabolism/Excretion – Itraconazole is extensively metabolized by the cytochrome P450 3A4 to several metabolites including the major metabolite hydroxyitraconazole. Fecal excretion of the parent drug varies between 3% and 18% of the dose. Renal excretion of the parent drug is < 0.03% of the dose. Itraconazole is not removed by hemodialysis.

The estimated mean half-life at steady-state of itraconazole after IV infusion was 35.4 hours.

Contraindications

CHF: Do not administer itraconazole capsules for the treatment of onychomycosis or dermatomycoses in patients with evidence of ventricular dysfunction such as CHF or a history of CHF.

Coadministration of pimozide, quinidine, dofetilide, cisapride, triazolam, or oral midazolam (see Warning Box and Drug Interactions); hypersensitivity to the drug or its excipients (there is no information regarding cross-hypersensitivity between itraconazole and other azole antifungal agents; use caution in prescribing to patients with hypersensitivity to other azoles); HMG-CoA reductase inhibitors metabolized by the CYP3A4 enzyme system (eg, lovastatin, simvastatin) during itraconazole therapy (see Drug Interactions); treatment of onychomycosis in pregnant women or in women contemplating pregnancy.

Warnings

Cardiac dysrhythmias: Life-threatening cardiac dysrhythmias or sudden death have occurred in patients using pimozide or quinidine concomitantly with itraconazole or other CYP3A4 inhibitors. Concomitant administration of these drugs with itraconazole is contraindicated.

CHF: Do not administer itraconazole for the treatment of onychomycosis or dermatomycoses in patients with evidence of ventricular dysfunction such as CHF or a history of CHF. Do not use itraconazole capsules for other indications in patients with evidence of ventricular dysfunction unless the benefit clearly outweighs the risk.

Itraconazole has been shown to have a negative inotropic effect, and has been associated with reports of CHF. Do not use itraconazole in patients with CHF or with a history of CHF unless the benefit clearly outweighs the risk. This individual benefit/risk assessment should take into consideration factors such as the severity of the indication, the dosing regimen, and the individual risk factors for CHF.

Hepatotoxicity: Itraconazole has been associated with rare cases of serious hepatotoxicity, including liver failure and death. Some of these cases had neither pre-existing liver disease, nor a serious underlying medical condition. If liver function tests are abnormal, discontinue treatment. In patients with raised liver enzymes or an active liver disease or who have experienced liver toxicity with other drugs, do not start treatment unless the expected benefit exceeds the risk of hepatic injury. In such cases, liver enzyme monitoring is necessary.

Bioequivalency: Do not use itraconazole capsules and oral solution interchangeably. Drug exposure is greater with the oral solution than with the capsules when the same dose of drug is given. Additionally, the topical effects of mucosal exposure may be different between the 2 formulations.

AIDS and neutropenic patients: Studies with itraconazole capsules in neutropenic and AIDS patients have indicated that itraconazole plasma concentrations are lower than those in healthy subjects (particularly in those patients who are achlorhydric). However, the bioavailability of itraconazole oral solution, when tested in AIDS patients, was found satisfactory and not altered by the stage of HIV infection.

Renal function impairment: Do not use itraconazole injection in patients with severe renal dysfunction (Ccr < 30 mL/min) because of prolonged elimination of hydroxypropyl-β-cyclodextrin.

Hepatic function impairment: Itraconazole is predominantly metabolized in the liver. The terminal half-life of itraconazole in cirrhotic patients is somewhat prolonged. A decrease in the oral bioavailability of itraconazole from itraconazole capsules was observed in cirrhotic patients; this can also be expected with the oral solution. It is advisable to monitor itraconazole plasma concentrations and to adapt the dose when necessary. In patients with raised liver enzymes or an active liver disease or who have experienced liver toxicity with other drugs, do not start treatment unless the expected benefit exceeds the risk of hepatic injury. In such cases, liver enzyme monitoring is necessary.

Elderly:

Oral solution – Since clinical data on the use of itraconazole oral solution in elderly patients is limited, it is advised to use the oral solution in these patients only if the potential benefit outweighs the potential risks.

Pregnancy: Category C.

Lactation: Itraconazole is excreted in breast milk.

Children: Safety and efficacy have not been established. A small number of patients from 3 to 16 years of age have been treated with 100 mg/day for systemic fungal infections and no serious adverse effects have been reported.

Precautions

Monitoring: Monitor plasma levels 3 to 4 hours after dosing in patients requiring treatment for > 1 month, in patients with systemic mycoses who have factors predisposing to poor absorption (eg, achlorhydria, renal insufficiency, neutropenia, AIDS) or in those who are taking drugs that may alter itraconazole absorption or metabolism (eg, rifampicin, phenytoin).

Monitor hepatic function periodically in all patients receiving continuous treatment for > 1 month or when a patient develops signs or symptoms suggestive of hepatitis (eg, anorexia, nausea, vomiting, fatigue, abdominal pain, dark urine). If tests are abnormal, terminate treatment.

Monitor serum potassium in patients at risk during high-dose itraconazole therapy.

Neuropathy: Discontinue if neuropathy occurs that may be attributable to itraconazole capsules or oral solution.

Decreased gastric acidity: Absorption of itraconazole from the capsules is impaired when gastric acidity is decreased. In patients also receiving acid-neutralizing medicines (eg, aluminum hydroxide), these should be given at least 2 hours after the intake of itraconazole capsules. In patients with achlorhydria, such as certain AIDS patients on acid secretion suppressors (eg, H_2 antagonists, proton pump inhibitors), it is advisable to give itraconazole capsules with a cola beverage.

Drug Interactions

Both itraconazole and its major metabolite, hydroxyitraconazole, are inhibitors of the cytochrome P450 3A4 enzyme system. Coadministration of itraconazole and drugs primarily metabolized by the cytochrome P450 3A4 enzyme system may result in increased plasma concentrations of the drugs that could increase or prolong both therapeutic and adverse effects.

Drugs that may affect itraconazole include antacids, didanosine, H_2 antagonists, macrolide antibiotics, phenytoin, protease inhibitors, proton pump inhibitors, and rifamycins.

Drugs that may be affected by itraconazole include benzodiazepines, buspirone, calcium blockers, cyclosporine, digoxin, tacrolimus, warfarin, alfentanil, zolpidem, vinca alkaloids, corticosteroids, protease inhibitors, HMG-CoA reductase inhibitors, triazolam, oral midazolam, alprazolam, carbamazepine, dofetilide, haloperidol, hydantoins (phenytoin), pimozide, polyenes, amphotericin B, quinidine, tolterodine, hypoglycemic agents, and rifamycins.

Adverse Reactions

Adverse reactions occurring in ≥ 3% of patients include the following: Nausea, vomiting, diarrhea, rash, hypokalemia, bilirubinemia, increased ALT.

LAMIVUDINE (3TC)

Tablets: 100 mg (*Rx*)	*Epivir-HBV* (GlaxoSmithKline)
Tablets: 150 mg (*Rx*)	*Epivir* (GlaxoSmithKline)
Oral solution: 5 mg/mL (*Rx*)	*Epivir-HBV* (GlaxoSmithKline)
Oral solution: 10 mg/mL (*Rx*)	*Epivir* (GlaxoSmithKline)

Warning:

Lactic acidosis and severe hepatomegaly with steatosis, including fatal cases, have been reported with the use of antiretroviral nucleoside analogs alone or in combination, including lamivudine and other antiretroviral agents (see Warnings).

Offer human immunodeficiency virus (HIV) counseling and testing to patients before beginning *Epivir-HBV* and periodically during treatment because *Epivir-HBV* tablets and oral solution contain a lower dose of the same active ingredient (lamivudine) as the *Epivir* tablets and oral solution used to treat HIV infection. If treatment with *Epivir-HBV* is prescribed for chronic hepatitis B for a patient with unrecognized or untreated HIV infection, rapid emergence of HIV resistance is likely because of subtherapeutic dose and inappropriate monotherapy.

Epivir tablets and oral solution (used to treat HIV infection) contain a higher dose of the active ingredient (lamivudine) than *Epivir-HBV* tablets and oral solution (used to treat chronic hepatitis B). Patients with HIV infection should receive only dosing forms appropriate for the treatment of HIV (see Warnings and Precautions).

Indications

HIV infection (Epivir): Lamivudine in combination with other antiretroviral agents is indicated for the treatment of HIV infection.

Chronic hepatitis B (Epivir-HBV): Treatment of chronic hepatitis B associated with evidence of hepatitis B viral replication and active liver inflammation.

Administration and Dosage

HIV infection:

Adults – 150 mg twice daily in combination with other antiretroviral agents. Lamivudine may be administered with or without food.

Children (3 months to ≤ 16 years of age) – 4 mg/kg twice daily (up to a maximum of 150 mg twice a day) administered with other antiretroviral agents.

Renal function impairment – Adjust lamivudine dose in accordance with renal function. Insufficient data are available to recommend a dosage of lamivudine in dialysis.

Adjustment of Lamivudine Dosage in HIV-Infected Adult and Adolescent Patients with Renal Function Impairment

Ccr (mL/min)	Recommended lamivudine dosage
≥ 50	150 mg twice daily
30 to 49	150 mg once daily
15 to 29	150 mg first dose, then 100 mg once daily
5 to 14	150 mg first dose, then 50 mg once daily
< 5	50 mg first dose, then 25 mg once daily

Chronic hepatitis B: 100 mg once daily in adults. Safety and efficacy of treatment > 1 year have not been established, and the optimum duration of treatment is not known.

Children (2 to 17 years of age) – 3 mg/kg once daily up to a maximum daily dose of 100 mg. Safety and effectiveness of treatment beyond 1 year have not been established, and the optimum duration of treatment is not known.

HIV co-infection – The formulation and dosage of lamivudine in *Epivir-HBV* are not appropriate for patients dually infected with HBV and HIV. If lamivudine is administered to such patients, use the higher dosage indicated for HIV therapy as part of an appropriate combination regimen.

Renal function impairment – Adjust the dose of lamivudine in accordance with renal function. No additional dosing of lamivudine is required after routine (4-hour) hemodialysis. Insufficient data are available to recommend a dosage of lamivudine in patients undergoing peritoneal dialysis.

Adjustment of Lamivudine Dosage in Chronic Hepatitis B Adult Patients with Renal Function Impairment	
Ccr (mL/min)	Recommended lamivudine dosage
≥ 50	100 mg once daily
30 to 49	100 mg first dose, then 50 mg once daily
15 to 29	100 mg first dose, then 25 mg once daily
5 to 14	35 mg first dose, then 15 mg once daily
< 5	35 mg first dose, then 10 mg once daily

Actions

Pharmacology: Lamivudine is a synthetic nucleoside analog with activity against HIV and hepatitis B virus (HBV). Lamivudine is phosphorylated intracellularly to lamivudine 5′-triphosphate (L-TP). Incorporation of the monophosphate form into viral DNA by HBV polymerase results in DNA chain termination. L-TP also inhibits the RNA- and DNA-dependent DNA polymerase activities of HIV-1 reverse transcriptase.

Pharmacokinetics:

Absorption/Distribution – Lamivudine is rapidly absorbed after oral administration in HIV- and HBV-infected patients and phosphorylated to its active form, L-TP. Absolute bioavailability as demonstrated in HIV-infected patients is 86% for the tablet and 87% for the oral solution. Although the solution demonstrates a slightly higher C_{max} than the tablet, no significant difference exists in AUC; therefore, the solution and tablet may be used interchangeably.

The apparent volume of distribution (V_d) is 1.3 L/kg suggesting distribution into extravascular spaces. C_{max} reported in HBV-infected patients was 0.5 to 2 hours. Binding of lamivudine to plasma proteins is < 36% and independent of dose.

Metabolism/Excretion – Metabolism is a minor route of elimination; the only known metabolite is the trans-sulfoxide metabolite. The mean elimination half-life of lamivudine ranges from 5 to 7 hours. In HIV-infected patients, renal clearance is 280.4 mL/min, representing 71% of total clearance; total clearance is 398.5 mL/min. The majority of the dose is eliminated in the urine as unchanged drug, with ≈ 5% excreted as the metabolite within 12 hours of dose administration.

Special populations:

Children – In HIV-infected pediatric patients ≈ 4 months to 16 years of age and chronic hepatitis B pediatric patients 2 to 12 years of age, lamivudine was rapidly absorbed with a T_{max} of 0.5 to 1 hour and an absolute bioavailability of 66%. After 8 mg/kg/day, C_{max} was 1.1 mcg/mL and half-life was 2 hours (vs 3.7 hours in adults). Weight-corrected oral clearances were higher, resulting in lower AUCs compared with adults. Total exposure to lamivudine, as reflected by mean AUC values, was comparable between pediatric patients receiving 8 mg/kg/day and adults receiving 4 mg/kg/day. Age-stratified oral clearance was highest at 2 years of age and declined from 2 to 12 years of age, where values were then similar to those seen in adults. In 8 patients, CSF lamivudine concentrations (0.04 to 0.3 mcg/mL) ranged from 5.6% to 30.9% of the concentration in a simultaneous serum sample.

Contraindications

Hypersensitivity to any of the components of the products.

Warnings

Lactic acidosis/severe hepatomegaly with steatosis: Lactic acidosis and severe hepatomegaly with steatosis, including fatal cases, have occurred with the use of antiretroviral nucleoside analogs alone or in combination, including lamivudine and other antiretrovirals. A majority of these cases have been in women. Obesity and prolonged nucleoside exposure may be risk factors. Most of these reports have described patients receiving nucleoside analogs for treatment of HIV infection, but there have been reports of lactic acidosis in patients receiving lamivudine for hepatitis B. Exercise caution when administering lamivudine to any patient, particularly to those with known risk factors for liver disease. Suspend treatment with lamivudine in any patient who develops clinical or laboratory findings suggestive of lactic acidosis or pronounced hepatotoxicity (which may include hepatomegaly and steatosis even in the absence of marked transaminase elevations).

HIV-HBV co-infection: *Epivir-HBV* tablets and oral solution contain a lower dose of the same active ingredient (lamivudine) as *Epivir* tablets and oral solution (and lamivudine/zidovudine tablets) used to treat HIV infection. The formulation and dosage of lamivudine in *Epivir-HBV* are not appropriate for patients infected with both HBV and HIV. If a decision is made to administer lamivudine to patients dually infected with HIV and HBV, *Epivir* tablets or oral solution or *Combivir* (lamivudine/zidovudine) tablets should be used as a part of an appropriate combination regimen and prescribing information should be consulted. *Combivir* (a fixed-dose combination tablet of lamivudine and zidovudine) should not be administered concomitantly with either *Epivir*, *Epivir-HBV*, or *Retrovir* (zidovudine).

Posttreatment exacerbations of hepatitis: Clinical and laboratory evidence of exacerbations of hepatitis have occurred after discontinuation of lamivudine (these have been primarily detected by serum ALT elevations in addition to the re-emergence of HBV DNA commonly observed after stopping treatment). Although most events appear to have been self-limited, fatalities have been reported in some cases. Similar events have been reported from postmarketing experience after changes from lamivudine-containing HIV treatment regimens to non-lamivudine-containing regimens in patients infected with both HIV and HBV. The causal relationship to discontinuation of lamivudine treatment is unknown. Closely monitor patients with clinical and laboratory follow-up for at least several months after stopping treatment. There is insufficient evidence to determine whether reinitiation of therapy alters the course of posttreatment exacerbations of hepatitis.

Elderly: Because elderly patients are more likely to have decreased renal function, take care in dose selection and monitor renal function.

Pregnancy: Category C.

Lamivudine has not affected the transmission of HBV from mother to infant; immunize infants appropriately to prevent neonatal acquisition of HBV.

Antiretroviral pregnancy registry – To monitor maternal-fetal outcomes of women exposed to lamivudine, an Antiretroviral Pregnancy Registry has been established. Physicians are encouraged to register patients by calling (800) 258-4263.

Lactation: Instruct mothers to discontinue nursing if they are receiving lamivudine, which is consistent with the CDC recommendation that HIV-infected mothers not breastfeed their infants to avoid risking postnatal transmission of HIV infection.

Children:

Hepatitis B – Safety and efficacy of lamivudine for treatment of chronic hepatitis B in children have been studied in pediatric patients from 2 to 17 years of age in a controlled clinical trial. Safety and efficacy in pediatric patients < 2 years of age have not been established.

HIV infection – The safety and effectiveness of lamivudine in combination with other antiretroviral agents have been established in pediatric patients ≥ 3 months of age.

Total exposure to lamivudine, as reflected by mean AUC values, was comparable between pediatric patients receiving an 8 mg/kg/day dose and adults receiving a 4 mg/kg/day dose.

Pancreatitis – Pancreatitis, which has been fatal in some cases, has been observed in antiretroviral nucleoside-experienced pediatric patients receiving lamivudine alone or in combination with other antiretroviral agents. Stop lamivudine treatment immediately if clinical signs, symptoms, or lab abnormalities suggestive of pancreatitis occur (see Adverse Reactions).

Precautions

Monitoring:

Epivir-HBV – Monitor patients regularly during treatment. The safety and efficacy of treatment with *Epivir-HBV* > 1 year have not been established. During treatment, combinations of events such as return of persistently elevated ALT, increasing levels of HBV DNA over time after an initial decline below assay limit, progression of clinical signs or symptoms of hepatic disease, and worsening of hepatic necroinflammatory findings may be considered as potentially reflecting loss of therapeutic response. Consider such observations when determining the advisability of continuing therapy.

Emergence of resistance-associated HBV mutations: Progression of hepatitis B, including death, has been reported in some patients with YMDD-mutant HBV, including patients from the liver transplant setting and from other clinical trials. The long-term clinical significance of YMDD-mutant HBV is not known. Increased clinical and laboratory monitoring may aid in treatment decisions if emergence of viral mutants is suspected.

Special risk: Safety and efficacy of *Epivir-HBV* have not been established in patients with decompensated liver disease or organ transplants; pediatric patients < 2 years of age (use appropriate infant immunizations to prevent HBV); patients dually infected with HBV and HCV, hepatitis delta, or HIV; or other populations not included in the principal Phase III controlled studies.

Drug Interactions

Drugs that may interact with lamivudine include zidovudine, zalcitabine, and trimethoprim/sulfamethoxazole.

Adverse Reactions

HIV – Adverse reactions occurring in ≥ 5% of patients include neuropathy, insomnia, dizziness, depression, nausea, diarrhea, vomiting, anorexia, abdominal pain/cramps, dyspepsia, myalgia, arthralgia, nasal symptoms, cough, headache, malaise, fatigue, fever, chills, and rash. Lab abnormalitites may include neutropenia, thrombocytopenia, anemia, and elevations in amylase, AST, ALT, and bilirubin.

Chronic hepatitis B – Adverse reactions occurring in ≥ 3% of patients include the following: Abdominal discomfort/pain; nausea/vomiting; diarrhea; myalgia; arthralgia; ear, nose, and throat infections; sore throat; malaise/fatigue; headache; fever or chills; rash. Lab abnormalitites may include platelets and elevations in ALT, serum lipase, and CPK.

Children – Adverse reactions in children are similar to adults and include pancreatitis, hepatomegaly, splenomegaly, stomatitis, and ear pain/swelling.

Pancreatitis, which has been fatal in some cases, has been observed in antiretroviral nucleoside-experienced pediatric patients receiving lamivudine alone or in combination with other antiretroviral agents. In 1 study, 14% of patients developed pancreatitis while receiving monotherapy with lamivudine. Three of these patients died of complications of pancreatitis. In a second study, 18% of patients developed pancreatitis.

Paresthesias and peripheral neuropathies were reported in < 1% to 15%.

In a 1-month pharmacokinetic study in children (2 to 12 years of age) and adolescents (13 to 17 years of age) with chronic hepatitis B receiving *Epivir-HBV*, the most commonly observed adverse events were malaise, fatigue, cough, fever, diarrhea, headache, and viral respiratory tract infections.

TENOFOVIR DISOPROXIL FUMARATE (PMPA)

Tablets: 300 mg (equivalent to 245 mg tenofovir disoproxil) *(Rx)*	*Viread* (Gilead Sciences)

Warning:

Lactic acidosis and severe hepatomegaly with steatosis, including fatal cases, have been reported with the use of nucleoside analogs alone or in combination with other antiretrovirals. A majority of these cases have been in women. Obesity and prolonged nucleoside exposure may be risk factors. Exercise particular caution when administering nucleoside analogs to any patient with known risk factors for liver disease. Cases also have been reported in patients with no known risk factors. Suspend treatment with tenofovir in any patient who develops clinical or laboratory findings suggestive of lactic acidosis or pronounced hepatotoxicity, which may include hepatomegaly and steatosis even in the absence of marked transaminase elevations.

Indications

HIV infection: In combination with other antiretroviral agents for the treatment of HIV-1 infection. This indication is based on studies conducted in treatment-experienced adults with evidence of HIV-1 viral replication despite ongoing antiretroviral therapy. Studies in antiretroviral naïve patients are ongoing. Consider the use of tenofovir for treating adult patients with HIV strains that are expected to be susceptible to tenofovir as assessed by laboratory testing or treatment history.

Administration and Dosage

The recommended dose is 300 mg once daily taken orally with a meal.

When administered with didanosine, give tenofovir 2 hours before or 1 hour after didanosine administration.

Actions

Pharmacology: Tenofovir disoproxil, an acyclic nucleoside phosphonate diester analog of adenosine monophosphate, inhibits the activity of HIV reverse transcriptase by competing with the natural substrate deoxyadenosine 5′-triphosphate and, after incorporation into DNA, by DNA chain termination.

Pharmacokinetics:

Absorption – The oral bioavailability of tenofovir in fasted patients is ≈ 25%. Maximum serum concentrations (C_{max}) are achieved in ≈ 1 hour. C_{max} and AUC values are ≈ 296 ng/mL and ≈ 2287 ng•hr/mL, respectively.

Administration of tenofovir disoproxil following a high-fat meal increases the oral biovavailability with an increase in tenofovir $AUC_{0-\infty}$ of ≈ 40% and an increase in C_{max} of ≈ 14%. Take tenofovir with a meal to enhance its bioavailability.

Distribution – In vitro binding of tenofovir to human plasma or serum proteins is < 0.7 and 7.2%, respectively. The volume of distribution at steady state is ≈ 1.3 L/kg.

Metabolism/Excretion – In vitro studies indicate that neither tenofovir disoproxil nor tenofovir are substrates of CYP450 enzymes. Tenofovir is eliminated by a combination of glomerular filtration and active tubular secretion. There may be competition for elimination with other compounds that are also renally eliminated.

Special populations –

Renal function impairment: Because tenofovir is primarily renally eliminated, tenofovir pharmacokinetics are likely to be affected by renal impairment.

Warnings

Lactic acidosis/severe hepatomegaly with steatosis: Lactic acidosis and severe hepatomegaly with steatosis, including fatal cases, have been reported with the use of nucleoside analogs alone or in combination with other antiretrovirals. A majority of these cases have been in women. Obesity and prolonged nucleoside exposure may be risk factors. Exercise particular caution when administering nucleoside analogs to any patient with known risk factors for liver disease. Cases also have been reported in patients with no known risk factors. Suspend treatment with tenofovir in any patient who develops clinical or laboratory findings suggestive of lactic acidosis or pronounced hepatotoxicity, which may include hepatomegaly and steatosis even in the absence of marked transaminase elevations (see Warning Box).

Renal function impairment: Do not administer tenofovir to patients with renal insufficiency (Ccr < 60 mL/min) until data become available describing the disposition of tenofovir in these patients.

Hepatic function impairment: The pharmacokinetics of tenofovir have not been studied in patients with hepatic impairment. Tenofovir pharmacokinetics may be altered in patients with hepatic insufficiency.

Mutagenesis: Tenofovir was mutagenic in the in vitro mouse lymphoma assay and negative in an in vitro bacterial mutagenicity test (Ames test).

Fertility impairment: In female rats, there was an alteration of the estrous cycle.

Elderly: In general, dose selection for the elderly patient should be cautious, keeping in mind the greater frequency of decreased hepatic, renal, or cardiac function, and of concomitant disease or other drug therapy.

Pregnancy: Category B.

Antiretroviral Pregnancy Registry – To monitor fetal outcomes of pregnant women exposed to tenofovir, an Antiretroviral Pregnancy Registry has been established. Health care providers are encouraged to register patients by calling (800) 258-4263.

Lactation: The Centers for Disease Control and Prevention recommend that HIV-infected mothers not breastfeed their infants to avoid risking postnatal transmission of HIV.

Precautions

Monitoring:

Bone toxicity – It is not known if long-term administration of tenofovir (> 1 year) will cause bone abnormalities. Therefore, if bone abnormalities are suspected, obtain appropriate consultation.

RIFAMPIN

Capsules: 150 and 300 mg (*Rx*)	Various, *Rifadin* (Aventis), *Rimactane* (Novartis)
Powder for injection: 600 mg (*Rx*)	*Rifadin* (Aventis)

Indications

Tuberculosis:

Oral – Oral treatment is for all forms of tuberculosis. A 3-drug regimen consisting of rifampin, isoniazid, and pyrazinamide is recommended in the initial phase of short-course therapy that is usually continued for 2 months.

IV – Initial treatment and retreatment of tuberculosis when the drug cannot be taken by mouth.

Neisseria meningitidis carriers: Treatment of asymptomatic carriers of *N. meningitidis* to eliminate meningococci from the nasopharynx. Not indicated for treatment of meningococcal infection.

Administration and Dosage

Oral: Administer once daily, either 1 hour before or 2 hours after meals.

Data is not available to determine dosage for children < 5 years of age.

Oral and IV:

Tuberculosis: Adults – 10 mg/kg in a single daily administration not to exceed 600 mg once daily.

Children – 10 to 20 mg/kg, not to exceed 600 mg/day.

The 2-month regimen: According to the MMWR, the 2-month daily regimen of rifampin and pyrazinamide is recommended in HIV-infected people. However, the drug toxicities may be increased.

The 4-month regimen: According to the MMWR, rifampin given daily for 3 months has resulted in better protection than placebo in treatment of LTBI in non-HIV patients with silicosis in a randomized prospective trial. However, because the patients receiving rifampin had a high rate of active tuberculosis (4%), experts have concluded that a 4-month regimen would be more prudent when using rifampin alone. This option may be useful for patients who cannot tolerate isoniazid or pyrazinamide.

The 6-month regimen: Ordinarily this consists of an initial 2-month phase of rifampin, isoniazid, and pyrazinamide and, if clinically indicated, streptomycin or ethambutol, followed by 4 months of rifampin and isoniazid. Reassess the need for a fourth drug when the results of susceptibility testing are known. If community rates of INH resistance are currently < 4%, an initial treatment regimen with < 4 drugs may be considered. Continue treatment for > 6 months if the patient is still sputum- or culture-positive, if resistant organisms are present, or if the patient is HIV positive.

Meningococcal carriers: Once daily for 4 consecutive days in the following doses:

Adults – 600 mg.

Children – 10 to 20 mg/kg, not to exceed 600 mg/day.

The following dosage has also been recommended –

Adults: 600 mg every 12 hours for 2 days.

Children (≥ 1 month of age): 10 mg/kg every 12 hours for 2 days.

Children (< 1 month of age): 5 mg/kg every 12 hours for 2 days.

Actions

Pharmacology: Rifampin inhibits DNA-dependent RNA polymerase activity in susceptible cells. Specifically, it interacts with bacterial RNA polymerase, but does not inhibit the mammalian enzyme. Cross-resistance has only been shown with other rifamycins. Rifampin at therapeutic levels has demonstrated bactericidal activity against intracellular and extracellular *Mycobacterium tuberculosis* organisms.

Pharmacokinetics:

Oral –

Absorption/Distribution: Rifampin is almost completely absorbed and achieves mean peak plasma levels within 1 to 4 hours. Absorption of rifampin is reduced by ≈ 30% when the drug is ingested with food.

Metabolism: Rifampin is metabolized in the liver by deacetylation; the metabolite is still active against *Mycobacterium tuberculosis*. About 40% is excreted in bile and undergoes enterohepatic circulation; however, the deacetylated metabolite is poorly absorbed. The half-life is ≈ 3 hours after a 600 mg oral dose, up to 5.1 after a 900 mg oral dose. With repeated administration, the half-life decreases and averages ≈ 2 to 3 hours.

Excretion: Elimination occurs mainly through the bile and, to a much lesser extent, the urine. Dosage adjustment is not necessary in renal failure, but is with hepatic dysfunction. Rifampin is not significantly removed by hemodialysis.

Contraindications

Hypersensitivity to any rifamycin.

Warnings

Hepatotoxicity: There have been fatalities associated with jaundice in patients with liver disease or patients receiving rifampin concomitantly with other hepatotoxic agents. Carefully monitor liver function, especially AST and ALT, prior to therapy and then every 2 to 4 weeks during therapy.

Hyperbilirubinemia: Hyperbilirubinemia, resulting from competition between rifampin and bilirubin for excretory pathways of the liver at the cell level, can occur in early days of treatment.

Porphyria: Isolated reports have associated porphyria exacerbation with rifampin administration.

Meningococci resistance: The possibility of rapid emergence of resistant meningococci restricts use to short-term treatment of asymptomatic carrier state. Not for treatment of meningococcal disease.

Hypersensitivity reactions: Hypersensitivity reactions have occurred during intermittent therapy or when treatment was resumed following accidental or intentional interruption and were reversible with rifampin discontinuation and appropriate therapy.

Hepatic function impairment: Dosage adjustment is necessary.

Pregnancy: Category C.

Lactation: Rifampin is excreted in breast milk.

Precautions

Monitoring: Perform baseline measurements of hepatic enzymes, bilirubin, serum creatinine, CBC, and platelet count (or estimate) in adults treated for tuberculosis with rifampin. Baseline tests are unnecessary in pediatric patients unless a complicating condition is known or clinically suspected.

Intermittent therapy: Intermittent therapy may be used if the patient cannot or will not self-administer drugs on a daily basis. Closely monitor patients on intermittent therapy for compliance, and caution against intentional or accidental interruption of prescribed therapy because of increased risk of serious adverse reactions.

Urine, feces, saliva, sputum, sweat, and tears may be colored red-orange. Soft contact lenses may be permanently stained. Advise patients of these possibilities.

IV: For IV infusion only. Must not be administered by IM or SC route.

Thrombocytopenia: Thrombocytopenia has occurred, primarily with high dose intermittent therapy, but has also been noted after resumption of interrupted treatment.

Cerebral hemorrhage and fatalities have occurred when rifampin administration has continued or resumed after appearance of purpura.

Drug Interactions

Rifampin is known to induce the hepatic microsomal enzymes that metabolize various drugs such as acetaminophen, oral anticoagulants, barbiturates, benzodiazepines, beta blockers, chloramphenicol, clofibrate, oral contraceptives, corticosteroids, cyclosporine, disopyramide, estrogens, hydantoins, mexiletine, quinidine, sulfones, sulfonylureas, theophyllines, tocainide, verapamil, digoxin, enalapril, morphine, nifedipine, ondansetron, progestins, protease inhibitors, buspirone, delavirdine, doxycycline, fluoroquinolones, losartan, macrolides, sulfonylureas, tacrolimus, thyroid hormones, TCAs, zolpidem, zidovudine, and ketoconazole. The therapeutic effects of these drugs may be decreased.

Enzyme induction properties: Rifampin has enzyme induction properties that can enhance the metabolism of endogenous substrates including adrenal hormones, thyroid hormones, and vitamin D. Rifampin and isoniazid have been reported to alter vitamin D metabolism. In some cases, reduced levels of circulating 25-hydroxy vitamin D and 1,25-dihydroxy vitamin D have been accompained by reduced serum calcium and phosphate, and elevated parathyroid hormone.

Drug/Lab test interactions: Therapeutic levels of rifampin inhibit standard assays for serum folate and vitamin B_{12}.

Transient abnormalities in liver function tests (eg, elevation in serum bilirubin, alkaline phosphatase, serum transaminases), and reduced biliary excretion of contrast media used for visualization of the gallbladder have also been observed.

Drug/Food interactions: Food interferes with the absorption of rifampin, possibly resulting in decreased peak plasma concentrations. Take on an empty stomach with a full glass of water.

Adverse Reactions

High doses of rifampin (> 600 mg) given once or twice weekly have resulted in a high incidence of adverse reactions including the following: "Flu-like" syndrome; hematopoietic reactions; cutaneous, GI, and hepatic reactions; shortness of breath; shock; renal failure; asymptomatic elevations of liver enzymes; rash.

GANCICLOVIR (DHPG)

Capsules: 250 and 500 mg (*Rx*) — *Cytovene* (Roche)
Powder for injection, lyophilized: 500 mg/vial ganciclovir (*Rx*)

Warning:

The clinical toxicity of ganciclovir includes granulocytopenia, anemia, and thrombocytopenia. In animal studies, ganciclovir was carcinogenic, teratogenic, and caused aspermatogenesis.

Ganciclovir IV is indicated for use only in the treatment of cytomegalovirus (CMV) retinitis in immunocompromised patients and for the prevention of CMV disease in transplant patients at risk for CMV disease.

Ganciclovir capsules are indicated only for prevention of CMV disease in patients with advanced HIV infection at risk for CMV disease and for maintenance treatment of CMV retinitis in immunocompromised patients.

Because oral ganciclovir is associated with a risk of more rapid rate of CMV retinitis progression, use only in those patients for whom this risk is balanced by the benefit associated with avoiding daily IV infusions.

Indications

IV:

CMV *retinitis* – Treatment of CMV retinitis in immunocompromised patients, including patients with AIDS.

CMV *disease* – Prevention of CMV disease in transplant recipients at risk for CMV disease.

Oral:

CMV *retinitis* – Alternative to the IV formulation for maintenance treatment of CMV retinitis in immunocompromised patients, including patients with AIDS, in whom retinitis is stable following appropriate induction therapy and for whom the risk of more rapid progression is balanced by the benefit associated with avoiding daily IV infusions.

CMV *disease* – Prevention of CMV disease in individuals with advanced HIV infection at risk for developing CMV disease.

Administration and Dosage

IV: Do not administer by rapid or bolus IV injection. The toxicity may be increased as a result of excessive plasma levels. Do not exceed the recommended infusion rate. IM or SC injection of reconstituted ganciclovir may result in severe tissue irritation because of high pH.

CMV *retinitis treatment (normal renal function):*

Induction – Recommended initial dose is 5 mg/kg (given IV at a constant rate of 1 hour) every 12 hours for 14 to 21 days. Do not use oral ganciclovir for induction.

Maintenance –

IV: Following induction, the recommended maintenance dose is 5 mg/kg given as a constant rate IV infusion over 1 hour once per day 7 days per week, or 6 mg/kg once per day 5 days/week.

Oral: Following induction, the recommended maintenance dose of oral ganciclovir is 1000 mg 3 times daily with food. Alternatively, the dosing regimen of 500 mg 6 times daily every 3 hours with food during waking hours may be used.

For patients who experience progression of CMV retinitis while receiving maintenance treatment with either formulation of ganciclovir, reinduction treatment is recommended.

Prevention of CMV disease in transplant recipients with normal renal function:

IV – The recommended initial dose of IV ganciclovir for patients with normal renal function is 5 mg/kg (given IV at a constant rate over 1 hour) every 12 hours for 7 to 14 days, followed by 5 mg/kg once daily 7 days/week or 6 mg/kg once daily 5 days/week.

Oral – The recommended prophylactic dosage is 1000 mg 3 times daily with food.

The duration of treatment with ganciclovir in transplant recipients is dependent on the duration and degree of immunosuppression. In controlled clinical trials in bone marrow allograft recipients, IV ganciclovir treatment was continued until day 100 to 120 posttransplantation. CMV disease occurred in several patients who discontinued treatment with IV ganciclovir prematurely. In heart allograft recipients, the onset of newly diagnosed CMV disease occurred after treatment with IV ganciclovir was stopped at day 28 post-transplant, suggesting that continued dosing may be necessary to prevent late occurrence of CMV disease in this patient population.

Prevention of CMV disease in patients with advanced HIV infection and normal renal function: The recommended dose of ganciclovir capsules is 1000 mg 3 times daily with food.

Renal function impairment:

IV – Refer to the table for recommended doses and adjust the dosing interval as indicated.

IV Ganciclovir Dose in Renal Impairment

Ccr (mL/min)	Ganciclovir induction dose (mg/kg)	Dosing interval (hours)	Ganciclovir maintenance dose (mg/kg)	Dosing interval (hours)
≥ 70	5	12	5	24
50 to 69	2.5	12	2.5	24
25 to 49	2.5	24	1.25	24
10 to 24	1.25	24	0.625	24
< 10	1.25	3 times/week following hemodialysis	0.625	3 times/week following hemodialysis

Hemodialysis: Dosing for patients undergoing hemodialysis should not exceed 1.25 mg/kg 3 times/week, following each hemodialysis session. Give shortly after completion of the hemodialysis session, since hemodialysis reduces plasma levels by ≈ 50%.

Oral: In renal impairment, modify the dose of oral ganciclovir as follows:

Oral Ganciclovir Dose in Renal Impairment

Ccr (mL/min)	Ganciclovir doses
≥ 70	1000 mg TID or 500 mg q3h, 6 times/day
50 to 69	1500 mg QD or 500 mg TID
25 to 49	1000 mg QD or 500 mg BID
10 to 24	500 mg QD
< 10	500 mg 3 times/week, following hemodialysis

Patient monitoring: Because of the frequency of granulocytopenia, anemia, and thrombocytopenia, it is recommended that CBCs and platelet counts be performed frequently, especially in patients in whom ganciclovir or other nucleoside analogs have previously resulted in cytopenia, or in whom neutrophil counts are < 1000/mcL at the beginning of treatment. Patients should have serum creatinine or Ccr values followed carefully to allow for dosage adjustment in renally impaired patients.

Reduction of dose: Dose reductions are required with IV therapy and should be considered with oral therapy for patients with renal impairment and for those with neutropenia, anemia, or thrombocytopenia. Do not administer in severe neutropenia (ANC < 500/mcL) or severe thrombocytopenia (platelets < 25,000/mcL).

Actions

Pharmacology: Ganciclovir, a synthetic guanine derivative active against CMV, is an acyclic nucleoside analog of 2'-deoxyguanosine that inhibits replication of herpes viruses both in vitro and in vivo. Sensitive human viruses include CMV, herpes simplex virus (HSV)-1 and -2, herpes virus type 6, Epstein-Barr virus, varicella-zoster virus, and hepatitis B virus.

Pharmacokinetics:

Absorption – Absolute bioavailability of oral ganciclovir under fasting conditions was ≈ 5%; following food it was 6% to 9%. When given with a high-fat meal, steady-state AUC increased and there was a significant prolongation of time to peak serum concentrations.

At the end of a 1-hour IV infusion of 5 mg/kg, total AUC and C_{max} ranged between 22.1 and 26.8 mcg•hr/mL and 8.27 and 9 mcg/mL, respectively.

Distribution – The steady-state volume of distribution after IV administration was 0.74 L/kg. Cerebrospinal fluid concentrations obtained 0.25 and 5.67 hours postdose in 3 patients who received 2.5 mg/kg ganciclovir IV every 8 or 12 hours ranged from 0.31 to 0.68 mcg/mL, representing 24% to 70% of the respective plasma concentrations. Binding to plasma proteins was 1% to 2% over ganciclovir concentrations of 0.5 and 51 mcg/mL.

Metabolism – Following oral administration of a single 1000 mg dose, 86% of the administered dose was recovered in the feces and 5% was recovered in the urine.

Excretion – When administered IV, ganciclovir exhibits linear pharmacokinetics over the range of 1.6 to 5 mg/kg and when administered orally, it exhibits linear kinetics up to a total daily dose of 4 g/day. Renal excretion of unchanged drug by glomerular filtration and active tubular secretion is the major route of elimination. In patients with normal renal function, 91.3% of IV ganciclovir was recovered unmetabolized in the urine. After oral administration, steady state is achieved within 24 hours. Renal clearance following oral administration was 3.1 mL/min/kg. Half-life was 3.5 hours following IV administration and 4.8 following oral use.

Children: At an IV dose of 4 or 6 mg/kg in 27 neonates (2 to 49 days of age), the pharmacokinetic parameters were, respectively, C_{max} of 5.5 and 7 mcg/mL, systemic clearance of 3.14 and 3.56 mL/min/kg and half-life of 2.4 hours for both.

Contraindications

Hypersensitivity to ganciclovir or acyclovir.

Warnings

CMV disease: Safety and efficacy have not been established for congenital or neonatal CMV disease, nor for the treatment of established CMV disease other than retinitis, nor for use in nonimmunocompromised individuals. The safety and efficacy of oral ganciclovir have not been established for treating any manifestation of CMV disease other than maintenance treatment of CMV retinitis.

Diagnosis of CMV retinitis: The diagnosis should be made by indirect ophthalmoscopy. Other conditions in the differential diagnosis of CMV retinitis include candidiasis, toxoplasmosis, histoplasmosis, retinal scars, and cotton wool spots, any of which may produce a retinal appearance similar to CMV. The diagnosis may be supported by a culture of CMV from urine, blood, or throat, but a negative CMV culture does not rule out CMV retinitis.

Retinal detachment: Retinal detachment has been observed in subjects with CMV retinitis both before and after initiation of therapy with ganciclovir. Its relationship to therapy is unknown. Patients with CMV retinitis should have frequent ophthalmologic evaluations to monitor the status of their retinitis and to detect any other retinal pathology.

Hematologic: Do not administer if the absolute neutrophil count is < 500/mm^3 or the platelet count is < 25,000/mm^3. Granulocytopenia (neutropenia), anemia, and thrombocytopenia have been observed in patients treated with ganciclovir. The frequency and severity of these events vary widely in different patient populations. Therefore, use with caution in patients with pre-existing cytopenias or with a history of cytopenic reactions to other drugs, chemicals, or irradiation. Granulocytopenia usually occurs during the first or second week of treatment, but may occur at any time during treatment. Cell counts usually begin to recover within 3 to

7 days of discontinuing the drug. Colony-stimulating factors have increased neutrophil and WBC counts in patients receiving IV ganciclovir for CMV retinitis.

Renal function impairment: Use ganciclovir with caution. Half-life and plasma/serum concentrations of ganciclovir will be increased because of reduced renal clearance (see Administration and Dosage).

If renal function is impaired, dosage adjustments are required for ganciclovir IV and should be considered for oral ganciclovir. Base such adjustments on measured or estimated Ccr values.

Hemodialysis reduces plasma levels of ganciclovir by ≈ 50%.

Carcinogenesis: Consider ganciclovir a potential carcinogen.

Mutagenesis: Because of the mutagenic and teratogenic potential of ganciclovir, advise women of childbearing potential to use effective contraception during treatment. Similarly, advise men to practice barrier contraception during and for at least 90 days following treatment with ganciclovir.

Fertility impairment: Although data in humans have not been obtained regarding this effect, it is considered probable that ganciclovir, at recommended doses, causes temporary or permanent inhibition of spermatogenesis.

Elderly: Pharmacokinetic profile in elderly patients is not established. Because elderly individuals frequently have a reduced glomerular filtration rate, pay particular attention to assessing renal function before and during ganciclovir therapy.

Pregnancy: Category C.

Lactation: It is not known whether ganciclovir is excreted in breast milk. The possibility of serious adverse reactions from ganciclovir in nursing infants is considered likely. Instruct mothers to discontinue nursing if they are receiving ganciclovir. The minimum interval before nursing can safely be resumed after the last dose of ganciclovir is unknown.

Children: Safety and efficacy in children have not been established. The use of ganciclovir in children warrants extreme caution to the probability of long-term carcinogenicity and reproductive toxicity. Administer to children only after careful evaluation and only if the potential benefits of treatment outweigh the risks. Oral ganciclovir has not been studied in children < 13 years of age.

There has been very limited clinical experience using ganciclovir for the treatment of CMV retinitis in patients < 12 years of age.

The spectrum of adverse reactions reported in 120 immunocompromised pediatric clinical trial participants with serious CMV infections receiving IV ganciclovir were similar to those reported in adults. Granulocytopenia (17%) and thrombocytopenia (10%) were most commonly reported.

Precautions

Monitoring: Because of the frequency of neutropenia, anemia, and thrombocytopenia in patients receiving ganciclovir, it is recommended that CBCs and platelet counts be performed frequently, especially in patients in whom ganciclovir or other nucleoside analogs have previously resulted in leukopenia, or in whom neutrophil counts are < $1000/mm^3$ at the beginning of treatment. Patients should also have serum creatinine or Ccr values followed carefully.

Large doses/rapid infusion: The maximum single dose administered was 6 mg/kg by IV infusion over 1 hour. Larger doses have resulted in increased toxicity. It is likely that more rapid infusions would also result in increased toxicity.

Phlebitis/Pain at injection site: Initially, reconstituted ganciclovir solutions have a high pH (pH 11). Despite further dilution in IV fluids, phlebitis or pain may occur at the site of IV infusion. Take care to infuse solutions containing ganciclovir only into veins with adequate blood flow to permit rapid dilution and distribution.

Hydration: Because ganciclovir is excreted by the kidneys and normal clearance depends on adequate renal function, administration of ganciclovir should be accompanied by adequate hydration.

Drug Interactions

Drugs that may affect ganciclovir include imipenem-cilastatin, nephrotoxic drugs, probenecid, didanosine, and zidovudine. Drugs that may be affected by ganciclovir include cytotoxic drugs, didanosine, and zidovudine.

Adverse Reactions

Adverse reactions occurring in ≥ 3% of AIDS patients include fever; infection; chills; sepsis; diarrhea; anorexia; vomiting; leukopenia; anemia; thrombocytopenia; neuropathy; sweating; pruritus.

VALGANCICLOVIR

Tablets: 450 mg (*Rx*)	*Valcyte* (Roche)

Warning:

The clinical toxicity of valganciclovir, which is metabolized to ganciclovir, includes granulocytopenia, anemia, and thrombocytopenia. In animal studies, ganciclovir was carcinogenic, teratogenic, and caused aspermatogenesis.

Indications

Cytomegalovirus (CMV) retinitis: For the treatment of CMV retinitis in patients with acquired immunodeficiency syndrome (AIDS).

Administration and Dosage

Strict adherence to dosage recommendations is essential to avoid overdose. Valganciclovir tablets cannot be substituted for ganciclovir capsules on a one-to-one basis.

CMV retinitis (normal renal function):

Induction – 900 mg (two 450 mg tablets) twice daily for 21 days with food.

Maintenance – Following induction treatment, or in patients with inactive CMV retinitis, the recommended dosage is 900 mg (two 450 mg tablets) once daily with food.

Renal impairment: Monitor serum creatinine or Ccr levels carefully. Dosage adjustment is required according to Ccr, as shown in the table below. Increased monitoring for cytopenias may be warranted in patients with renal impairment.

Oral Valganciclovir in Renal Impairment

Ccr (mL/min)[1]	Induction dose	Maintenance dose
≥ 60	900 mg twice daily	900 mg once daily
40 to 59	450 mg twice daily	450 mg once daily
25 to 39	450 mg once daily	450 mg every 2 days
10 to 24	450 mg every 2 days	450 mg twice weekly

[1] An estimated creatinine clearance can be related to serum creatinine by the following formulas: Males: $\frac{\text{Weight (kg)} \times (140 - \text{age})}{72 \times \text{serum creatinine (mg/dL)}} = \text{Ccr}$

Females: 0.85 × above value

Hemodialysis patients: Do not prescribe valganciclovir to patients receiving hemodialysis.

Handling and disposal: Exercise caution in the handling of valganciclovir tablets. Do not break or crush tablets. Because valganciclovir is considered a potential teratogen and carcinogen in humans, observe caution in handling broken tablets. Avoid direct contact of broken or crushed tablets with skin or mucous membranes. If such contact occurs, wash thoroughly with soap and water, and rinse eyes thoroughly with plain water.

Because ganciclovir shares some of the properties of antitumor agents (ie, carcinogenicity and mutagenicity), consider handling and disposing according to guidelines issued for antineoplastic drugs.

Actions

Pharmacology: Valganciclovir is an L-valyl ester (prodrug) of ganciclovir that exists as a mixture of 2 diastereomers. After oral administration, both diastereomers are rapidly converted to ganciclovir by intestinal and hepatic esterases.

Drug resistance – Viruses resistant to ganciclovir can arise after prolonged treatment with valganciclovir.

Pharmacokinetics:

Absorption – Valganciclovir is well absorbed from the GI tract and rapidly metabolized in the intestinal wall and liver to ganciclovir. The absolute bioavailability of ganciclovir from valganciclovir tablets following administration with food was ≈ 60%. Ganciclovir median T_{max} following administration of 450 to 2625 mg valganciclovir tablets ranged from 1 to 3 hours. Systemic exposure to the prodrug, valganciclovir, is transient and low, and the AUC_{24} and C_{max} values are ≈ 1% and 3% of those of ganciclovir, respectively.

Distribution – Plasma protein binding of ganciclovir is 1% to 2%. When ganciclovir was administered IV, the steady-state volume of distribution of ganciclovir was ≈ 0.703 L/kg (n = 69).

Metabolism – Valganciclovir is rapidly hydrolyzed to ganciclovir; no other metabolites have been detected.

Excretion – The major route of elimination of valganciclovir is by renal excretion as ganciclovir through glomerular filtration and active tubular secretion. Systemic clearance of IV administered ganciclovir was ≈ 3.07 mL/min (n = 68) while renal clearance was ≈ 2.99 mL/min/kg (n = 16).

The terminal half-life of ganciclovir following oral administration of valganciclovir tablets to either healthy or HIV-positive/CMV-positive subjects was ≈ 4.08 hours (n = 73), and that following administration of IV ganciclovir was ≈ 3.81 hours (n = 69).

Special populations –

Renal function impairment: Because the major elimination pathway for ganciclovir is renal, dosage reductions according to creatinine clearance are required for valganciclovir tablets.

Decreased renal function results in decreased clearance of ganciclovir from valganciclovir, and a corresponding increase in terminal half-life. Therefore, dosage adjustment is required for patients with impaired renal function.

Hemodialysis – Hemodialysis reduces plasma concentrations of ganciclovir by ≈ 50% following valganciclovir administration. Patients receiving hemodialysis (Ccr < 10 mL/min) cannot use valganciclovir tablets because the daily dose of valganciclovir tablets required for these patients is < 450 mg (see Administration and Dosage).

Liver transplant patients – In liver transplant patients, the ganciclovir $AUC_{0\text{-}24\ hr}$ achieved with 900 mg valganciclovir was ≈ 41.7 mcg•hr/mL (n = 28) and the $AUC_{0\text{-}24\ hr}$ achieved with the approved dosage of 5 mg/kg IV ganciclovir was ≈ 48.2 mcg•hr/mL (n = 27).

Contraindications

Hypersensitivity to valganciclovir or ganciclovir.

Warnings

Toxicity: The clinical toxicity of valganciclovir, which is metabolized to ganciclovir, includes granulocytopenia, anemia, and thrombocytopenia. In animal studies, ganciclovir was carcinogenic, teratogenic, and caused aspermatogenesis.

Hematologic: Valganciclovir tablets should not be administered if the absolute neutrophil count is < 500 cells/mm^3, the platelet count is < 25,000/mm^3, or the hemoglobin is < 8 g/dL.

Severe leukopenia, neutropenia, anemia, thrombocytopenia, pancytopenia, bone marrow depression, and aplastic anemia have been observed in patients treated with valganciclovir tablets (and ganciclovir) (see Precautions and Adverse Reactions).

Cytopenia may occur at any time during treatment and may increase with continued dosing. Cell counts usually begin to recover within 3 to 7 days of discontinuing drug.

Renal function impairment: If renal function is impaired, dosage adjustments are required for valganciclovir.

Carcinogenesis: Like ganciclovir, valganciclovir is a potential carcinogen.

Mutagenesis: Valganciclovir increases mutations in mouse lymphoma cells.

Fertility impairment: It is considered probable that in humans, valganciclovir at the recommended doses may cause temporary or permanent inhibition of spermatogenesis. Animal data also indicate that suppression of fertility in females may occur.

Because of the mutagenic and teratogenic potential of ganciclovir, advise women of childbearing potential to use effective contraception during treatment. Similarly, advise men to practice barrier contraception during and for at least 90 days following treatment with valganciclovir.

Elderly: The pharmacokinetic characteristics of valganciclovir in elderly patients have not been established. Since elderly individuals frequently have a reduced glomerular filtration rate, pay particular attention to assessing renal function before and during administration of valganciclovir.

Pregnancy: *Category* C.

Lactation: It is not known whether ganciclovir or valganciclovir is excreted in human milk. Because of potential for serious adverse events in nursing infants, mothers should be instructed not to breastfeed if they are receiving valganciclovir tablets. In addition, the Centers for Disease Control and Prevention recommend that HIV-infected mothers not breastfeed their infants to avoid risking postnatal transmission of HIV.

Children: Safety and efficacy of valganciclovir in pediatric patients have not been established.

Precautions

Monitoring: Because of the frequency of neutropenia, anemia, and thrombocytopenia in patients receiving valganciclovir tablets, it is recommended that complete blood counts and platelet counts be performed frequently, especially in patients in whom ganciclovir or other nucleoside analogs have previously resulted in leukopenia, or in whom neutrophil counts are < 1000 cell/mm^3 at the beginning of treatment. Increased monitoring for cytopenias may be warranted if therapy with oral ganciclovir is changed to oral valganciclovir, because of increased plasma concentrations of ganciclovir after valganciclovir administration.

Increased serum creatinine levels have been observed in trials evaluating valganciclovir tablets. Patients should have serum creatinine or Ccr values monitored carefully to allow for dosage adjustments in renally impaired patients. The mechanism of impairment of renal function is not known.

Drug Interactions

No in vivo drug interaction studies were conducted with valganciclovir. However, because valganciclovir is rapidly and extensively converted to ganciclovir, interactions associated with ganciclovir will be expected for valganciclovir tablets (see Ganciclovir monograph).

Drugs that may affect valganciclovir include imipenem-cilastin, nephrotoxic drugs, probenecid, didanosine, and zidovudine. Drugs that may be affected by valganciclovir include cytotoxic drugs, didanosine, and zidovudine.

Drug/Food interactions: When valganciclovir tablets were administered with a high-fat meal containing ≈ 600 total calories (31.1 g fat, 51.6 g carbohydrates, and 22.2 g protein) at a dose of 875 mg once daily to 16 HIV-positive subjects, the steady-state ganciclovir AUC increased by 30% (95% CI 12% to 51%), and the C_{max} increased by 14% (95% CI 5% to 36%), without any prolongation in time to peak plasma concentrations (T_{max}). Administer valganciclovir tablets with food.

Adverse Reactions

Adverse reactions occurring in ≥ 3% of patients include the following: Headache, insomnia, peripheral neuropathy, paresthesia, diarrhea, nausea, vomiting, abdominal pain, neutropenia, anemia, thrombocytopenia, pyrexia, retinal detachment.

ACYCLOVIR (Acycloguanosine)

Tablets: 400 and 800 mg (*Rx*) — *Zovirax* (GlaxoWellcome)
Capsules: 200 mg (*Rx*)
Suspension: 200 mg/5 mL (*Rx*)
Powder for injection: 500 and 1000 mg/vial (as sodium) (*Rx*)

Indications

Parenteral: Treatment of initial and recurrent mucosal and cutaneous herpes simplex virus (HSV)-1 and -2 and varicella-zoster (shingles) infections in immunocompromised patients.

Herpes simplex encephalitis in patients > 6 months of age.

Severe initial clinical episodes of genital herpes in patients who are not immunocompromised.

Oral: Treatment of initial episodes and management of recurrent episodes of genital herpes in certain patients. Severity of the disease depends upon the immune status of the patient, frequency and duration of episodes, and degree of cutaneous or systemic involvement.

Acute treatment of herpes zoster (shingles) and chickenpox (varicella).

Administration and Dosage

Parenteral: For IV infusion only. Avoid rapid or bolus IV, IM, or SC injection. Administer over at least 1 hour to prevent renal tubular damage. Initiate therapy as soon as possible following onset of signs and symptoms.

IV Acyclovir Dosage/Management Guidelines

Indication	Dosage	
	Adults	Children (< 12 years)
Mucosal and cutaneous HSV infections in immunocompromised patients	5 mg/kg infused at a constant rate over 1 hour every 8 hours (15 mg/kg/day) for 7 days[1]	250 mg/m^2 infused at a constant rate over 1 hour every 8 hours (750 mg/m^2/day) for 7 days[1]
Varicella-zoster infections (shingles) in immunocompromised patients[2]	10 mg/kg infused at a constant rate over 1 hour every 8 hours for 7 days[3]	500 mg/m^2 infused at a constant rate over at least 1 hour every 8 hours for 7 days[3]
Herpes simplex encephalitis	10 mg/kg infused at a constant rate over at least 1 hour every 8 hours for 10 days	500 mg/m^2 infused at a constant rate over at least 1 hour every 8 hours for 10 days[4]

[1] For severe initial clinical episodes of herpes genitalis, use the same dose for 5 days.
[2] Base dosage for obese patients on ideal body weight (10 mg/kg).
[3] Do not exceed 500 mg/m^2 every 8 hours.
[4] > 6 months of age.

Renal function impairment, acute or chronic – Adjust the dosing interval as indicated below:

Parenteral Acyclovir Dosage in Renal Function Impairment

Ccr (mL/min/1.73 m^2)	Percent of recommended dose	Dosing interval (hours)
> 50	100%	8
25 to 50	100%	12
10 to 25	100%	24
0 to 10	50%	24

Hemodialysis – The mean plasma half-life of acyclovir during hemodialysis is ≈ 5 hours; a 60% decrease in plasma concentrations follows a 6-hour dialysis period. Therefore, administer a dose after each dialysis.

Oral:

Herpes simplex –

Initial genital herpes: 200 mg every 4 hours 5 times daily for 10 days. In patients with extremely severe episodes in which prostration, CNS involvement, urinary retention, or inability to take oral medication requires hospitalization and more aggressive management, initiate therapy with IV acyclovir (see above).

Chronic suppressive therapy for recurrent disease: 400 mg 2 times daily for up to 12 months, followed by reevaluation. Reevaluate the frequency and severity of the patient's HSV after 1 year of therapy to assess the need for continuation of therapy; frequency and severity of episodes of untreated genital herpes may change over time. Reevaluation usually requires a trial off acyclovir to assess the need for reinstitution of suppressive therapy. Some patients, such as those with very frequent or severe episodes before treatment, may warrant uninterrupted suppression for > 1 year.

Alternative regimens have included doses ranging from 200 mg 3 times daily to 200 mg 5 times daily.

Intermittent therapy: 200 mg every 4 hours 5 times daily for 5 days. Initiate therapy at the earliest sign or symptom (prodrome) of recurrence.

Herpes zoster, acute treatment – 800 mg every 4 hours 5 times daily for 7 to 10 days.

Chickenpox – 20 mg/kg (not to exceed 800 mg) 4 times daily for 5 days. Initiate at earliest sign or symptom.

Renal impairment, acute or chronic –

Oral Acyclovir Dosage in Renal Function Impairment

Normal dosage regimen (5× daily)	Ccr (mL/min/1.73 m^2)	Adjusted dosage regimen	
		Dose (mg)	Dosing interval
200 mg every 4 hours	> 10 0 to 10	200 200	Every 4 hours, 5× daily Every 12 hours
400 mg every 12 hours	> 10 0 to 10	400 200	Every 12 hours Every 12 hours
800 mg every 4 hours	> 25 10 to 25 0 to 10	800 800 800	Every 4 hours, 5× daily Every 8 hours Every 12 hours

Hemodialysis – For patients that require hemodialysis, adjust dosing schedule so that a dose is administered after each dialysis. No supplemental dose is necessary after peritoneal dialysis.

Actions

Pharmacology: A synthetic acyclic purine nucleoside analog, acyclovir has in vitro inhibitory activity against HSV-1 and HSV-2, varicella zoster, Epstein-Barr, and cytomegalovirus. Acyclovir is preferentially taken up and selectively converted to the active triphosphate form by HSV-infected cells. Acyclovir triphosphate interferes with HSV DNA polymerase and inhibits viral DNA replication. In vitro, acyclovir triphosphate can be incorporated into growing chains of DNA by viral DNA polymerase and, to a much smaller extent, by cellular DNA polymerase. When incorporation occurs, the DNA chain is terminated.

Pharmacokinetics:

Absorption/Distribution – When acyclovir was administered to adults at 5 mg/kg (≈ 250 mg/m^2) by 1 hour infusions every 8 hours, mean steady-state peak and trough concentrations were 9.8 mcg/mL (5.5 to 13.8 mcg/mL) and 0.7 mcg/mL (0.2 to 1 mcg/mL), respectively. Similar concentrations are achieved in children > 1 year of age when doses of 250 mg/m^2 are given every 8 hours. Oral acyclovir is slowly and incompletely absorbed from the GI tract. Peak concentrations are reached in 1.5 to 2 hours; absorption is unaffected by food. Bioavailability is between 15% and 30% and decreases with increasing doses. Concentrations achieved in CSF are

≈ 50% of plasma values. Plasma protein binding is 9% to 33%. Acyclovir is widely distributed in tissues and body fluids, including brain, kidney, lung, liver, muscle, spleen, uterus, vaginal mucosa, vaginal secretions, CSF, and herpetic vesicular fluid.

Metabolism/Excretion – Renal excretion of unchanged drug by glomerular filtration and tubular secretion following IV use accounts for 62% to 91% of the dose. Mean renal excretion of unchanged drug following oral use is 14.4% (8.6% to 19.8%). The only major urinary metabolite may account for up to 14% of the dose in patients with normal renal function. An insignificant amount is recovered in feces and expired CO_2; there is no evidence of tissue retention.

Half-life and total body clearance depend on renal function:

Acyclovir Half-Life and Total Body Clearance Based on Renal Function

Ccr (mL/min/1.73 m^2)	Half-life (hr)	Total body clearance (mL/min/1.73 m^2)
> 80	2.5	327
50 to 80	3	248
15 to 50	3.5	190
0 (Anuric)	19.5	29

The half-life and total body clearance of acyclovir in pediatric patients > 1 year of age is similar to those in adults with normal renal function.

Contraindications

Hypersensitivity to acyclovir or any component of the formulation.

Warnings

Pregnancy: Category C.

Lactation: Acyclovir concentrations in breast milk in women following oral administration have ranged from 0.6 to 4.1 times corresponding plasma levels. These concentrations would potentially expose the nursing infant to a dose of acyclovir up to 0.3 mg/kg/day.

Children: Safety and efficacy of oral acyclovir in children < 2 years of age have not been established.

Precautions

Diagnosis: Proof of HSV infection rests on viral isolation and identification in tissue culture. Although the cutaneous vesicular lesions associated with HSV are often characteristic, other etiologic agents can cause similar lesions.

Genital herpes: Avoid sexual intercourse when visible lesions are present.

Herpes zoster infections: Adults ≥ 50 years of age tend to have more severe shingles, and acyclovir treatment showed more significant benefit for older patients. Treatment was more useful if started within the first 48 hours of rash onset.

Chickenpox: Although chickenpox in otherwise healthy children is usually a self-limited disease of mild to moderate severity, adolescents and adults tend to have more severe disease. Treatment was initiated within 24 hours of the typical chickenpox rash in the controlled studies, and there is no information regarding the effects of treatment begun later in the disease course. It is unknown whether the treatment of chickenpox in childhood has any effect on long-term immunity. However, there is no evidence to indicate that acyclovir treatment of chickenpox would have any effect on either decreasing or increasing the incidence or severity of subsequent recurrences of herpes zoster (shingles) later in life.

Do not exceed: Do not exceed the recommended dosage, frequency, or length of treatment. Base dosage adjustments on estimated Ccr.

Renal effects: Precipitation of acyclovir crystals in renal tubules can occur if the maximum solubility of free acyclovir is exceeded or if the drug is administered by bolus injection. Serum creatinine and BUN rise and Ccr decreases.

Bolus administration of the drug leads to a 10% incidence of renal dysfunction, while infusion of 5 mg/kg (250 mg/m^2) over an hour was associated with a lower frequency (4.6%). Concomitant use of other nephrotoxic drugs, pre-existing renal disease and dehydration make further renal impairment with acyclovir more likely. In most instances, alterations of renal function were transient and resolved spontaneously or with improvement of water and electrolyte balance, with drug dosage adjustments, or with drug discontinuation. However, these changes may progress to acute renal failure.

Hydration: Accompany IV infusion by adequate hydration. Because maximum urine concentration occurs within the first 2 hours following infusion, establish sufficient urine flow during that period to prevent precipitation in renal tubules.

Encephalopathic changes: Patients (1%) receiving acyclovir IV have manifested encephalopathic changes characterized by either lethargy, obtundation, tremors, confusion, hallucinations, agitation, seizures, or coma. Use with caution in those patients who have underlying neurologic abnormalities; those with serious renal, hepatic, or electrolyte abnormalities or significant hypoxia; and those who have manifested prior neurologic reactions to cytotoxic drugs.

Resistance: Exposure of HSV isolates to acyclovir in vitro can lead to the emergence of less sensitive viruses. In severely immunocompromised patients, prolonged or repeated courses of acyclovir may result in resistant viruses that may not fully respond to continued acyclovir therapy.

Drug Interactions

Drugs that may affect acyclovir include probenecid and zidovudine.

Adverse Reactions

Adverse reactions (parenteral) occurring in ≥ 3% of patients include inflammation or phlebitis at injection site, transient elevations of serum creatinine or BUN, and nausea or vomiting.

Adverse reactions (oral) occurring in ≥ 3% of patients include malaise, nausea, and headache.

FAMCICLOVIR

Tablets: 125, 250, and 500 mg (*Rx*) — *Famvir* (GlaxoSmithKline)

Indications

Acute herpes zoster: Management of acute herpes zoster (shingles).

Genital herpes: Treatment of recurrent episodes of genital herpes.

Administration and Dosage

Herpes zoster: The recommended dosage is 500 mg every 8 hours for 7 days. Initiate therapy promptly as soon as herpes zoster is diagnosed.

Genital herpes (recurrent episodes): The recommended dosage is 125 mg twice daily for 5 days. Initiate therapy at the first sign or symptom if medical management of a genital herpes recurrence is indicated.

Famciclovir Dosage in Renal Function Impairment

Ccr (mL/min)	Dose regimen
Herpes zoster	
≥ 60	500 mg q 8 h
40 to 59	500 mg q 12 h
20 to 39	500 mg q 24 h
< 20	250 mg q 48 h
Recurrent genital herpes	
≥ 40	125 mg q 12 h
20 to 39	125 mg q 24 h
< 20	125 mg q 48 h

Hemodialysis patients: The recommended dose of famciclovir is 250 mg (herpes zoster) or 125 mg (genital herpes) administered following each dialysis treatment.

Actions

Pharmacology: Famciclovir undergoes rapid biotransformation to the active antiviral compound penciclovir, which has inhibitory activity against herpes simplex virus types 1 (HSV-1) and 2 (HSV-2), and varicella-zoster virus (VZV). In HSV-1-, HSV-2-, and VZV-infected cells, viral thymidine kinase phosphorylates penciclovir to a monophosphate form that, in turn, is converted to penciclovir triphosphate by cellular kinases. In vitro, penciclovir triphosphate inhibits HSV-2 polymerase competitively with deoxyguanosine triphosphate. Consequently, herpes viral DNA synthesis and, therefore, replication are selectively inhibited.

Pharmacokinetics:

Absorption – The absolute bioavailability of famciclovir is 77%. The area under the plasma concentration-time curve (AUC) was 8.6 mcg•hr/mL. The maximum concentration (C_{max}) was 3.3 mcg/mL and the time to C_{max} (T_{max}) was 0.9 hours.

After a 1-hour IV infusion of penciclovir at doses of 5 to 20 mg/kg, the volume of distribution (Vd_b) of penciclovir was 83.1 and 125 L, respectively. Penciclovir is < 20% bound to plasma proteins over the concentration range of 0.1 to 20 mcg/mL. The blood/plasma ratio of penciclovir is ≈ 1.

Metabolism – Famciclovir given orally is deacetylated and oxidized to form penciclovir. Inactive metabolites include 6-deoxy penciclovir, monoacetylated penciclovir, and 6-deoxy monoacetylated penciclovir (each < 0.5% of the dose). Cytochrome P450 does not play an important role in famciclovir metabolism.

Excretion – Following a single 500 mg oral dose of radio-labeled famciclovir, 73% and 27% of administered radioactivity were recovered in urine and feces over 72 hours, respectively. Penciclovir accounted for 82% and 6-deoxy penciclovir accounted for 7% of the radioactivity excreted in the urine. Approximately 60% of the administered radiolabeled dose was collected in urine in the first 6 hours.

Renal clearance of penciclovir following the oral administration of a single 500 mg dose of famciclovir was 27.7 L/hr.

The plasma elimination half-life of penciclovir was 2 hours after IV penciclovir and 2.3 hours after 500 mg oral famciclovir. The half-life in 7 herpes zoster patients was 3 hours.

Contraindications

Hypersensitivity to famciclovir.

Warnings

Renal function impairment: Apparent plasma clearance, renal clearance, and the plasma-elimination rate constant of penciclovir decreased linearly with reductions in renal function. After a single 500 mg oral famciclovir dose to healthy volunteers and to volunteers with varying degrees of renal insufficiency, the following results were obtained.

Pharmacokinetics of Famciclovir in Patients with Renal Function Impairment

Parameter (mean)	Ccr ≥ 60 (mL/min; n = 15)	Ccr 40 to 59 (mL/min; n = 5)	Ccr 20 to 39 (mL/min; n = 4)	Ccr < 20 (mL/min; n = 3)
Ccr (mL/min)	88.1	49.3	26.5	12.7
CL_R (L/hr)	30.1	13[1]	4.2	1.6
CL/F[2] (L/hr)	66.9	27.3	12.8	5.8
Half-life (hr)	2.3	3.4	6.2	13.4

[1] n = 4

[2] CL/F consists of bioavailability factor and famciclovir to penciclovir conversion factor.

Dosage adjustment is recommended in renal insufficiency (see Administration and Dosage).

Hepatic function impairment: Well-compensated chronic liver disease (chronic hepatitis, chronic ethanol abuse, or primary biliary cirrhosis) had no effect on extent of availability (AUC) of penciclovir following a single dose of 500 mg famciclovir. However, there was a 44% decrease in penciclovir mean maximum plasma level and the time to maximum plasma concentration was increased by 0.75 hours in patients with hepatic insufficiency compared with normal volunteers. No dosage adjustment is recommended in well-compensated hepatic impairment. Penciclovir pharmacokinetics have not been evaluated in severe uncompensated hepatic impairment.

Elderly: Mean penciclovir AUC was 40% larger and penciclovir renal clearance was 22% lower after the oral administration of famciclovir in elderly volunteers (65 to 79 years of age) compared with younger volunteers.

Pregnancy: Category B.

Lactation: It is not known whether famciclovir is excreted in breast milk. Because of the potential for tumorigenicity shown for famciclovir in rats, discontinue nursing or the drug, taking into account the importance of the drug to the mother.

Children: Safety and efficacy in children < 18 years of age have not been established.

Drug Interactions

The conversion of 6-deoxy penciclovir to penciclovir is catalyzed by aldehyde oxidase. Interactions with other drugs metabolized by this enzyme could occur.

Drugs that may affect famciclovir include cimetidine, probenecid, and theophylline.

Drugs that may be affected by famciclovir include digoxin.

Drug/Food interactions: When famciclovir was administered with food, penciclovir C_{max} decreased ≈ 50%. Because the systemic availability of penciclovir (AUC) was not altered, it appears that famciclovir may be taken without regard to meals.

Adverse Reactions

Adverse reactions occurring in ≥ 3% of patients include dizziness, diarrhea, abdominal pain, dyspepsia, constipation, vomiting, fatigue, fever, pruritus.

The most frequent adverse events were headache and nausea.

RIBAVIRIN

Capsules: 200 mg (*Rx*)	*Rebetol* (Schering)
Lyophilized powder for aerosol reconstitution: 6 g ribavirin/100 mL vial. Contains 20 mg/mL when reconstituted with 300 mL sterile water (*Rx*)	*Virazole* (ICN)

Warning:

Capsules: Ribavirin monotherapy is not effective for the treatment of chronic hepatitis C virus infection and should not be used alone for this indication.

The primary toxicity of ribavirin is hemolytic anemia. The anemia associated with ribavirin therapy may result in worsening of cardiac disease that has led to fatal and nonfatal MIs. Do not treat patients with a history of significant or unstable cardiac disease with ribavirin.

Significant teratogenic or embryocidal effects have been demonstrated in all animal species exposed to ribavirin. In addition, ribavirin has a multiple-dose half-life of 12 days, and it may persist in nonplasma compartments for as long as 6 months. Therefore, ribavirin therapy is contraindicated in women who are pregnant and in the male partners of women who are pregnant. Extreme care must be taken to avoid pregnancy during therapy and for 6 months after completion of treatment in both female patients and in female partners of male patients who are taking ribavirin. At least 2 reliable forms of effective contraception must be utilized during treatment and during the 6-month posttreatment follow-up period.

Aerosol: In patients requiring mechanical ventilator assistance, pay strict attention to procedures that minimize the accumulation of drug precipitate that can result in mechanical ventilator dysfunction and associated increased pulmonary pressures.

Sudden deterioration of respiratory function has been associated with initiation of aerosolized ribavirin use in infants. Carefully monitor respiratory function during treatment. If initiation of aerosolized ribavirin treatment appears to produce sudden deterioration of respiratory function, stop treatment and reinstitute only with extreme caution, continuous monitoring, and consideration of concomitant administration of bronchodilators (see Warnings).

Ribavirin aerosol is not indicated for use in adults. Physicians and patients should be aware that ribavirin has been shown to produce testicular lesions in rodents and to be teratogenic in all animal species in which adequate studies have been conducted.

Indications

Capsules:

Chronic hepatitis C – Only in combination with *Intron* A (interferon alfa-2b, recombinant) injection for the treatment of chronic hepatitis C in patients with compensated liver disease previously untreated with alpha interferon or who have relapsed following alpha interferon therapy.

Aerosol:

Severe lower respiratory tract infections – Treatment of hospitalized infants and young children with severe lower respiratory tract infections caused by respiratory syncytial virus (RSV).

Administration and Dosage

Capsules: The recommended dose of ribavirin capsules depends on the patient's body weight.

Recommended Dosing	
Body weight	Ribavirin capsules
≤ 75 kg	2 × 200 mg capsules AM, 3 × 200 mg capsules PM daily PO
> 75 kg	3 × 200 mg capsules AM, 3 × 200 mg capsules PM daily PO

Ribavirin may be administered without regard to food but should be administered in a consistent manner with respect to food intake.

Treatment duration – The recommended duration of treatment for patients previously untreated with interferon is 24 to 48 weeks. Individualize the duration of treatment depending on baseline disease characteristics, response to therapy, and tolerability of the regimen. Assess virologic response after 24 weeks of treatment. Consider treatment discontinuation in any patient who has not achieved an HCV-RNA below the limit of detection by 24 weeks. There are no safety and efficacy data on treatment for > 48 weeks in the previously untreated patient population.

In patients who relapse following interferon therapy, the recommended duration of treatment is 24 weeks. There are no safety and efficacy data on treatment for > 24 weeks in the relapse patient population.

Dose modifications – In clinical trials, ≈ 26% of patients required modification of their dose of ribavirin capsules, *Intron A* injection, or both agents. If severe adverse reactions or laboratory abnormalities develop during combination therapy, modify or discontinue the dose, if appropriate, until the adverse reactions abate. If intolerance persists after dose adjustment, discontinue combination therapy.

A permanent dose reduction is required for patients with a history of stable cardiovascular disease if the hemoglobin decreases by ≥ 2 g/dL during any 4-week period. In addition, discontinue combination therapy in cardiac history patients if the hemoglobin remains < 12 g/dL after 4 weeks on a reduced dose.

It is recommended that a patient whose hemoglobin level falls below 10 g/dL have his/her ribavirin dose reduced to 600 mg daily (1 × 200 mg capsule AM, 2 × 200 mg capsules PM). Permanently discontinue ribavirin therapy in patients whose hemoglobin level falls below 8.5 g/dL.

Guidelines for Dose Modifications and Discontinuation for Anemia Based on Hemoglobin Levels		
	Dose reduction ribavirin capsules 600 mg daily	Permanent discontinuation of ribavirin treatment
No cardiac history	< 10 g/dL	< 8.5 g/dL
Cardiac history patients	≥ 2 g/dL decrease during any 4-wk period during treatment	< 12 g/dL after 4 wks of dose reduction

Special populations: Do not use ribavirin in patients with Ccr < 50 mL/min. Administer ribavirin with caution to patients with pre-existing cardiac disease. Assess patients before commencement of therapy and appropriately monitor them during therapy. Stop therapy if there is any deterioration of cardiovascular status.

Aerosol: For aerosol administration only. Ribavirin aerosol is not to be administered with any other aerosol-generating device or together with other aerosolized medications.

The recommended treatment regimen is 20 mg/mL as the starting solution in the drug reservoir of the Small Particle Aerosol Generator (SPAG-2) unit. Treatment is carried out for 12 to 18 hours/day for 3 to 7 days.

Mechanically ventilated infants – The recommended dose and administration schedule for infants who require mechanical ventilation is the same as for those who do not. Either a pressure or volume cycle ventilator may be used in conjunction with the

SPAG-2. In either case, suction endotracheal tubes every 1 to 2 hours and monitor pulmonary pressures frequently (every 2 to 4 hours). For both pressure and volume ventilators, heated wire connective tubing and bacteria filters in series in the expiratory limb of the system (which must be changed frequently, eg, every 4 hours) must be used to minimize the risk of ribavirin precipitation in the system and the subsequent risk of ventilator dysfunction. Use water column pressure release valves in the ventilator circuit for pressure-cycled ventilators. They also may be used with volume-cycled ventilators.

Nonmechanically ventilated infants – The aerosol is delivered to an infant oxygen hood from the SPAG-2 aerosol generator. Administration by face mask or oxygen tent may be necessary if a hood cannot be used. However, the volume and condensation area are larger in a tent, and this may alter the drug's delivery dynamics.

Reconstitution – Reconstitute drug with a minimum of 75 mL of Sterile Water for Injection or Inhalation in the original 100 mL vial. Shake well. Transfer to the clean, sterilized 500 mL wide-mouth Erlenmeyer flask (SPAG-2 Reservoir) and further dilute to a final volume of 300 mL with Sterile Water for Injection or Inhalation. The final concentration should be 20 mg/mL.

Important: This water should not have any antimicrobial agent or other substance added. Discard solutions placed in the SPAG-2 unit at least every 24 hours and when the liquid level is low before adding newly reconstituted solution. Using the recommended drug concentration of 20 mg/mL ribavirin as the starting solution in the SPAG-2 unit's drug reservoir, the average aerosol concentration for a 12-hour period is 190 mcg/L of air.

Actions

Pharmacology:

Antiviral effects – Ribavirin has antiviral inhibitory activity in vitro against RSV, influenza virus, and herpes simplex virus. The mechanism of action is unknown.

Immunologic effects – Neutralizing antibody responses to RSV were decreased in ribavirin-treated infants compared with placebo-treated infants; clinical significance of this observation is unknown.

Pharmacokinetics:

Absorption –

Capsules: Ribavirin was rapidly and extensively absorbed following oral administration. However, because of first-pass metabolism, the absolute bioavailability averaged 64%.

Aerosol: Ribavirin administered by aerosol is absorbed systemically. The plasma half-life was 9.5 hours.

Distribution –

Capsules: Following oral dosing with 600 mg twice daily, steady-state was reached by ≈ 4 weeks.

Aerosol: Bioavailability of the aerosol is unknown and may depend on mode of delivery. After aerosol use, peak plasma concentrations are less than the concentration that reduced RSV plaque formation in tissue culture by 85% to 98%. Respiratory tract secretions are likely to contain ribavirin in concentrations many times higher than those required to reduce plaque formation. However, RSV is an intracellular virus and serum concentrations may better reflect intracellular concentrations in the respiratory tract than respiratory secretion concentrations.

Accumulation of drug or metabolites in red blood cells occurs, with plateauing in red cells in ≈ 4 days. Accumulation gradually declines with an apparent half-life of 40 days.

Metabolism –

Capsules: Ribavirin is metabolized by a reversible phosphorylation pathway and a degradative pathway involving deribosylation and amide hydrolysis.

Excretion –

Capsules: Ribavirin and its metabolites are excreted renally. After oral administration of 600 mg ribavirin, ≈ 61% and 12% was eliminated in the urine and feces. Upon discontinuaton of dosing, the mean half-life was 298 hours.

Contraindications

Capsules: May cause birth defects or death of the exposed fetus. Ribavirin capsules are contraindicated in women who are pregnant or in men whose female partners are pregnant (see Warnings), and in patients with a history of hypersensitivity to ribavirin or any component of the capsule.

Patients with autoimmune hepatitis must not be treated with combination *Rebetol/Intron* A therapy because using these medicines can make the hepatitis worse.

Aerosol: Hypersensitivity to the drug or its components; pregnancy or the potential for pregnancy during exposure to the drug (see Warnings).

Warnings

Capsules:

Monotherapy – Ribavirin monotherapy is not effective for the treatment of chronic hepatitis C virus infection. Therefore, ribavirin capsules must not be used alone. The safety and efficacy of ribavirin capsules have only been established when used together with *Intron* A (interferon alfa-2b, recombinant) as *Rebetron* combination therapy.

Adverse events – There are significant adverse events caused by *Rebetol/Intron* A, including severe depression and suicidal ideation, hemolytic anemia, suppression of bone marrow function, pulmonary dysfunction, pancreatitis, and diabetes. Review the *Rebetron* combination therapy package insert in its entirety prior to initiation of combination treatment for additional safety information.

Hemoglobinopathies – Do not treat patients with hemoglobinopathies (eg, thalassemia major, sickle-cell anemia) with ribavirin.

Pancreatitis – Suspend ribavirin therapy in patients with signs and symptoms of pancreatitis and discontinue in patients with confirmed pancreatitis.

Renal function impairment – The multiple-dose pharmacokinetics of ribavirin cannot be accurately predicted in patients with renal dysfunction. Ribavirin is not effectively removed by hemodialysis. Do not treat patients with Ccr < 50 mL/min with ribavirin.

Hepatic function impairment – The mean C_{max} values increased with severity of hepatic dysfunction and was 2-fold greater in subjects with severe hepatic dysfunction when compared with control subjects.

Aerosol:

Underlying conditions – The presence of underlying conditions such as prematurity, immunosuppression, or cardiopulmonary disease may increase the severity of the infection and its risk to the patient.

Assisted ventilation – Some subjects requiring assisted ventilation have experienced serious difficulties because of inadequate ventilation and gas exchange. Drug precipitation within the ventilatory apparatus, including the endotracheal tube, has resulted in increased positive and expiratory pressure and increased positive inspiratory pressure. Accumulation of fluid in tubing ("rain out") also has been noted.

Respiratory function – Carefully monitor respiratory function during treatment. If ribavirin aerosol treatment produces sudden deterioration of respiratory function, stop treatment and reinstitute only with extreme caution, continuous monitoring, and consideration of concomitant administration of bronchodilators.

Deaths – Deaths during or shortly after treatment with aerosolized ribavirin have been reported in 20 cases.

Anemia: Although anemia has not been reported with aerosol use, it occurs frequently with oral and IV ribavirin.

Capsules – The primary toxicity of ribavirin is hemolytic anemia, which was observed in ≈ 10% of *Rebetol/Intron* A-treated patients in clinical trials. The anemia associated with ribavirin capsules occurs within 1 to 2 weeks of initiation of therapy. It is advised that hemoglobin or hematocrit be obtained pretreatment and at week 2 and 4 of therapy, or more frequently if clinically indicated. Then follow patients as clinically appropriate.

Mutagenesis:

Capsules – Ribavirin demonstrated increased incidences of mutation and cell transformation in multiple genotoxicity assays.

Fertility impairment:

Capsules – Use ribavirin with caution in fertile men. In studies in mice to evaluate the time course and reversibility of ribavirin-induced testicular degeneration at 0.1 to 0.8 × the maximum human 24-hour dose of ribavirin administered for 3 or 6 months, abnormalities in sperm occurred. Upon cessation of treatment, essentially total recovery from ribavirin-induced testicular toxicity was apparent within 1 or 2 spermatogenesis cycles.

Elderly:

Capsules – In clinical trials, elderly subjects had a higher frequency of anemia (67%) than did younger patients (28%) (see Warnings).

In general, cautiously administer ribavirin capsules to elderly patients, starting at the lower end of the dosing range, reflecting the greater frequency of decreased hepatic, renal, or cardiac function, and of concomitant disease or other drug therapy.

Monitor renal function and make dosing adjustments accordingly. Do not use ribavirin in elderly patients with Ccr < 50 mL/min.

Pregnancy: Category X.

Lactation: Ribavirin is toxic to lactating animals and their offspring.

It is not known whether ribavirin is excreted in human milk. Because of the potential for serious adverse reactions from the drug in nursing infants, a decision should be made whether to discontinue nursing or to delay or discontinue ribavirin.

Children:

Capsules – Safety and effectiveness in pediatric patients have not been established.

Precautions

Monitoring:

Capsules – The recommended monitoring for all patients treated with ribavirin prior to beginning treatment and then periodically thereafter:

- Standard hematologic tests: Including hemoglobin (pretreatment, week 2 and week 4 of therapy, and as clinically appropriate) (see Warnings), complete and differential white blood cell counts, and platelet count.
- Blood chemistries: Liver function tests and TSH.
- Pregnancy: Including monthly monitoring for women of childbearing potential.

Aerosol – Monitor respiratory function and fluid status during treatment.

Health care personnel:

Aerosol – Health care workers directly providing care to patients receiving aerosolized ribavirin should be aware that ribavirin is teratogenic in all animal species in which adequate studies have been conducted.

Health care workers who are pregnant should consider avoiding direct care of patients receiving aerosolized ribavirin. If close patient contact cannot be avoided, take precautions to limit exposure.

Drug Interactions

Drugs that may interact with ribavirin capsules include antacids.

Adverse Reactions

Aerosol: Adverse reactions may include bacterial pneumonia; pneumothorax; apnea; ventilator dependence; cardiac arrest; hypotension; digitalis toxicity; rash; conjunctivitis; reticulocytosis; dyspnea; bigeminy; bradycardia; tachycardia; bronchospasm; pulmonary edema; hypoventilation; cyanosis; atelectasis; worsening of respiratory status.

Healthcare workers: Headache (51%); conjunctivitis (32%); rhinitis, nausea, rash, dizziness, pharyngitis, lacrimation (10% to 20%).

Capsules: Adverse reactions occurring in ≥ 3% of patients include headache; dizziness; nausea; anorexia; dyspepsia; vomiting; myalgia; arthralgia; musculoskeletal pain; insomnia; irritability; depression; emotional lability; concentration impaired; nervousness; dyspnea; sinusitis; alopecia; rash; pruritus; injection site inflammation; injection site reaction; fatigue; rigors; fever; influenza-like symptoms; asthenia; chest pain; taste perversion.

FOSCARNET SODIUM (Phosphonoformic acid)

Injection: 24 mg/mL (*Rx*)	*Foscavir* (Astra)

Warning:

Renal impairment, the major toxicity, occurs to some degree in most patients. Continual assessment of a patient's risk and frequent monitoring of serum creatinine with dose adjustment for changes in renal function are imperative.

Seizures related to alterations in plasma minerals and electrolytes have been associated with foscarnet treatment. Therefore, patients must be carefully monitored for such changes and their potential sequelae. Mineral and electrolyte supplementation may be required.

Foscarnet causes alterations in plasma minerals and electrolytes that have led to seizures. Monitor patients frequently for such changes and their potential sequelae.

Indications

Cytomegalovirus (CMV) retinitis: Treatment of CMV retinitis in patients with AIDS.

Combination: Combination therapy with ganciclovir for patients who have relapsed after monotherapy with either drug.

Herpes simplex virus (HSV) infections: Treatment of acyclovir-resistant mucocutaneous HSV infections in immunocompromised patients.

Administration and Dosage

HSV infections: Foscarnet is not a cure for HSV infections. While complete healing may occur, relapse occurs in most patients.

Caution: Do not administer by rapid or bolus IV injection. Toxicity may be increased as a result of excessive plasma levels. An infusion pump must be used.

It is recommended that 750 to 1000 mL of normal saline or 5% dextrose solution be given prior to the first infusion of foscarnet to establish diuresis. With subsequent infusions, 750 to 1000 mL of hydration fluid should be given with 90 to 120 mg/kg of foscarnet, and 500 mL with 40 to 60 mg/kg of foscarnet. Hydration fluid may need to be decreased if clinically warranted. After the first dose, administer the hydration fluid concurrently with each infusion of foscarnet.

Induction treatment: The recommended initial dose for patients with normal renal function is 60 mg/kg, adjusted for individual patients' renal function, given IV at a constant rate over a minimum of 1 hour every 8 hours for 2 to 3 weeks, depending on clinical response.

Maintenance treatment: 90 to 120 mg/kg/day (individualized for renal function) as an IV infusion over 2 hours. It is recommended that most patients be started on maintenance treatment with 90 mg/kg/day. Escalation to 120 mg/kg/day may be considered should early reinduction be required because of retinitis progression.

Patients who experience progression of retinitis while receiving maintenance therapy may be retreated with the induction and maintenance regimens above.

Dose adjustment in renal impairment:

Foscarnet Dosing Guide Based on Ccr for Induction			
	HSV: Equivalent to		CMV: Equivalent to
Ccr (mL/min/kg)	80 mg/kg/day	120 mg/kg/day	180 mg/kg/day
> 1.4	40 q 12 hr	40 q 8 hr	60 q 8 hr
> 1 to 1.4	30 q 12 hr	30 q 8 hr	45 q 8 hr
> 0.8 to 1	20 q 12 hr	35 q 12 hr	50 q 12 hr
> 0.6 to 0.8	35 q 24 hr	25 q 12 hr	40 q 12 hr
> 0.5 to 0.6	25 q 24 hr	40 q 24 hr	60 q 24 hr
≥ 0.4 to 0.5	20 q 24 hr	35 q 24 hr	50 q 24 hr
< 0.4	Not recommended	Not recommended	Not recommended

Foscarnet Dosing Guide Based on Ccr for Maintenance		
Ccr (mL/min/kg)	CMV: Equivalent to	
	90 mg/kg/day	120 mg/kg/day
> 1.4	90 q 24 hr	120 q 24 hr
> 1 to 2.4	70 q 24 hr	90 q 24 hr
> 0.8 to 1	50 q 24 hr	65 q 24 hr
> 0.6 to 0.8	80 q 48 hr	105 q 48 hr
> 0.5 to 0.6	60 q 48 hr	30 q 48 hr
≥ 0.4 to 0.5	50 q 48 hr	65 q 48 hr
< 0.4	Not recommended	Not recommended

Actions

Pharmacology: Foscarnet exerts its antiviral activity by a selective inhibition at the pyrophosphate binding site on virus-specific DNA polymerases and reverse transcriptases at concentrations that do not affect cellular DNA polymerases. CMV strains resistant to ganciclovir may be sensitive to foscarnet. Acyclovir- or ganciclovir-resistant mutants may be resistant to foscarnet.

Pharmacokinetics: Foscarnet is 14% to 17% bound to plasma protein at plasma drug concentrations of 1 to 1000 mcM.

Approximately 80% to 90% of IV foscarnet is excreted unchanged in the urine of patients with normal renal function. Both tubular secretion and glomerular filtration account for urinary elimination of foscarnet.

Plasma half-life increases with the severity of renal impairment. Half-lives of 2 to 8 hours occurred in patients having estimated or measured 24-hour Ccr of 44 to 90 mL/min.

The foscarnet terminal half-life determined by urinary excretion was 87.5 ± 41.8 hours, possibly because of release of foscarnet from bone. Postmortem data provide evidence that foscarnet does accumulate in bone in humans.

Variable penetration into cerebrospinal fluid (CSF) has been observed. Disease-related defects in the blood-brain barrier may be responsible for the variations seen.

Contraindications

Hypersensitivity to foscarnet.

Warnings

Mineral and electrolyte imbalances: Foscarnet has been associated with changes in serum electrolytes including hypocalcemia (15%), hypophosphatemia (8%) and hyperphosphatemia (6%), hypomagnesemia (15%), and hypokalemia (16%). Foscarnet is associated with a transient, dose-related decrease in ionized serum calcium, which may not be reflected in total serum calcium.

Accidental exposure: Accidental skin and eye contact with foscarnet sodium solution may cause local irritation and burning sensation. Flush the exposed area with water.

Other CMV infections: Safety and efficacy have not been established for the treatment of other CMV infections (eg, pneumonitis, gastroenteritis); congenital or neonatal CMV disease; nonimmunocompromised individuals.

Neurotoxicity and seizures: Foscarnet was associated with seizures in AIDS patients.

Statistically significant risk factors associated with seizures were low baseline absolute neutrophil count (ANC), impaired baseline renal function, and low total serum calcium. Several cases of seizures were associated with death.

Renal function impairment: The major toxicity of foscarnet is renal impairment, which occurs to some degree in most patients. Approximately 33% of 189 patients with AIDS and CMV retinitis who received IV foscarnet in clinical studies developed significant impairment of renal function, manifested by a rise in serum creatinine concentration to ≥ 2 mg/dL.

Elderly: Because these individuals frequently have reduced glomerular filtration, pay particular attention to assessing renal function before and during administration.

Pregnancy: Category C.

Lactation: It is not known whether foscarnet is excreted in breast milk.

Children: The safety and efficacy of foscarnet in children have not been studied.

Precautions

Monitoring: The majority of patients will experience some decrease in renal function due to foscarnet administration. Therefore, it is recommended that Ccr be determined at baseline, 2 to 3 times/week during induction therapy, and at least once every 1 to 2 weeks during maintenance therapy, with foscarnet dose adjusted accordingly. More frequent monitoring may be required for some patients. It also is recommended that a 24-hour Ccr be determined at baseline and periodically thereafter to ensure correct dosing. Discontinue if Ccr drops to < 0.4 mL/min/kg.

Because of foscarnet's propensity to chelate divalent metal ions and alter levels of serum electrolytes, closely monitor patients for such changes. It is recommended that a schedule similar to that recommended for serum creatinine be used to monitor serum calcium, magnesium, potassium, and phosphorus.

Careful monitoring and appropriate management of creatinine are of particular importance in patients with conditions that may predispose them to seizures.

Diagnosis of CMV retinitis: Diagnosis of CMV retinitis should be established by an ophthalmologist familiar with the retinal presentation of these conditions.

Toxicity/Local irritation: The maximum single-dose administered was 120 mg/kg by IV infusion over 2 hours. It is likely that larger doses, or more rapid infusions, would result in increased toxicity. Infuse solutions containing foscarnet only into veins with adequate blood flow to permit rapid dilution and distribution, and avoid local irritation. Local irritation and ulcerations of penile epithelium have occurred in patients receiving foscarnet, possibly because of drug in urine. Adequate hydration with close attention to personal hygiene may minimize the occurrence of such events.

Anemia: Anemia occurred in 33% of patients. Granulocytopenia occurred in 17% of patients.

Drug Interactions

Drugs that may interact with foscarnet include nephrotoxic drugs (eg, aminoglycosides, amphotericin B, IV pentamidine), pentamidine, and zidovudine.

Foscarnet decreases serum levels of ionized calcium. Exercise particular caution when other drugs known to influence serum calcium levels are used concurrently.

Adverse Reactions

Adverse reactions occurring in ≥ 3% of patients include fever; nausea; anemia; diarrhea; abnormal renal function including acute renal failure, decreased Ccr and increased serum creatinine; vomiting; headache; seizure; death; marrow suppression; injection site pain or inflammation; paresthesia; dizziness; involuntary muscle contractions; hypoesthesia; neuropathy; sensory disturbances; influenza-like symptoms; bacterial/fungal infections; rectal hemorrhage; dry mouth; melena; flatulence; ulcerative stomatitis; pancreatitis; granulocytopenia; leukopenia; thrombocytopenia; platelet abnormalities; thrombosis; WBC abnormalities; lymphadenopathy; electrolyte abnormalities; neurotoxicity; renal impairment; decreased weight; increased alkaline phosphatase, LDH and BUN; acidosis; cachexia; thirst; depression; confusion; anxiety; aggressive reaction; hallucination; coughing; dyspnea; pneumonia; sinusitis; pharyngitis; rhinitis; respiratory disorders or insufficiency; pulmonary infiltration; stridor; pneumothorax; hemoptysis; bronchospasm; rash; increased sweating; pruritus; skin ulceration; seborrhea; erythematous rash; maculopapular rash; vision abnormalities; taste perversions; eye abnormalities; eye pain; conjunctivitis; hypertension; palpitations; ECG abnormalities.

ADEFOVIR DIPIVOXIL

Tablets: 10 mg (*Rx*) *Hepsera* (Gilead Sciences)

Warning:

Severe acute exacerbations of hepatitis have been reported in patients who have discontinued anti-hepatitis B therapy, including adefovir. Closely monitor hepatic function in patients who discontinue anti-hepatitis B therapy.

In patients at risk of or having renal dysfunction, chronic administration of adefovir may result in nephrotoxicity. Closely monitor for renal function and adjust dose as required.

Human immunodeficiency virus (HIV) resistance may emerge in chronic hepatitis B patients with unrecognized or untreated HIV infection treated with anti-hepatitis B therapies, such as adefovir.

Lactic acidosis and severe hepatomegaly with steatosis, including fatal cases, have been reported with the use of nucleoside analogs alone or in combination with other antiretrovirals.

Indications

Chronic hepatitis B: Treatment of chronic hepatitis B in adults with active viral replication and persistent elevations in serum aminotransferases (ALT or AST) or histologically active disease.

Administration and Dosage

The recommended dose is 10 mg once daily without regard to food.

Dosage adjustment in renal impairment:

Adefovir Dosage Adjustment in Renal Impairment				
	Ccr (mL/min)			
	≥ 50	20 to 49	10 to 19	Hemodialysis patients
Recommended dose and dosing interval	10 mg q 24 h	10 mg q 48 h	10 mg q 72 h	10 mg q 7 days following dialysis

The pharmacokinetics of adefovir have not been evaluated in nonhemodialysis patients with Ccr below 10 mL/min; therefore, no dosing recommendation is available for these patients.

Actions

Pharmacology: Adefovir is an acyclic nucleotide analog of adenosine monophosphate.

Pharmacokinetics:

Absorption – The oral bioavailability of adefovir is 59%. Adefovir may be taken without regard to food.

Distribution – Binding of adefovir to plasma or proteins is less than or equal to 4%.

Metabolism/Excretion – Elimination half-life is approximately 7.48 hours. Adefovir is renally excreted.

Special populations –

Renal impairment: In subjects with impaired renal function or with end-stage renal disease requiring hemodialysis, C_{max}, AUC, and $T_{½}$ were increased. It is recommended that the dosing interval of adefovir be modified in these patients.

Contraindications

Previously demonstrated hypersensitivity to any of the components of the product.

Warnings

Exacerbations of hepatitis after discontinuation of treatment: Severe acute exacerbation of hepatitis has been reported in patients who have discontinued anti-hepatitis B therapy, including adefovir. Monitor patients who discontinue adefovir for hepatic function.

Nephrotoxicity: Nephrotoxicity characterized by a delayed onset of gradual increases in serum creatinine and decreases in serum phosphorus was shown to be the treatment-limiting toxicity of adefovir therapy at higher doses in HIV-infected patients (60 and 120 mg/day) and in chronic hepatitis B patients (30 mg/day). Chronic administration of adefovir (10 mg once daily) may result in nephrotoxicity. The overall risk of nephrotoxicity in patients with normal renal function is low. This is of special importance in patients at risk of or having renal dysfunction and patients taking concomitant nephrotoxic agents (eg, cyclosporine, tacrolimus, aminoglycosides, vancomycin, nonsteroidal anti-inflammatory drugs).

Lactic acidosis/severe hepatomegaly with steatosis: Lactic acidosis and severe hepatomegaly with steatosis, including fatal cases, have been reported with nucleoside analogs alone or in combination with antiretrovirals. A majority of these cases have been in women. Obesity and prolonged nucleoside exposure may be risk factors. Suspend treatment with adefovir in any patient who develops clinical or laboratory findings of lactic acidosis or hepatotoxicity (which may include hepatomegaly and steatosis even in the absence of marked transaminase elevations).

Elderly: Exercise caution in elderly patients who may have a greater frequency of decreased renal or cardiac function caused by concomitant disease or other drug therapy.

Pregnancy: Category C. To monitor fetal outcomes of pregnant women exposed to adefovir, a pregnancy registry has been established. Health care providers are encouraged to register patients by calling (800) 258-4263.

Lactation: It is not known whether adefovir is excreted in human milk. Instruct mothers not to breastfeed if they are taking adefovir.

Precautions

Monitoring:

Renal function – Monitor renal function in all patients during treatment with adefovir, particularly for those with pre-existing or other risks for renal impairment. Patients with renal insufficiency at baseline or during treatment may require dose adjustment. Evaluate the risks and benefits of adefovir treatment prior to discontinuing adefovir in a patient with treatment-emergent nephrotoxicity.

HIV resistance – Prior to initiating adefovir, offer HIV antibody testing to all patients. Treatment with anti-hepatitis B therapies, such as adefovir, that have activity against HIV in a chronic hepatitis B patient with unrecognized or untreated HIV infection may result in emergence of HIV resistance.

Drug coadministration – Closely monitor patients when adefovir is coadministered with drugs that are excreted renally or with other drugs known to affect renal function.

Drug Interactions

Drugs that may interact with adefovir include ibuprofen.

Coadministration of adefovir with drugs that reduce renal function or compete for active tubular secretion may increase serum concentrations of adefovir or these coadministered drugs.

Adverse Reactions

Adverse reactions may include the following: Asthenia, headache, abdominal pain, nausea, flatulence, diarrhea, dyspepsia. Laboratory abnormalities may include the following: Increased ALT or AST, hematuria, increased creatine kinase, increased amylase, glycosuria, increased serum creatinine greater than or equal to 0.3 mg/dL from baseline 4% (compared with 2% placebo).

CIDOFOVIR

Injection: 75 mg/mL (*Rx*) — *Vistide* (Gilead Sciences)

Warning:

Renal impairment is the major toxicity of cidofovir. Cases of acute renal failure resulting in dialysis or contributing to death have occurred with as few as 1 or 2 doses of cidofovir. To minimize possible nephrotoxicity, IV prehydration with normal saline and administration of probenecid must be used with each cidofovir infusion. Monitor renal function (serum creatinine and urine protein) within 48 hours prior to each dose of cidofovir and modify the dose for changes in renal function as appropriate. Cidofovir is contraindicated in patients who are receiving other nephrotoxic agents.

Neutropenia has been observed in association with cidofovir treatment. Monitor neutrophil counts during cidofovir therapy.

Cidofovir is indicated only for the treatment of cytomegalovirus (CMV) retinitis in patients with acquired immunodeficiency syndrome (AIDS).

In animal studies, cidofovir was carcinogenic, teratogenic, and caused hypospermia.

Indications

CMV *retinitis:* For the treatment of CMV retinitis in patients with AIDS.

Administration and Dosage

Do not administer by intraocular injection.

The recommended dosage, frequency, or infusion rate must not be exceeded. Cidofovir must be diluted in 100 mL 0.9% normal saline solution prior to administration. To minimize potential nephrotoxicity, probenecid and IV saline prehydration must be administered with each cidofovir infusion.

Induction treatment: The recommended dose of cidofovir for patients with a serum creatinine of ≤ 1.5 mg/dL, a Ccr > 55 mL/min, and a urine protein < 100 mg/dL (equivalent to < 2+ proteinuria) is 5 mg/kg body weight (given as an IV infusion at a constant rate over 1 hour) administered once weekly for 2 consecutive weeks. Because serum creatinine in patients with advanced AIDS and CMV retinitis may not provide a complete picture of the patient's underlying renal status, it is important to utilize the Cockcroft-Gault formula to more precisely estimate Ccr. As Ccr is dependent on serum creatinine and patient weight, it is necessary to calculate clearance prior to initiation of cidofovir. Calculate Ccr (mL/min) according to the following formula:

$$\text{Males: } \frac{\text{Weight (kg)} \times (140 - \text{age})}{72 \times \text{serum creatinine (mg/dL)}} = \text{Ccr}$$

Females: $0.85 \times$ above value

Maintenance treatment: The recommended maintenance dose of cidofovir is 5 mg/kg body weight (given as an IV infusion at a constant rate over 1 hour) administered once every 2 weeks.

Probenecid: Probenecid must be administered orally with each cidofovir dose. Administer 2 g 3 hours prior to the cidofovir dose and administer 1 g at 2 hours and again at 8 hours after completion of the 1-hour cidofovir infusion (for a total of 4 g).

Ingestion of food prior to each dose of probenecid may reduce drug-related nausea and vomiting. Administration of an antiemetic may reduce the potential for nausea associated with probenecid ingestion. In patients who develop allergic or hypersensitivity reactions to probenecid, consider the use of an appropriate prophylactic or therapeutic antihistamine or acetaminophen.

Zidovudine should be temporarily discontinued or decreased by 50% when coadministered with probenecid on the day of cidofovir infusion.

Hydration: Patients must receive a total of 1 L of 0.9% normal saline solution IV with each infusion of cidofovir. Infuse the saline solution over a 1- to 2-hour period immediately before the cidofovir infusion. Patients who can tolerate the additional fluid load should receive a second liter. If administered, initiate the second liter of saline at the start of the cidofovir infusion or immediately afterwards, and infuse over a 1- to 3-hour period.

Changes in renal function during therapy: For increases in serum creatinine (0.3 to 0.4 mg/dL), reduce the cidofovir dose from 5 to 3 mg/kg. Discontinue cidofovir therapy for an increase in serum creatinine of ≥ 0.5 mg/dL above baseline or development of ≥ 3+ proteinuria.

Pre-existing renal impairment: Cidofovir is contraindicated in patients with a serum Ccr > 1.5 mg/dL, a calculated Ccr of ≤ 55 mL/min, or a urine protein ≥ 100 mg/dL (equivalent to ≥ 2+ proteinuria).

Actions

Pharmacology: Cidofovir is a nucleotide analog that suppresses CMV replication by selective inhibition of viral DNA synthesis.

Resistance – Consider the possibility of viral resistance for patients who show a poor clinical response or experience recurrent retinitis progression during therapy.

Cross resistance – Ganciclovir or ganciclovir/foscarnet-resistant isolates that are cross-resistant to cidofovir have been obtained from drug-naive patients and from patients following ganciclovir or ganciclovir/foscarnet therapy. To date, all clinical isolates that exhibit high level resistance to ganciclovir, because of mutations in the DNA polymerase and UL97 genes, have been shown to be cross-resistant to cidofovir. Cidofovir is active against some, but not all, CMV isolates that are resistant to foscarnet. The incidence of foscarnet-resistant isolates that are resistant to cidofovir is not known.

Pharmacokinetics: Cidofovir must be administered with probenecid. Renal tubular secretion contributes to the elimination of cidofovir.

Cidofovir Pharmacokinetic Parameters Following 3 and 5 mg/kg Infusions With and Without Probenecid

	Cidofovir administered without probenecid		Cidofovir administered with probenecid	
Parameters	3 mg/kg	5 mg/kg	3 mg/kg	5 mg/kg
AUC (mcg•hr/mL)	≈ 20	28.3	≈ 25.7	≈ 40.8
C_{max} (end of infusion) (mcg/mL)	≈ 7.3	11.5	≈ 9.8	≈ 19.6
Vd_{ss} (mL/kg)	≈ 537		≈ 410	
Clearance (mL/min/1.73 m^2)	≈ 179		≈ 148	
Renal clearance (mL/min/1.73 m^2)	≈ 150		≈ 98.6	

In vitro, cidofovir was < 6% bound to plasma or serum proteins over the cidofovir concentration range 0.25 to 25 mcg/mL. CSF concentrations of cidofovir following IV infusion of cidofovir 5 mg/kg with concomitant probenecid and IV hydration were undetectable (< 0.1 mcg/mL, assay detection threshold) at 15 minutes after the end of a 1-hour infusion in 1 patient whose corresponding serum concentration was 8.7 mcg/mL.

Contraindications

Initiation of therapy in patients with a serum creatinine of > 1.5 mg/dL, a calculated Ccr of ≤ 55 mL/min, or a urine protein ≥ 100 mg/dL (equivalent to ≥ 2+ proteinuria); patients receiving agents with a nephrotoxic potential (such agents must be discontinued ≥ 7 days prior to starting cidofovir therapy); hypersensitivity to cidofovir; a history of clinically severe hypersensitivity to probenecid or other sulfa-containing medications; direct intraocular injection.

Warnings

Other CMV infections: The safety and efficacy of cidofovir have not been established for treatment of other CMV infections, congenital or neonatal CMV disease, or CMV disease in non-HIV-infected individuals.

Direct intraocular injection: May be associated with iritis, ocular hypotony, and permanent impairment of vision.

Nephrotoxicity: Dose-dependent nephrotoxicity is the major dose-limiting toxicity related to cidofovir administration. Monitor renal function (serum creatinine and urine protein) within 48 hours prior to each dose of cidofovir. Dose adjustment or discontinuation is required for changes in renal function while on therapy. Proteinuria may be an early indicator of cidofovir-related nephrotoxicity. Continued administration of cidofovir may lead to additional proximal tubular cell injury that may result in glycosuria; decreases in serum phosphate, uric acid, and bicarbonate; elevations in serum creatinine; or acute renal failure, in some cases, resulting in the need for dialysis. Patients with these adverse events occurring concurrently and meeting a criteria of Fanconi's syndrome have been reported. Renal function that did not return to baseline after drug discontinuation has been observed in clinical studies of cidofovir.

Because of the potential for increased nephrotoxicity, doses greater than the recommended dose must not be administered and the frequency or rate of administration must not be exceeded.

Hematological toxicity: Neutropenia may occur during cidofovir therapy. Monitor neutrophil count while receiving cidofovir therapy.

Metabolic acidosis: Decreased serum bicarbonate associated with proximal tubule injury and renal wasting syndrome (including Fanconi's syndrome) have been reported in patients receiving cidofovir. Cases of metabolic acidosis in association with liver dysfunction and pancreatitis resulting in death have been reported in patients receiving cidofovir.

Decreased intraocular pressure (OPV)/ocular hypotony: Monitor OPV during cidofovir therapy.

Fertility impairment: Studies showed inhibition of spermatogenesis in rats and monkeys. However, no adverse effects on fertility or reproduction were seen following once-weekly IV injections of cidofovir in male rats for 13 consecutive weeks.

Elderly: No studies of the safety and efficacy of cidofovir in patients > 60 years of age have been conducted. Because elderly individuals frequently have reduced glomerular filtration, pay particular attention to assessing renal function before and during cidofovir administration.

Pregnancy: *Category* C. Use cidofovir during pregnancy only if the potential benefit justifies the potential risk to the fetus.

Lactation: The US Public Health Service Centers for Disease Control and Prevention advises HIV-infected women not to breastfeed to avoid postnatal transmission of HIV to a child who may not be infected.

Children: Safety and efficacy in children have not been studied. The use of cidofovir in children with AIDS warrants extreme caution because of the risk of long-term carcinogenicity and reproductive toxicity. Administer cidofovir to children only after careful evaluation and only if the potential benefits of treatment outweigh the risks.

Precautions

Monitoring: Monitor serum creatinine and urine protein within 48 hours prior to each dose, and white blood cell counts with differential prior to each dose. In patients with proteinuria, administer IV hydration and repeat the test. Periodically monitor intraocular pressure, visual acuity, and ocular symptoms.

Uveitis/Iritis: Monitor patients for signs and symptoms of uveitis/iritis during cidofovir therapy.

Drug Interactions

Nephrotoxic agents: Concomitant administration of cidofovir and agents with nephrotoxic potential (eg, IV aminoglycosides [eg, tobramycin, gentamicin, amikacin], amphotericin B, foscarnet, IV pentamidine, vancomycin, and nonsteroidal anti-inflammatory agents) is contraindicated. Such agents must be discontinued ≥ 7 days prior to starting therapy with cidofovir.

Adverse Reactions

In clinical trials, cidofovir was withdrawn because of adverse events in 39% of patients treated with 5 mg/kg every other week as maintenance therapy.

Adverse reactions reported in more than 15% of patients include the following: Proteinuria (≥ 30 mg/dL), nausea/vomiting, fever, neutropenia (< 750 cells/mm^3), asthenia, headache, rash, infection, alopecia, diarrhea, pain, creatinine elevation (> 1.5 mg/dL), anemia, anorexia, dyspnea, chills, increased cough, oral moniliasis. Adverse reactions reported in more than 5% of patients include the following: Proteinuria (≥ 100 mg/dL), neutropenia (< 500 cells/mm^3), decreased intraocular pressure, decreased serum bicarbonate (≤ 16 mEq/L), fever, infection, creatinine elevation (≥ 2 mg/dL), pneumonia, dyspnea, nausea with vomiting. Renal toxicity and decrease from baseline IOP also were reported.

BILE ACID SEQUESTRANTS

CHOLESTYRAMINE	
Powder: 4 g anhydrous cholestyramine resin/9 g powder (*Rx*)	Various, *LoCHOLEST* (Warner Chilcott), *Questran* (Bristol-Myers Squibb)
4 g anhydrous cholestyramine resin/dose (*Rx*)	Various
4 g anhydrous cholestyramine resin/5.7 g powder (*Rx*)	*LoCHOLEST Light* (Warner Chilcott)
4 g anhydrous cholestyramine resin/5.5 g powder (*Rx*)	*Prevalite* (Upsher Smith)
4 g anhydrous cholestyramine resin/6.4 g powder (*Rx*)	*Questran Light* (Bristol-Myers Squibb)
COLESEVELAM HCl	
Tablets: 625 mg (*Rx*)	*Welchol* (Sankyo Parke Davis)
COLESTIPOL HCl	
Tablets: 1g (*Rx*)	*Colestid* (Pharmacia)
Granules: 5 g colestipol HCl/dose, 5 g colestipol HCl/7.5 g powder (*Rx*)	

Indications

Hyperlipoproteinemia: Adjunctive therapy for the reduction of elevated serum cholesterol in patients with primary hypercholesterolemia (elevated LDL) who do not respond adequately to diet.

Biliary obstruction (cholestyramine only): Relief of pruritus associated with partial biliary obstruction.

Administration and Dosage

Although generally given 3 to 4 times daily, there appears to be no advantage to dosing more frequently than twice daily.

CHOLESTYRAMINE:

Powder –

Adults: 4 g 1 to 2 times daily.

Maintenance dose: 8 to 16 g/day divided into 2 doses. Use gradual increases in dose with periodic assessment of lipid/lipoprotein levels at intervals of ≥ 4 weeks. Maximum recommended daily dose is 24 g.

Suggested time of administration is at mealtime but may be modified to avoid interference with absorption of other medications. Although the recommended dosing schedule is twice daily, it may be given in 1 to 6 per day.

COLESEVELAM: Take with liquid.

Monotherapy – The recommended starting dose is 3 tablets taken twice daily with meals or 6 tablets once daily with a meal. The dose can be increased to 7 tablets depending on desired therapeutic effect.

Combination therapy – For maximal therapeutic effect in combination with an HMG-CoA reductase inhibitor, the recommended dose of colesevalam is 3 tablets taken twice daily with meals or 6 tablets taken once daily with a meal. Doses of 4 to 6 tablets/day have been shown to be safe and effective when coadministered with an HMG-CoA reductase inhibitor or when the 2 drugs are dosed apart.

COLESTIPOL HCl:

Granules –

Adults: 5 to 30 g colestipol per day given once or in divided doses. The starting dose should be 5 g once or twice daily with a daily increment of 5 g at 1- or 2-month intervals.

Tablets – 2 to 16 g/day given once or in divided doses. The starting dose should be 2 g once or twice daily. Dosage increases of 2 g, once or twice daily, should occur at 1 or 2 month intervals.

Swallow tablets whole; do not cut, chew, or crush.

Actions

Pharmacology: Bile acid sequestering resins bind bile acids in the intestine to form an insoluble complex, which is excreted in the feces. This results in a partial removal of bile acids from the enterohepatic circulation, preventing their absorption. The lipid-lowering effect of 4 g cholestyramine equals 5 g colestipol.

Contraindications

Hypersensitivity to bile acid sequestering resins or any components of the products; complete biliary obstruction.

Warnings

Powder: To avoid accidental inhalation or esophageal distress, do not take powder or granules dry. Mix with fluids.

Pregnancy: These agents are not absorbed systemically and are not expected to cause fetal harm when given during pregnancy in recommended doses.

Lactation: Exercise caution when administering to a nursing woman. The possible lack of proper vitamin absorption may have an effect on nursing infants.

Children: Dosage schedules have not been established.

Precautions

Malabsorption: Because they sequester bile acids, these resins may interfere with normal fat absorption and digestion and may prevent absorption of fat-soluble vitamins such as A, D, E, and K.

Chronic use of resins may be associated with increased bleeding tendency due to hypoprothrombinemia associated with vitamin K deficiency.

Reduced folate: Reduction of serum or red cell folate has been reported over long-term administration of cholestyramine. Consider supplementation with folic acid.

Hyperchloremic acidosis: Prolonged use may cause hyperchloremic acidosis, especially in younger and smaller patients where relative dosage may be higher.

Constipation: These agents may produce or severely worsen preexisting constipation. Fecal impaction may occur and hemorrhoids may be aggravated.

Drug Interactions

These resins may delay or reduce the absorption of concomitant oral medication by binding the drugs in the gut. Take other drugs ≥ 1 hour before or 4 to 6 hours after these agents.

Drugs that may be affected by bile acid sequestrants include anticoagulants, aspirin, clindamycin, clofibrate, diclofenac, digitalis glycosides, furosemide, gemfibrozil, glipizide, hydrocortisone, imipramine, iopanoic acid, methyldopa, mycophenolate, nicotinic acid (niacin), penicillin G, phenytoin, phosphate supplements, piroxicam, propranolol, tetracyclines, thiazide diuretics, thyroid hormones, tolbutamide, ursodiol, and vitamins A, D, E, and K.

Adverse Reactions

GI:

Most common – Constipation; infection; flatulence.

Less frequent – Abdominal pain/distention/cramping; GI bleeding; belching; bloating; nausea; vomiting; diarrhea; loose stools; indigestion; dyspepsia; heartburn; anorexia; steatorrhea; rhinitis; pharyngitis.

Miscellaneous: Transient and modest elevations of AST, ALT, and alkaline phosphatase, (colestipol); liver function abnormalities (cholestyramine); pain, flu syndrome, accidental injury, asthenia (colesevelam); headache (including migraine and sinus); anxiety; vertigo; dizziness; lightheadedness; insomnia; fatigue; tinnitus; syncope; drowsiness; urticaria; dermatitis; asthma; wheezing; rash; backache; muscle/joint pains; hematuria; dysuria; burnt odor to urine; diuresis; uveitis; anorexia; weight loss/gain; increased libido; swollen glands; edema; weakness; shortness of breath; swelling of hands/feet.

CEPHALOSPORINS AND RELATED ANTIBIOTICS

CEFACLOR	
Tablets, extended release: 375 and 500 mg (*Rx*)	*Ceclor CD* (Eli Lilly)
Capsules: 250 and 500 mg (*Rx*)	Various, *Ceclor Pulvules* (Eli Lilly)
Powder for oral suspension: 125, 187, 250, and 375 mg/5 mL (*Rx*)	Various, *Ceclor* (Eli Lilly)
CEFADROXIL	
Capsules: 500 mg (as monohydrate) (*Rx*)	Various, *Duricef* (Bristol-Myers Squibb)
Tablets: 1 g (as monohydrate) (*Rx*)	Various, *Duricef* (Bristol-Myers Squibb)
Powder for oral suspension: 125, 250, and 500 mg/5 mL (*Rx*)	Various, *Duricef* (Bristol-Myers Squibb)
CEFAMANDOLE NAFATE	
Powder for injection: 1 g/10 mL and 2 g/20 mL (*Rx*)	*Mandol* (Lilly)
CEFAZOLIN SODIUM	
Powder for injection: 250 and 500 mg, 1, 5, 10, and 20 g (*Rx*)	Various, *Ancef* (GlaxoSmithKline), *Zolicef* (Apothecon), *Kefzol* (Eli Lilly)
Injection: 500 mg or 1 g (*Rx*)	*Ancef* (GlaxoSmithKline), *Kefzol* (Eli Lilly)
CEFDINIR	
Capsules: 300 mg (*Rx*)	*Omnicef* (Parke-Davis)
Oral suspension: 125 mg/5 mL (*Rx*)	*Omnicef* (Parke-Davis)
CEFDITOREN PIVOXIL	
Tablets: 200 mg (*Rx*)	*Spectracef* (TAP Pharm.)
CEFEPIME HCl	
Powder for injection: 500 mg, 1 and 2 g (*Rx*)	*Maxipime* (Dura)
CEFIXIME	
Tablets: 200 and 400 mg (*Rx*)	*Suprax* (Lederle)
Powder for oral suspension: 100 mg/5 mL (*Rx*)	*Suprax* (Lederle)
CEFMETAZOLE SODIUM	
Powder for injection: 1 and 2 g (*Rx*)	*Zefazone* (Pharmacia)
Injection: 1 and 2 g/50 mL (*Rx*)	*Zefazone* (Pharmacia)
CEFONICID SODIUM	
Powder for injection: 1 and 10 g (*Rx*)	*Monocid* (GlaxoSmithKline)
CEFOPERAZONE SODIUM	
Powder for injection: 1 and 2 g (*Rx*)	*Cefobid* (Roerig)
Injection: 1, 2, and 10 g (*Rx*)	*Cefobid* (Roerig)
CEFOTAXIME SODIUM	
Powder for injection: 500 mg, 1, 2, and 10 g (*Rx*)	*Claforan* (Aventis)
Injection: 1 and 2 g (*Rx*)	*Claforan* (Aventis)
CEFOTETAN DISODIUM	
Powder for injection: 1, 2, and 10 g (*Rx*)	*Cefotan* (AstraZeneca)
Injection: 1 and 2 g/50 mL (*Rx*)	*Cefotan* (AstraZeneca)
CEFOXITIN SODIUM	
Powder for injection: 1, 2, and 10 g (*Rx*)	*Mefoxin* (Merck)
Injection: 1 and 2 g (*Rx*)	*Mefoxin* (Merck)
CEFPODOXIME PROXETIL	
Tablets: 100 and 200 mg (*Rx*)	*Vantin* (Pharmacia)
Granules for suspension: 50 and 100 mg/5 mL (*Rx*)	*Vantin* (Pharmacia)
CEFPROZIL	
Tablets: 250 and 500 mg (as anhydrous) (*Rx*)	*Cefzil* (Bristol-Myers Squibb)
Powder for oral suspension: 125 and 250 mg (as anhydrous)/5 mL (*Rx*)	*Cefzil* (Bristol-Myers Squibb)
CEFTAZIDIME	
Powder for injection: 500 mg, 1, 2, 6, and 10 g (*Rx*)	*Fortaz* (GlaxoSmithKline), *Tazidime* (Eli Lilly), *Ceptaz* (GlaxoSmithKline), *Tazicef* (GlaxoSmithKline/Bristol-Myers Squibb)
Injection: 1 and 2 g (*Rx*)	*Fortaz* (GlaxoSmithKline), *Tazicef* (GlaxoSmithKline/Bristol-Myers Squibb)

CEFTIBUTEN	
Capsules: 400 mg (*Rx*)	*Cedax* (Schering-Plough)
Powder for oral suspension: 90 and 180 mg/5 mL (*Rx*)	*Cedax* (Schering-Plough)
CEFTIZOXIME SODIUM	
Powder for injection: 500 mg, 1, 2, and 10 g (as sodium) (*Rx*)	*Cefizox* (Fujisawa)
Injection: 1 and 2 g (as sodium) (*Rx*)	*Cefizox* (Fujisawa)
CEFTRIAXONE SODIUM	
Powder for injection: 250 and 500 mg, 1, 2, and 10 g (*Rx*)	*Rocephin* (Roche)
Injection: 1 and 2 g (*Rx*)	*Rocephin* (Roche)
CEFUROXIME	
Tablets: 125, 250, and 500 mg (*Rx*)	*Ceftin* (GlaxoSmithKline)
Suspension: 125 and 250 mg (as axetil)/5 mL (when reconstituted) (*Rx*)	*Ceftin* (GlaxoSmithKline)
Powder for injection: 750 mg, 1.5 and 7.5 g (as sodium)/vial (*Rx*)	Various, *Zinacef* (GlaxoSmithKline), *Kefurox* (Lilly)
Injection: 750 mg and 1.5 g (as sodium) (*Rx*)	*Zinacef* (GlaxoSmithKline)
CEPHALEXIN	
Capsules: 250 and 500 mg (*Rx*)	Various, *Keflex* (Dista), *Biocef* (Inter Ethical Labs)
Tablets: 250 and 500 mg and 1 g (*Rx*)	Various
Powder for oral suspension: 125 and 250 mg/5 mL (*Rx*)	Various, *Biocef* (Inter. Ethical Labs), *Keflex* (Dista)
CEPHALEXIN HCl MONOHYDRATE	
Tablets: 500 mg (*Rx*)	*Keftab* (Dista)
CEPHAPIRIN SODIUM	
Powder for injection: 1 g (*Rx*)	*Cefadyl* (Apothecon)
CEPHRADINE	
Capsules: 250 and 500 mg (*Rx*)	Various, *Velosef* (Bristol-Myers Squibb)
Powder for oral suspension: 125 and 250 mg/5 mL (when reconstituted) (*Rx*)	Various, *Velosef* (Bristol-Myers Squibb)
Powder for injection: 250 and 500 mg, 1 and 2 g (*Rx*)	*Velosef* (Bristol-Myers Squibb)
LORACARBEF	
Pulvules (capsules): 200 and 400 mg (*Rx*)	*Lorabid* (Eli Lilly)
Powder for oral suspension: 100 and 200 mg/5 mL (*Rx*)	*Lorabid* (Eli Lilly)

Indications

For approved indications, refer to the Administration and Dosage section.

Administration and Dosage

Duration of therapy: Continue administration for a minimum of 48 to 72 hours after fever abates or after evidence of bacterial eradication has been obtained.

Perioperative prophylaxis: Discontinue prophylactic use within 24 hours after the surgical procedure. In surgery where infection may be particularly devastating, prophylactic use may be continued for 3 to 5 days following surgery completion.

CEFACLOR:

Adults – Usual dosage is 250 mg every 8 hours. In severe infections or those caused by less susceptible organisms, dosage may be doubled.

Capsules: Food does not affect the extent of absorption.

Tablets, extended release: Administer with food to enhance absorption. Do not cut, crush, or chew.

Acute bacterial exacerbations of chronic bronchitis – 500 mg/12 hours for 7 days.

Secondary bacterial infection of acute bronchitis – 500 mg/12 hours for 7 days.

Pharyngitis or tonsillitis – 375 mg/12 hours for 10 days.

Uncomplicated skin and skin structure infections – 375 mg/12 hours for 7 to 10 days.

Children – Give 20 mg/kg/day in divided doses, every 8 hours. In more serious infections, otitis media, and infections caused by less susceptible organisms, administer 40 mg/kg/day, with a maximum dosage of 1 g/day.

Twice-daily treatment option: For otitis media and pharyngitis, the total daily dosage may be divided and administered every 12 hours.

CEFADROXIL: Can be given without regard to meals.

Urinary tract infections – For uncomplicated lower urinary tract infection (eg, cystitis), the usual dosage is 1 or 2 g/day in single or 2 divided doses. For all other urinary tract infections, the usual dosage is 2 g/day in 2 divided doses.

Skin and skin structure infections – 1 g/day in single or 2 divided doses.

Pharyngitis and tonsillitis –

Group A β-hemolytic streptococci: 1 g/day in single or 2 divided doses for 10 days.

Children –

Urinary tract infections, skin and skin structure infections: 30 mg/kg/day in divided doses every 12 hours.

Pharyngitis, tonsillitis: 30 mg/kg/day in single or 2 divided doses. For β-hemolytic streptococcal infections, continue treatment for at least 10 days.

Renal impairment – Adjust dosage according to Ccr rates to prevent drug accumulation.

Initial adult dose: 1 g: The maintenance dose (based on Ccr rate, mL/min/1.73 m^2) is 500 mg at the intervals below:

Cefadroxil Dosage in Renal Impairment	
Ccr (mL/min)	Dosage interval (hours)
0 to 10	36
10 to 25	24
25 to 50	12
> 50	No adjustment

CEFAMANDOLE NAFTATE:

Adults – Usual dosage range is 500 mg to 1 g every 4 to 8 hours; 500 mg every 6 hours is adequate in uncomplicated skin and skin structure infections. In uncomplicated urinary tract infections, 500 mg every 8 hours; in more serious urinary tract infections, the dose may be increased to 1 g every 8 hours. In severe infections, administer 1 g at 4- to 6-hour intervals. In life-threatening infections or infections caused by less susceptible organisms, up to 2 g every 4 hours may be needed.

Infants and children – 50 to 100 mg/kg/day in equally divided doses every 4 to 8 hours is effective for most infections susceptible to cefamandole. This may be increased to 150 mg/kg/day (not to exceed the maximum adult dose) for severe infections.

Perioperative prophylaxis –

Adults: 1 or 2 g IM or IV, ½ to 1 hour prior to the surgical incision, followed by 1 or 2 g every 6 hours for 24 to 48 hours.

Children (3 months of age and older): 50 to 100 mg/kg/day in equally divided doses by the routes and schedule designated above.

Renal function impairment – Reduce dosages and monitor the serum levels. After an initial dose of 1 to 2 g (depending on the severity of infection), follow maintenance dosage in table.

Maintenance Cefamandole Dosage Guide for Patients with Renal Impairment			
Renal function impairment	Ccr (mL/min/ 1.73 m^2)	Life-threatening infections (Maximum dosage)	Less severe infections
Normal	> 80	2 g q 4 h	1 to 2 g q 6 h
Mild	50 to 80	1.5 g q 4 h or 2 g q 6 h	0.75 to 1.5 g q 6 h
Moderate	25 to 50	1.5 g q 6 h or 2 g q 8 h	0.75 to 1.5 g q 8 h
Sever e	10 to 25	1 g q 6 h or 1.25 g q 8 h	0.5 to 1 g q 8 h
Marked	2 to 10	0.67 g q 8 h or 1 g q 12 h	0.5 to 0.75 g q 12 h
None	< 2	0.5 g q 8 h or 0.75 g q 12 h	0.25 to 0.5 g q 12 h

CEFAZOLIN SODIUM: Total daily dosages are the same for IM and IV administration.

Mild infections caused by susceptible gram-positive cocci – 250 to 500 mg every 8 hours.

Moderate-to-severe infections – 500 mg to 1 g every 6 to 8 hours.

Pneumococcal pneumonia – 500 mg every 12 hours.

Severe, life-threatening infections (eg, endocarditis, septicemia) – 1 to 1.5 g every 6 hours. Rarely, 12 g/day have been used.

Acute uncomplicated urinary tract infections – 1 g every 12 hours.

Perioperative prophylaxis –

Preoperative: 1 g IV or IM, ½ to 1 hour prior to surgery.

Intraoperative (≥ 2 hrs): 0.5 to 1 g IV or IM during surgery at appropriate intervals.

Postoperative: 0.5 to 1 g IV or IM every 6 to 8 hours for 24 hours after surgery.

Renal function impairment – All reduced dosage recommendations apply after an initial loading dose appropriate to the severity of the infection.

Cefazolin Dosage in Renal Impairment

Serum Creatinine (mg %)	Ccr (mL/min)	Dose		Dosage interval (hrs)
		≤ 1.5	≥ 55	
≤ 1.5	55	250 to 500	500 to 1000	6 to 8
1.6 to 3	35 to 54	250 to 500	500 to 1000	≥ 8
3.1 to 4.5	11 to 34	125 to 250	250 to 500	12
≥ 4.6	10	125 to 250	250 to 500	18 to 24

Children –

Mild to moderately severe infections: A total daily dosage of 25 to 50 mg/kg (≈ 10 to 20 mg/lb) in 3 or 4 equal doses.

Severe infections: Total daily dosage may be increased to 100 mg/kg (45 mg/lb).

CEFDINIR:

Adults/Adolescents – Capsules may be taken without regard to meals.

Cefdinir Dosage in Adults and Adolescents (≥ 13 years of age)

Type of infection	Dosage	Duration
Community-acquired pneumonia	300 mg q 12 hrs	10 days
Acute exacerbations of chronic bronchitis	300 mg q 12 hrs or 600 mg q 24 hrs	10 days 10 days
Acute maxillary sinusitis	300 mg q 12 hrs or 600 mg q 24 hrs	10 days 10 days
Pharyngitis/Tonsillitis	300 mg q 12 hrs or 600 mg q 24 hrs	5 to 10 days 10 days
Uncomplicated skin and skin structure infections	300 mg q 12 hrs	10 days

Children –

Powder for oral suspension: The recommended dosage in pediatric patients is 14 mg/kg, up to a maximum dose of 600 mg/day. Oral suspension may be administered without regard to meals.

Cefdinir Dosage in Pediatric Patients (6 Months Through 12 Years of Age)

Type of infection	Dosage	Duration
Acute bacterial otitis media	7 mg/kg q 12 h or 14 mg/kg q 24 h	10 days 10 days
Acute maxillary sinusitis	7 mg/kg q 12 h or 14 mg/kg q 24 h	10 days 10 days

Cefdinir Dosage in Pediatric Patients (6 Months Through 12 Years of Age)		
Type of infection	Dosage	Duration
Pharyngitis/Tonsillitis	7 mg/kg q 12 h or 14 mg/kg q 24 h	5 to 10 days 10 days
Uncomplicated skin and skin structure infections	7 mg/kg q 12 h	10 days

Cefdinir for Oral Suspension Pediatric Dosage Chart		
Weight		
kg	lb	125 mg/5 mL
9	20	2.5 mL (½ tsp) q 12 h or 5 mL (1 tsp) q 24 h
18	40	5 mL (1 tsp) q 12 h or 10 mL (2 tsp) q 24 h
27	60	7.5 mL (1½ tsp) q 12 h or 15 mL (3 tsp) q 24 h
36	80	10 mL (2 tsp) q 12 h or 20 mL (4 tsp) q 24 h
≥ 43[1]	95	12 mL (2½ tsp) q 12 h or 24 mL (5 tsp) q 24 h

[1] Pediatric patients who weigh ≥ 43 kg should receive the maximum daily dose of 600 mg.

Renal function impairment – For adult patients with Ccr < 30 mL/min, the dose of cefdinir should be 300 mg given once daily.

For pediatric patients with a Ccr of < 30 mL/min/1.73 m^2, the dose of cefdinir should be 7 mg/kg (≤ 300 mg) given once daily.

Hemodialysis – Hemodialysis removes cefdinir from the body. In patients maintained on chronic hemodialysis, the recommended initial dosage regimen is a 300 mg or 7 mg/kg dose every other day. At the conclusion of each hemodialysis session, give 300 mg (or 7 mg/kg). Subsequent doses (300 mg or 7 mg/kg) are then administered every other day.

CEFDITOREN PIVOXIL:

Cefditoren Dosage and Administration in Adults and Adolescents ≥ 12 Years of Age[1]		
Type of infection	Dosage	Duration (days)
Acute bacterial exacerbation of chronic bronchitis	400 mg BID	
Pharyngitis/Tonsillitis		10
Uncomplicated skin and skin structure infections	200 mg BID	

[1] Take with meals.

Renal impairment – It is recommended that ≤ 200 mg twice daily be administered to patients with moderate renal impairment (Ccr 30 to 49 mL/min/1.73 m^2) and 200 mg every day be administered to patients with severe renal impairment (Ccr < 30 mL/min/1.73 m^2).

CEFEPIME:

Recommended Dosage Schedule for Cefepime			
Site and type of infection	Dose	Frequency	Duration (days)
Mild to moderate uncomplicated or complicated urinary tract infections, including pyelonephritis, caused by *Escherichia coli, Klebsiella pneumoniae*, or *Proteus mirabilis*.[1]	0.5 to 1 g IV/IM[2]	q 12 hrs	7 to 10
Severe uncomplicated or complicated urinary tract infections, including pyelonephritis, caused by *E. coli* or *K. pneumoniae*.[1]	2 g IV	q 12 hrs	10

Recommended Dosage Schedule for Cefepime			
Site and type of infection	Dose	Frequency	Duration (days)
Moderate to severe pneumonia caused by *Streptococcus pneumoniae*,[1] *Pseudomonas aeruginosa, K. pneumoniae*, or *Enterobacter* sp.	1 to 2 g IV	q 12 hrs	10
Moderate to severe uncomplicated skin and skin structure infections caused by *Staphylococcus aureus* or *Streptococcus pyogenes*.	2 g IV	q 12 hrs	10
Empiric therapy for febrile neutropenic patients.	2 g IV	q 8 hrs	7[3]
Complicated intra-abdominal infections (used in combination with metronidazole) caused by *E. coli*, viridans group streptococci, *P. aeruginosa, K. pneumoniae, Enterobacter* species, or *Bacteroides fragilis*.	2 g IV	q 12 hrs	7 to 10

[1] Including cases associated with concurrent bacteremia.

[2] IM route of administration is indicated only for mild to moderate, uncomplicated, or complicated UTIs caused by *E. coli* when the IM route is a more appropriate route of drug administration.

[3] Or until resolution of neutropenia. In patients whose fever resolves but who remain neutropenic for > 7 days, frequently re-evaluate the need for continued antimicrobial therapy.

Empiric therapy for febrile neutropenic patients – As monotherapy for empiric treatment of febrile neutropenic patients. In patients at high risk for severe infection (including patients with a history of recent bone marrow transplantation, with hypotension at presentation, with an underlying hematologic malignancy, or with severe or prolonged neutropenia), antimicrobial monotherapy may not be appropriate. Insufficient data exist to support the efficacy of cefepime monotherapy in such patients.

Complicated intra-abdominal infections – In combination with metronidazole for complicated intra-abdominal infections caused by *E. coli*, viridans group streptococci, *P. aeruginosa, K. pneumoniae, Enterobacter* sp., or *B. fragilis*.

Pediatric patients (2 months to 16 years of age) – Treatment of uncomplicated and complicated urinary tract infections (including pyelonephritis), uncomplicated skin and skin structure infections, pneumonia, and as empiric therapy for febrile neutropenic patients.

Renal function impairment – In patients with impaired renal function (Ccr < 60 mL/min), adjust the dose of cefepime to compensate for the slower rate of renal elimination. The recommended initial dose should be the same as in patients with normal renal function.

In patients undergoing hemodialysis, ≈ 68% of the total amount of cefepime present in the body at the start of dialysis will be removed during a 3-hour dialysis period. Give a repeat dose, equivalent to the initial dose, at the completion of each dialysis session.

In elderly patients with renal insufficiency, adjust dosage and administration.

In patients undergoing continuous ambulatory peritoneal dialysis, administer cefepime at normal recommended doses at a dosage interval of every 48 hours.

<table>
<tr><th colspan="5">Recommended Cefepime Maintenance Schedule in Patients with Renal Impairment</th></tr>
<tr><th>Ccr (mL/min)</th><th colspan="4">Recommended maintenance schedule</th></tr>
<tr><td>> 60</td><td>500 mg q 12 h [1]</td><td>1 g q 12 h</td><td>2 g q 12 h</td><td>2 g q 8 h</td></tr>
<tr><td>30 to 60</td><td rowspan="2">500 mg q 24 h</td><td>1 g q 24 h</td><td>2 g q 24 h</td><td>2 g q 12 h</td></tr>
<tr><td>11 to 29</td><td>500 mg q 24 h</td><td>1 g q 24 h</td><td>2 g q 24 h</td></tr>
<tr><td>≤ 11</td><td>250 mg q 24 h</td><td>250 mg q 24 h</td><td>500 mg q 24 h</td><td>1 g q 24 h</td></tr>
</table>

[1] Normal recommended dosing schedule.

IV administration – Administer over ≈ 30 minutes. Reconstitute with 50 or 100 mL of a compatible IV fluid. Cefepime is compatible at concentrations of 1 to 40 mg/

mL with 0.9% Sodium Chloride Injection, 5% and 10% Dextrose Injection, M/6 Sodium Lactate Injection, 5% Dextrose and 0.9% Sodium Chloride Injection, Lactated Ringers and 5% Dextrose Injection, *Normosol-R* or *Normosol-M* in 5% Dextrose injection.

Cefepime Admixture Stability

Cefepime concentration (mg/mL)	Admixture and concentration	IV Infusion solutions	Stability time for RT/L[1] (20° to 25°C) (hours)	Stability time for refrigeration (2° to 8°C)
40	Amikacin 6 mg/mL	NS[2] or D5W[3]	24	7 days
40	Ampicillin 1 mg/mL	D5W[3]	8	8 hrs
40	Ampicillin 10 mg/mL	D5W[3]	2	8 hrs
40	Ampicillin 1 mg/mL	NS[2]	24	48 hrs
40	Ampicillin 10 mg/mL	NS[2]	8	48 hrs
4	Ampicillin 40 mg/mL	NS[2]	8	8 hrs
4 to 40	Clindamycin phosphate 0.25 to 6 mg/mL	NS[2] or D5W[3]	24	7 days
4	Heparin 10 to 50 units/mL	NS[2] or D5W[3]	24	7 days
4	Potassium chloride 10 to 40 mEq/L	NS[2] or D5W[3]	24	7 days
4	Theophylline 0.8 mg/mL	D5W[3]	24	7 days
1 to 4	na	*Aminosyn II* 4.25% with electrolytes and calcium	8	3 days
0.125 to 0.25	na	*Inpersol* with 4.25% dextrose	24	7 days

[1] Ambient room temperature and light.
[2] 0.9% sodium chloride injection.
[3] 5% dextrose injection.

Admixture compatibility/incompatibility: Intermittent IV infusion with a Y-type administration set can be accomplished with compatible solutions; however, during infusion of a solution containing cefepime, it is desirable to discontinue the other solution.

Solutions of cefepime, like those of most β-lactam antibiotics, should not be added to solutions of ampicillin at a concentration > 40 mg/mL, and should not be added to metronidazole, vancomycin, gentamicin, tobramycin, netilmicin sulfate, or aminophylline because of potential interaction. However, if concurrent therapy with cefepime is indicated, each of these antibiotics can be administered separately.

IM administration: Reconstitute cefepime with the following diluents: Sterile Water for Injection, 0.9% Sodium Chloride, 5% Dextrose Injection, 0.5% or 1% lidocaine HCl, or Sterile Bacteriostatic Water for Injection with parabens or benzyl alcohol.

Pediatric dosing: The usual recommended daily dosage in pediatric patients up to 40 kg in weight is 50 mg/kg/dose administered every 12 hours (every 8 hours for febrile neutropenic patients), for 7 to 10 days, depending on the indication and severity of infection. The maximum dose for pediatric patients (2 months to 16 years of age) should not exceed the recommended adult dose.

Renal impairment – Data in pediatric patients with impaired renal function are not available; however, because cefepime pharmacokinetics are similar in adult and pediatric patients, changes in dosing regimen similar to those in adults are recommended for pediatric patients.

CEFIXIME:

Adults – 400 mg/day as a single 400 mg tablet (recommended for gonococcal infections) or as 200 mg every 12 hours.

Children – 8 mg/kg/day suspension as a single daily dose or as 4 mg/kg every 12 hours. Treat children > 50 kg or > 12 years of age with the recommended adult dose.

Treat otitis media with the suspension.

For *S. pyogenes* infections, administer cefixime for ≥ 10 days.

Renal function impairment –

Cefixime Dosing in Renal Impairment	
Ccr (mL/min)	Dosage
> 60	Standard
21 to 60 or renal hemodialysis	75% of standard
≤ 20 or continuous ambulatory peritoneal dialysis	50% of standard

CEFMETAZOLE SODIUM:

Adults –

General guidelines: 2 g IV every 6 to 12 hours for 5 to 14 days.

Prophylaxis –

Cefmetazole Dosing Regimen for Prophylaxis	
Surgery	Dosing Regimen
Vaginal hysterectomy	2 g single dose 30 to 90 min before surgery or 1 g doses 30 to 90 min before surgery and repeated 8 and 16 hrs later.
Abdominal hysterectomy	1 g doses 30 to 90 min before surgery and repeated 8 and 16 hrs later.
Cesarean section	2 g single dose after clamping cord or 1 g doses after clamping cord; repeated at 8 and 16 hrs.
Colorectal surgery	2 g single dose 30 to 90 min before surgery or 2 g doses 30 to 90 min before surgery and repeated 8 to 16 hrs later.
Cholecystectomy (high risk)	1 g doses 30 to 90 min before surgery and repeated 8 and 16 hrs later.

Renal function impairment –

Cefmetazole Dosage Guidelines in Renal Function Impairment			
Renal function	Ccr (mL/min/1.73 m^2)	Dose (g)	Frequency (hrs)
Mild impairment	50 to 90	1 to 2	q 12
Moderate impairment	30 to 49	1 to 2	q 16
Severe impairment	10 to 29	1 to 2	q 24
Essentially no function	< 10	1 to 2	q 48[1]

[1] Administered after hemodialysis.

CEFONICID SODIUM:

Adults – Usual dose is 1 g/24 hours, IV or by deep IM injection. Doses > 1 g/day are rarely necessary; however, up to 2 g/day have been well tolerated.

General Cefonicid Dosage Guidelines (IM or IV)		
Type of infection	Daily dosage (g)	Frequency
Uncomplicated urinary tract	0.5	once every 24 hrs
Mild to moderate	1	once every 24 hrs
Severe or life-threatening	2[1]	once every 24 hrs
Surgical prophylaxis	1	1 hr preoperatively

[1] When administering 2 g IM doses once daily, divide dose in half and give each half in a different large muscle mass.

Preoperative prophylaxis – Administer 1 g 1 hour prior to appropriate surgical procedures to provide protection from most infections caused by susceptible organisms for ≈ 24 hours after administration.

Renal function impairment – Renal function impairment requires modification of dosage. Following an initial loading dosage of 7.5 mg/kg, IM or IV, follow maintenance schedule below. It is not necessary to administer additional dosage following dialysis.

Cefonicid Dosage in Adults with Reduced Renal Function		
Ccr (mL/min/ 1.73^2)	Mild to moderate infections	Severe infections
60 to 79	10 mg/kg q 24 hr	25 mg/kg q 24 hr
40 to 59	8 mg/kg q 24 hr	20 mg/kg q 24 hr
20 to 39	4 mg/kg q 24 hr	15 mg/kg q 24 hr
10 to 19	4 mg/kg q 48 hr	15 mg/kg q 48 hr
5 to 9	4 mg/kg q 3 to 5 days	15 mg/kg q 3 to 5 days
< 5	3 mg/kg q 3 to 5 days	4 mg/kg q 3 to 5 days

CEFOPERAZONE SODIUM: Administer IM or IV.

Usual adult dose is 2 to 4 g/day administered in equally divided doses every 12 hours.

In severe infections or infections caused by less sensitive organisms, the total daily dose or frequency may be increased. Patients have been successfully treated with a total daily dosage of 6 to 12 g divided into 2, 3, or 4 administrations ranging from 1.5 to 4 g/dose. A total daily dose of 16 g by constant infusion has been given without complications.

Hepatic disease or biliary obstruction – In general, total daily dosage > 4 g should not be necessary.

Renal function impairment –

Hemodialysis: The half-life is reduced slightly during hemodialysis. Thus, schedule dosing to follow a dialysis period.

CEFOTAXIME SODIUM:

Adults – Administer IV or IM. Maximum daily dosage should not exceed 12 g.

Cefotaxime Dosage Guidelines for Adults		
Type of infection	Daily dosage (g)	Frequency and route
Gonococcal urethritis/cervicitis in males and females	0.5	0.5 g IM (single dose)
Rectal gonorrhea in females	0.5	0.5 g IM (single dose)
Rectal gonorrhea in males	1	1 g IM (single dose)
Uncomplicated infections	2	1 g every 12 hrs IM or IV
Moderate to severe infections	3 to 6	1 to 2 g every 8 hrs IM or IV
Infections commonly needing higher dosage (eg, septicemia)	6 to 8	2 g every 6 to 8 hrs IV
Life-threatening infections	≤ 12	2 g every 4 hrs IV

Perioperative prophylaxis: 1 g IV or IM, 30 to 90 minutes prior to surgery.

Cesarean section: Administer the first 1 g dose IV as soon as the umbilical cord is clamped. Administer the second and third doses as 1 g IV or IM at 6- and 12-hour intervals after the first dose.

Children –

Cefotaxime Dosage Guidelines in Pediatrics			
Age	Weight (kg)	Dosage schedule	Route
0 to 1 week	-	50 mg/kg every 12 hrs	IV
1 to 4 weeks	-	50 mg/kg every 8 hrs	IV
1 month to 12 years	< 50[1]	50 to 180 mg/kg/day in 4 to 6 divided doses[2]	IV or IM

[1] For children ≥ 50 kg, use adult dosage.
[2] Use higher doses for more severe or serious infections including meningitis.

Renal function impairment – In patients with estimated Ccr < 20 mL/min/1.73 m^2, reduce dosage by ½.

When only serum creatinine is available, the following formula may be used to convert this value into Ccr. The serum creatinine should represent steady-state renal function.

CDC-recommended treatment schedules for gonorrhea –

Disseminated gonococcal infection: Give 1 g IV every 8 hours.

Gonococcal ophthalmia in adults: For penicillinase-producing *Neisseria gonorrhoeae* (PPNG), give 500 mg IV 4 times/day.

CEFOTETAN DISODIUM:

Adults – The usual dosage is 1 or 2 g IV or IM every 12 hours for 5 to 10 days. Determine proper dosage and route of administration by the condition of the patient, severity of the infection and susceptibility of the causitive organism.

General Cefotetan Dosage Guidelines		
Type of Infection	Daily Dose	Frequency and Route
Urinary tract	1 to 4 g	500 mg every 12 hrs IV or IM 1 or 2 g every 24 hrs IV or IM 1 or 2 g every 12 hrs IV or IM
Skin/Skin structure		2 g q 24 hrs IV
Mild to moderate[2]	2 g	1 g q 12 hrs IV or IM
Severe	4 g	2 g q 12 hrs IV
Other sites	2 to 4 g	1 or 2 g every 12 hrs IV or IM
Severe	4 g	2 g every 12 hrs IV
Life-threatening	6 g[1]	3 g every 12 hrs IV

[1] Maximum daily dosage should not exceed 6 g.
[2] Treat *K. pneumoniae* skin and skin structure infections with 1 or 2 g every 12 hours IV or IM.

Prophylaxis – To prevent postoperative infection in clean contaminated or potentially contaminated surgery in adults, give a single 1 or 2 g IV dose 30 to 60 minutes prior to surgery. In patients undergoing cesarean section, give the dose as soon as the umbilical cord is clamped.

Renal function impairment – Reduce the dosage schedule using the following guidelines:

Cefotetan Dosage in Renal Impairment		
Ccr (mL/min)	Dose	Frequency
> 30	Usual recommended dose[1]	Every 12 hrs
10 to 30	Usual recommended dose[1]	Every 24 hrs
< 10	Usual recommended dose[1]	Every 48 hrs

[1] Dose determined by the type and severity of infection and susceptibility of the causitive organism.

Alternatively, the dosing interval may remain constant at 12-hour intervals, but reduce dose by ½ for patients with a Ccr of 10 to 30 mL/min, and by ¼ for patients with a Ccr < 10 mL/min.

Dialysis – Cefotetan is dialyzable; for patients undergoing intermittent hemodialysis, give ¼ of the usual recommended dose every 24 hours on days between dialysis and ½ of the usual recommended dose on the day of dialysis.

CEFOXITIN SODIUM:

Adult – Adult dosage range is 1 to 2 g every 6 to 8 hours.

Cefoxitin Dosage Guidelines

Type of infection	Daily dosage	Frequency and route
Uncomplicated (pneumonia, urinary tract, cutaneous)[1]	3 to 4 g	1 g every 6 to 8 hrs IV or IM
Moderately severe or severe	6 to 8 g	1 g every 4 hrs or 2 g every 6 to 8 hrs IV
Infections commonly requiring higher dosage (eg, gas gangrene)	12 g	2 g every 4 hrs or 3 g every 6 hrs IV

[1] Including patients in whom bacteremia is absent or unlikely.

Uncomplicated gonorrhea – 2 g IM with 1 g oral probenecid given concurrently or up to 30 minutes before cefoxitin.

Prophylactic use, surgery – Administer 2 g IV or IM 30 to 60 minutes prior to surgery followed by 2 g every 6 hours after the first dose for no more than 24 hours.

Prophylactic use, cesarean section – Administer 2 g IV as soon as the umbilical cord is clamped. If a 3-dose regimen is used, give the second and third 2 g dose IV, 4 and 8 hours after the first dose.

Prophylactic use, transurethral prostatectomy – Administer 1 g prior to surgery; 1 g every 8 hours for up to 5 days.

Renal function impairment –

Adults: Initial loading dose is 1 to 2 g. Mantenance doses:

Maintenance Cefoxitin Dosage in Renal Impairment

Renal function	Ccr (mL/min/1.73 m^2)	Dose (g)	Frequency (hrs)
Mild impairment	30 to 50	1 to 2	8 to 12
Moderate impairment	10 to 29	1 to 2	12 to 24
Severe impairment	5 to 9	0.5 to 1	12 to 24
Essentially no function	< 5	0.5 to 1	24 to 48

Hemodialysis – Administer a loading dose of 1 to 2 g after each hemodialysis. Give the maintenance dose as indicated in the table above.

Infants and children ≥ 3 months: 80 to 160 mg/kg/day divided every 4 to 6 hours. Use higher dosages for more severe or serious infections. Do not exceed 12 g/day.

Prophylactic use (≥ 3 months) – 30 to 40 mg/kg/dose every 6 hours

Renal function impairment – Modify consistent with recommendation for adults.

CDC recommended treatment schedules for acute pelvic inflammatory disease (PID) – 2 g IV every 6 hours plus 100 mg doxycycline IV or orally every 12 hours.

CEFPODOXIME PROXETIL: Administer with food to enhance absorption.

Dosage/Duration of Cefpodoxime

Type of infection	Total daily dose	Dose frequency	Duration
Adults ≥ 13 years of age			
Acute community-acquired pneumonia	400 mg	200 mg every 12 hrs	14 days
Acute bacterial exacerbations of chronic bronchitis (tablets)	400 mg	200 mg every 12 hrs	10 days
Uncomplicated gonorrhea (men and women) and rectal gonococcal infections (women)	200 mg	single dose	
Skin and skin structure	800 mg	400 mg every 12 hrs	7 to 14 days
Pharyngitis/Tonsillitis	200 mg	100 mg every 12 hrs	5 to 10 days

Dosage/Duration of Cefpodoxime			
Type of infection	Total daily dose	Dose frequency	Duration
Uncomplicated urinary tract infection	200 mg	100 mg every 12 hrs	7 days
Children (5 months through 12 years of age):[1]			
Acute otitis media	10 mg/kg/day (max 400 mg/day)	10 mg/kg every 24 hrs (max 400 mg/dose) or 5 mg/kg every 12 hrs (max 200 mg/dose)	10 days
Pharyngitis/Tonsillitis	10 mg/kg/day (max 200 mg/day)	5 mg/kg every 12 hrs (max 100 mg/dose)	5 to 10 days

[1] Do not exceed adult recommended doses.

Renal dysfunction – For patients with severe renal impairment (Ccr < 30 mL/min), increase the dosing intervals to every 24 hours. In patients maintained on hemodialysis, use a frequency of 3 times/week after hemodialysis.

CEFPROZIL:

Cefprozil Dosage and Duration		
Population/Infection	Dosage (mg)	Duration (days)
Adults (≥ 13 years of age)		
Pharyngitis/Tonsillitis	500 q 24 hrs	10[1]
Acute sinusitis (use higher dose for moderate to severe infections)	250 q 12 hrs or 500 q 12 hrs	10
Secondary bacterial infection of acute bronchitis and acute bacterial exacerbation of chronic bronchitis	500 q 12 hrs	10
Uncomplicated skin and skin structure infections	250 q 12 hrs, 500 q 24 hrs, or 500 q 12 hrs	10
Children (2 to 12 years of age)[2]		
Pharyngitis/Tonsillitis	7.5 mg/kg q 12 hrs	10[1]
Uncomplicated skin and skin structure infections	20 mg/kg q 24 hrs	10
Infants and children (6 months to 12 years of age)[2]		
Otitis media	15 mg/kg q 12 hrs	10
Acute sinusitis (use higher dose for moderate to severe infections)	7.5 mg/kg q 12 hrs or 15 mg/kg q 12 hrs	10

[1] For infections caused by *S. pyogenes*, administer for ≥ 10 days.
[2] Not to exceed adult recommended doses.

Renal function impairment – For Ccr of 30 to 120 mL/min, use standard dosage and dosing interval. For Ccr < 30 mL/min, use a dosage 50% of standard at the standard dosing interval.

Cefprozil is in part removed by hemodialysis; therefore, administer after the completion of hemodialysis.

CEFTAZIDIME:

Ceftazidime Dosage Guidelines		
Patient/Infection site	Dose	Frequency
Adults Usual recommended dose	1 g IV or IM	q 8 to 12 h
Uncomplicated urinary tract infections	250 mg IV or IM	q 12 h
Complicated urinary tract infections	500 mg IV or IM	q 8 to 12 h
Uncomplicated pneumonia; mild skin and skin structure infections	500 mg to 1 g IV or IM	q 8 h

Ceftazidime Dosage Guidelines		
Patient/Infection site	Dose	Frequency
Bone and joint infections	2 g IV	q 12 h
Serious gynecological and intra-abdominal infections		
Meningitis	2 g IV	q 8 h
Very severe life-threatening infections, especially in immunocompromised patients		
Pseudomonal lung infections in cystic fibrosis patients w/normal renal function[1]	30 to 50 mg/kg IV up to 6 g/day	q 8 h
Neonates (0 to 4 weeks)	30 mg/kg IV	q 12 h
Infants and children (1 month to 12 years of age)	30 to 50 mg/kg IV up to 6 g/day[2]	q 8 h

[1] Although clinical improvement has been shown, bacteriological cures cannot be expected in patients with chronic respiratory disease and cystic fibrosis.
[2] Reserve the higher dose for immunocompromised children or children with cystic fibrosis or meningitis.

Renal function impairment – Ceftazidime is excreted by the kidneys, almost exclusively by glomerular filtration. In patients with impaired renal function (glomerular filtration rate (GFR) < 50 mL/min), reduce dosage to compensate for slower excretion. In patients with suspected renal insufficiency, give an initial loading dose of 1 g. Estimate GFR to determine the appropriate maintenance dose.

Ceftazidime Dosage in Renal Impairment		
Ccr (mL/min)	Recommended unit dose of ceftazidime	Frequency of dosing
31 to 50	1 g	q 12 h
16 to 30	1 g	q 24 h
6 to 15	500 mg	q 24 h
≤ 5	500 mg	q 48 h

In patients with severe infections who normally receive 6 g ceftazidime daily were it not for renal insufficiency, the unit dose given in the table above may be increased by 50% or the dosing frequency increased appropriately.

Dialysis – Give a 1 g loading dose, followed by 1 g after each hemodialysis period.

Ceftazidime also can be used in patients undergoing intraperitoneal dialysis (IPD) and continuous ambulatory peritoneal dialysis (CAPD). Give a loading dose of 1 g, followed by 500 mg every 24 hours. In addition to IV use, ceftazidime can be incorporated in the dialysis fluid at a concentration of 250 mg per 2 L of dialysis fluid.

CEFTIBUTEN: Ceftibuten suspension must be administered ≥ 2 hours before or 1 hour after a meal.

Ceftibutin Dosage and Duration			
Type of infection	Daily maximum dose	Dose and frequency	Duration
Adults ≥ 12 years of age			
Acute bacterial exacerbations of chronic bronchitis caused by *H. influenzae*, *M. catarrhalis*, or *Streptococcus pneumoniae*	400 mg	400 mg/day	10 days
Pharyngitis and tonsillitis caused by *S. pyogenes*			
Acute bacterial otitis media caused by *H. influenzae*, *M. catarrhalis*, or *S. pyogenes*			

Ceftibutin Dosage and Duration			
Type of infection	Daily maximum dose	Dose and frequency	Duration
Children			
Pharyngitis and tonsillitis caused by *S. pyogenes*	400 mg	9 mg/kg/day	10 days
Acute bacterial otitis media caused by *H. influenzae*, *M. catarrhalis*, or *S. pyogenes*			

Ceftibuten Oral Suspension Pediatric Dosage Chart[1]			
Weight			
kg	lb	90 mg/5 mL	180 mg/5 mL
10	22	5 mL (1 tsp)/day	2.5 mL (½ tsp)/day
20	44	10 mL (2 tsp)/day	5 mL (1 tsp)/day
40	88	20 mL (4 tsp)/day	10 mL (2 tsp)/day

[1] Children > 45 kg should receive the maximum daily dose of 400 mg.

Renal function impairment – Ceftibuten may be given at normal doses in impaired renal function with creatinine clearance of ≥ 50 mL/min. Dosing recommendations for patients with varying degrees of renal insufficiency are presented in the following table.

Ceftibuten Dosage in Renal Impairment	
Ccr (mL/min)	Recommended dosing schedules
> 50	9 mg/kg or 400 mg q 24 h (normal dosing schedule)
30 to 49	4.5 mg/kg or 200 mg q 24 h
5 to 29	2.25 mg/kg or 100 mg q 24 h

Hemodialysis patients – In patients undergoing hemodialysis 2 or 3 times weekly, a single 400 mg dose of ceftibuten capsules or a single dose of 9 mg/kg (maximum of 400 mg) oral suspension may be given at the end of each hemodialysis session.

CEFTIZOXIME SODIUM:

Adults – Usual dosage is 1 or 2 g every 8 to 12 hours.

Ceftizoxime Dosage Guidelines in Adults		
Type of infection	Daily dose (g)	Frequency and route
Uncomplicated urinary tract	1	500 mg every 12 hrs IM or IV
Pelvic inflammatory disease (PID)[1]	6	2 g every 8 hrs IV
Other sites	2 to 3	1 g every 8 to 12 hrs IV or IM
Severe or refractory	3 to 6	1 g every 8 hours IM or IV 2 g every 8 to 12 hrs IM [1] or IV
Life-threatening[2]	9 to 12	3 to 4 g every 8 hrs IV

[1] Dosages up to 2 g every 4 hours have been given.
[2] Divide 2 g IM doses and give in different large muscle masses.

Urinary tract infections – Higher dosage is recommended.

Gonorrhea, uncomplicated – A single 1 g IM injection is the usual dose.

Life-threatening infections – The IV route may be preferable for patients with bacterial septicemia, localized parenchymal abscesses (such as intra-abdominal abscess), peritonitis or other severe or life-threatening infections.

In those patients with normal renal function, the IV dosage is 2 to 12 g daily. In conditions such as bacterial septicemia, 6 to 12 g/day IV may be given initially for several days, and the dosage gradually reduced according to clinical response and laboratory findings.

Pediatric –

Children (≥ 6 months): 50 mg/kg every 6 to 8 hours. Dosage may be increased to 200 mg/kg/day. Do not exceed the maximum adult dose for serious infection.

Renal function impairment: Renal function impairment requires modification of dosage. Following an initial loading dose of 500 mg to 1 g IM or IV, use the maintenance dosing schedule in the following table.

Hemodialysis – No additional supplemental dosing is required following hemodialysis; give the dose (according to the table below) at the end of dialysis.

Ceftizoxime Dosage in Adults with Renal Impairment			
Renal function	Ccr (mL/min)	Less severe infections	Life-threatening infections
Mild impairment	50 to 79	500 mg q 8 h	750 mg to 1.5 g q 8 h
Moderate to severe impairment	5 to 49	250 to 500 mg q 12 h	500 mg to 1 g q 12 h
Dialysis patients	0 to 4	500 mg q 48 h or 250 mg q 24 h	500 mg to 1 g q 48 h or 500 mg q 24 h

CEFTRIAXONE SODIUM: Administer IV or IM.

Adults – Usual daily dosage is 1 to 2 g once a day (or in equally divided doses twice a day) depending on type and severity of infection. Do not exceed a total daily dose of 4 g.

Uncomplicated gonococcal infections: Give a single IM dose of 250 mg.

Surgical prophylaxis: Give a single 1 g dose ½ to 2 hours before surgery.

Children – To treat serious infections other than meningitis, administer 50 to 75 mg/kg/day (not to exceed 2 g) in divided doses every 12 hours.

Meningitis: 100 mg/kg/day (not to exceed 4 g). Thereafter, a total daily dose of 100 mg/kg/day (not to exceed 4 g/day) is recommended. May give daily dose once per day or in equally divided doses every 12 hours. Usual duration is 7 to 14 days.

Skin and skin structure infections: Give 50 to 75 mg/kg once daily (or in equally divided doses twice daily), not to exceed 2 g.

CDC-recommended treatment schedules for chancroid, gonorrhea, and acute PID –

Chancroid (Haemophilus ducreyi infection): 250 mg IM as a single dose.

Gonococcal infections:

Uncomplicated – 125 mg IM in a single dose plus 1 g azithromycin in single oral dose or 100 mg doxycycline twice a day for 7 days.

Conjunctivitis – 1 g IM single dose.

Disseminated – 1 g IM or IV every 24 hours.

Meningitis/Endocarditis – 1 to 2 g IV every 12 hours for 10 to 14 days (meningitis) or for ≥ 4 weeks (endocarditis).

Children (< 45 kg) – With bacteremia or arthritis, use 50 mg/kg (maximum, 1 g) IM or IV in a single dose for 7 days. For meningitis, increase duration to 10 to 14 days and maximum dose to 2 g.

Infants – 25 to 50 mg/kg/day IV or IM in a single daily dose, not to exceed 125 mg. For disseminated infection, continue for 7 days, with a duration of 7 to 14 days with documented meningitis.

Acute PID (ambulatory): 250 mg IM plus doxycycline.

CEFUROXIME:

Oral – Tablets and suspension are not bioequivalent and not substitutable on a mg/mg basis.

Tablets: The tablets may be given without regard to meals.

Suspension: Administer with food.

Dosage for Cefuroxime Axetil Tablets		
Population/Infection	Dosage	Duration (days)
Adults (≥ 13 years of age)		
Pharyngitis/Tonsillitis	250 mg bid	10
Acute bacterial exacerbations of chronic bronchitis[1]	250 or 500 mg bid	10
Secondary bacterial infections of acute bronchitis		5 to 10
Uncomplicated skin and skin structure infections	250 or 500 mg bid	10
Uncomplicated urinary tract infections	125 or 250 mg bid	7 to 10
Uncomplicated gonorrhea	1000 mg once	single dose
Early Lyme disease	500 mg bid	20
Children who can swallow tablets whole[2]		
Pharyngitis/Tonsillitis	125 mg bid	10
Acute otitis media	250 mg bid	10

[1] Safety and efficacy of drug administered < 10 days in patients with acute exacerbations of chronic bronchitis have not been established.
[2] Do not exceed adult recommended doses.

Dosage for Cefuroxime Axetil Suspension			
Population/Infection	Dosage	Daily maximum dose	Duration (days)
Infants and children (3 months to 12 years of age)			
Pharyngitis/Tonsillitis	20 mg/kg/day divided bid	500 mg	10
Acute otitis media	30 mg/kg/day divided bid	1000 mg	10
Impetigo	30 mg/kg/day divided bid	1000 mg	10

Renal failure: Because cefuroxime is renally eliminated, its half-life will be prolonged in patients with renal failure.

Parenteral –

Dosage:

Adults – 750 mg to 1.5 g IM or IV every 8 hours, usually for 5 to 10 days.

Cefuroxime Dosage Guidelines		
Type of infection	Daily dosage (g)	Frequency
Uncomplicated urinary tract, skin and skin structure, disseminated gonococcal, uncomplicated pneumonia	2.25	750 mg every 8 hrs
Severe or complicated	4.5	1.5 g every 8 hrs
Bone and joint	4.5	1.5 g every 8 hrs
Life-threatening or caused by less susceptible organisms	6	1.5 g every 6 hrs
Bacterial meningitis	9	≤ 3 g every 8 hrs
Uncomplicated gonococcal	1.5 g IM[1]	single dose

[1] Administered at 2 different sites together with 1 g oral probenecid.

Preoperative prophylaxis: For clean-contaminated or potentially contaminated surgical procedures, administer 1.5 g IV prior to surgery (≈ ½ to 1 hour before). Thereafter, give 750 mg IV or IM every 8 hours when the procedure is prolonged.

For preventative use during open heart surgery, give 1.5 g IV at the induction of anesthesia and every 12 hours thereafter for a total of 6 g.

Renal function impairment: Reduce dosage.

Parenteral Cefuroxime Dosage in Renal Impairment (Adults)	
Ccr (mL/min)	Dose and frequency
> 20	750 mg to 1.5 g every 8 hrs
10 to 20	750 mg every 12 hrs
< 10	750 mg every 24 hrs [1]

[1] Because cefuroxime is dialyzable, give patients on hemodialysis a further dose at the end of the dialysis.

Infants and children (> 3 months) – 50 to 100 mg/kg/day in equally divided doses every 6 to 8 hours. Use 100 mg/kg/day (not to exceed maximum adult dose) for more severe or serious infections.

Bone and joint infections: 150 mg/kg/day (not to exceed maximum adult dose) in equally divided doses every 8 hours.

Bacterial meningitis: Initially, 200 to 240 mg/kg/day IV in divided doses every 6 to 8 hours.

In renal insufficiency, modify dosage frequency per adult guidelines.

CEPHALEXIN:

Adults – 1 to 4 g/day in divided doses.

Usual dose: 250 mg every 6 hours.

Streptococcal pharyngitis, skin and skin structure infections, uncomplicated cystitis in patients > 15 years: 500 mg every 12 hours.

May need larger doses for more severe infections or less susceptible organisms. If dose is > 4 g/day, use parenteral drugs.

Children – Do not exceed adult recommended doses.

Monohydrate: 25 to 50 mg/kg/day in divided doses. For streptococcal pharyngitis in patients > 1 year of age and for skin and skin structure infections, divide total daily dose and give every 12 hours. In severe infections, double the dose.

Otitis media – 75 to 100 mg/kg/day in 4 divided doses.

β-hemolytic streptococcal infections – Continue treatment for ≥ 10 days.

HCl monohydrate – Safety and efficacy not established for use in children.

CEPHAPIRIN SODIUM:

Adults – 500 mg to 1 g every 4 to 6 hours IM or IV. The lower dose is adequate for certain infections, such as skin and skin structure and most urinary tract infections; the higher dose is recommended for more serious infections.

Serious or life-threatening infections – Up to 12 g daily. Use the IV route when high doses are indicated.

Renal function impairment: Patients with reduced renal function (moderately severe oliguria or serum creatinine > 5 mg/100 mL) may be treated adequately with a lower dose, 7.5 to 15 mg/kg every 12 hours. Patients who are to be dialyzed should receive the same dose just prior to dialysis and every 12 hours thereafter.

Perioperative prophylaxis: 1 to 2 g IM or IV administered ½ to 1 hour prior to the start of surgery; 1 to 2 g during surgery (administration modified depending on duration of operation); 1 to 2 g IV or IM every 6 hours for 24 hours postoperatively.

Children – Recommended total daily dose is 40 to 80 mg/kg (20 to 40 mg/lb) administered in 4 equally divided doses.

Infants – Cephapirin has not been extensively studied in infants; therefore, in the treatment of children < 3 months of age, consider the relative benefit to risk.

CEPHRADINE:

Oral – May be given without regard to meals.

Adults:

Skin, skin structure, and respiratory tract infections (other than lobar pneumonia) – Usual dose is 250 mg every 6 hours or 500 mg every 12 hours.

Lobar pneumonia – 500 mg every 6 hours or 1 g every 12 hours.

Uncomplicated urinary tract infections – The usual dose is 500 mg every 12 hours. In more serious infections and prostatitis, 500 mg every 6 hours or 1 g every 12 hours. Severe or chronic infections may require larger doses (up to 1 g every 6 hours).

Children: No adequate information is available on the efficacy of twice a day regimens in children < 9 months of age. For children > 9 months, the usual dose is 25 to 50 mg/kg/day, in equally divided doses every 6 or 12 hours. For otitis media caused by *H. influenzae*, 75 to 100 mg/kg/day in equally divided doses every 6 or 12 hours is recommended; do not exceed 4 g/day.

All patients regardless of age and weight: Larger doses (up to 1 g 4 times/day) may be given for severe or chronic infections.

Parenteral – Parenteral therapy may be followed by oral. To minimize pain and induration, inject IM deep into a large muscle mass.

Adults: Daily dose is 2 to 4 g in equally divided doses 4 times/day, IM or IV. In bone infections, the usual dosage is 1 g IV 4 times/day. A dose of 500 mg 4 times/day is adequate in uncomplicated pneumonia, skin and skin structure infections, and most urinary tract infections. In severe infections, dose may be increased by giving every 4 hours or by increasing dose up to a maximum of 8 g/day.

Perioperative prophylaxis – Recommended doses are 1 g IV or IM administered 30 to 90 minutes prior to the start of surgery, followed by 1 g every 4 to 6 hours after the first dose for 1 or 2 doses, or for up to 24 hours postoperatively.

Cesarean section – Give 1 g IV as soon as the umbilical cord is clamped. Give the second and third doses as 1 g IM or IV at 6 to 12 hours after the first dose.

Infants and children – 50 to 100 mg/kg/day in 4 equally divided doses; determine by age, weight, and infection severity.

Renal impairment dosage –

Patients not on dialysis:

Cephradine Dosage in Renal Impairment		
Ccr (mL/min)	Dose (mg)	Time interval (hours)
> 20	500	6
5 to 20	250	6
< 5	250	12

Patients on chronic, intermittent dialysis: 250 mg initially; repeat at 12 hours and after 36 to 48 hours.

LORACARBEF: Administer ≥ 1 hour before or 2 hours after a meal.

Dosage/Duration of Loracarbef		
Population/Infection	Dosage (mg)	Duration (days)
Adults ≥ 13 years of age		
Lower respiratory tract		
Secondary bacterial infection of acute bronchitis	200 to 400 q 12 hrs	7
Acute bacterial exacerbation of chronic bronchitis	400 q 12 hrs	7
Pneumonia	400 q 12 hrs	14
Upper respiratory tract		
Pharyngitis/Tonsillitis	200 q 12 hrs	10[1]
Sinusitis	400 q 12 hrs	10
Skin and skin structure		
Uncomplicated	200 q 12 hrs	7
Urinary tract		
Uncomplicated cystitis	200 q 24 hrs	7
Uncomplicated pyelonephritis	400 q 12 hrs	14
Infants and children (6 months to 12 years)[2]		
Upper respiratory tract		
Acute otitis media[3]	30 mg/kg/day in divided doses q 12 hrs	10
Acute maxillary sinusitis		
Pharyngitis/Tonsillitis	15 mg/kg/day in divided doses q 12 hrs	10[1]

Dosage/Duration of Loracarbef		
Population/Infection	Dosage (mg)	Duration (days)
Skin and skin structure		
Impetigo	15 mg/kg/day in divided doses q 12 hrs	7

[1] In treatment of infections caused by *S. pyogenes*, administer for ≥ 10 days.
[2] Do not exceed adult recommended doses.
[3] Use suspension; it is more rapidly absorbed than capsules, resulting in higher peak plasma concentrations when given at the same dose.

Renal function impairment – Use usual dose and schedule in patients with Ccr levels ≥ 50 mL/min. Patients with Ccr between 10 and 49 mL/min may be given half the recommended dose at the usual dosage interval. Patients with Ccr levels < 10 mL/min may receive recommended dose given every 3 to 5 days; patients on hemodialysis should receive another dose following dialysis.

Actions

Pharmacology: Cephalosporins are structurally and pharmacologically related to penicillins. **Cefoxitin** and **cefotetan** (cephamycins) and **loracarbef** (a carbacephem) are included because of their similarity.

Cephalosporins inhibit mucopeptide synthesis in the bacterial cell wall, making it defective and osmotically unstable. The drugs are usually bactericidal, depending on organism susceptibility, dose, tissue concentrations, and the rate at which organisms are multiplying. They are more effective against rapidly growing organisms forming cell walls.

Pharmacokinetics:

Pharmacokinetic Parameters of Cephalosporins										
			Half-Life							
	Drug	Routes	Normal renal function (minutes)	ESRD[1] (hours)	Hemodialysis (hours)	Protein bound (%)	Recovered unchanged in urine (%)	Peak serum level 1 g IV dose (mcg/mL)	Sodium (mEq/g)
First	Cefadroxil	Oral	78-96	20-25	3-4	20	> 90	—	—
First	Cefazolin	IM-IV	90–120	3-7	9-14	80-86	60-80	185	2-2.1
First	Cephalexin	Oral	50-80	19-22	4-6	10	> 90	—	—
First	Cephapirin	IM-IV	36	1.8-4	1.8	44-50	70	73	2.4
First	Cephradine	Oral/IM-IV	48-80	8-15	—	8-17	> 90	86	6[2]
Second	Cefaclor	Oral	35-54	2-3	1.6-2.1	25	60-85	—	—
Second	Cefamandole	IM-IV	30-60	8-11	7	70	65-85	139	3.3
Second	Cefmetazole	IM-IV	72-90	—	—	65	85	—	2
Second	Cefonicid	IM-IV	270	11	—	90	99	221.3	3.7
Second	Cefotetan	IM-IV	180-276	13-35	5	88-90	51-81	158	3.5
Second	Cefoxitin	IV	40-60	20	4	73	85	110	2.3
Second	Cefprozil	Oral	78	5.2-5.9	decreased	36	60	—	—
Second	Cefuroxime	Oral/IM-IV	80	16-22[3]	3.5	50	66-100	100[4]	2.4[3]
Second	Loracarbef	Oral	60	32	4	25	> 90	—	—

Pharmacokinetic Parameters of Cephalosporins

	Drug	Routes	Half-Life			Protein bound (%)	Recovered unchanged in urine (%)	Peak serum level 1 g IV dose (mcg/mL)	Sodium (mEq/g)
			Normal renal function (minutes)	ESRD[1] (hours)	Hemodialysis (hours)				
Third	Cefdinir	Oral	100	16	3.2	60-70	12-18	—	—
	Cefepime	IM-IV	102-138	17-21	11-16	20	85	79	—
	Cefixime	Oral	180-240	11.5	—	65	50	—	—
	Cefoperazone	IM-IV	120	1.3-2.9	2	82-93	20-30	73-153	1.5
	Cefotaxime	IM-IV	60	3-11	2.5	30-40	60	42-102	2.2
	Cefpodoxime[5]	Oral	120-180	9.8	—	21-29	29-33	—	—
	Ceftazidime	IM-IV	114-120	14-30	—	< 10	80-90	69-90	2.3
	Ceftibuten	Oral	144	13.4-22.3	2-4	65	56	—	—
	Ceftizoxime	IM-IV	102	25-30	6	30	80	60-87	2.6
	Ceftriaxone	IM-IV	348-522	15.7	14.7	85-95	33-67	151	3.6

[1] ESRD = End stage renal disease (Ccr < 10 mL/min/1.73 m^2).
[2] Also available in sodium-free form.
[3] Injection only.
[4] Following 1.5 g IV dose.
[5] Extended spectrum agent.

Cephalexin, cephradine, cefaclor, cefixime, cefprozil, cefadroxil, ceftibuten, and **loracarbef** are well absorbed from the GI tract. Cephalosporins are widely distributed to most tissues and fluids. First and second generation agents do not readily enter cerebrospinal fluid (CSF), except **cefuroxime**, even when meninges are inflamed. Third generation compounds (little data for cefixime) readily diffuse into the CSF of patients with inflamed meninges. However, CSF levels of **cefoperazone** are relatively low. Most cephalosporins and metabolites are primarily excreted renally.

Microbiology:

Organisms Generally Susceptible to Cephalosporins																											
Organisms		First Generation					Second Generation									Third Generation										Organisms	
✓ = generally susceptible ‡ = demonstrated in vitro activity		Cefadroxil	Cefazolin	Cephalexin	Cephapirin	Cephradine	Cefaclor	Cefamandole	Cefonicid	Cefoxitin	Cefuroxime	Cefmetazole	Cefotetan	Cefprozil	Loracarbef	Cefdinir	Cefepime[1]	Cefixime	Cefoperazone	Cefotaxime	Cefpodoxime[2]	Ceftazidime	Ceftibuten	Ceftizoxime	Ceftriaxone	✓ = generally susceptible ‡ = demonstrated in vitro activity	
Gram-positive	*Staphylococci*[3]	✓	✓	✓[4]	✓	✓	✓[4]		✓[4]	✓	✓	✓	✓	✓	✓	✓[5]	✓[6]		✓	✓[5]	✓[4]	✓		✓	✓	*Staphylococci*[3]	Gram-positive
	Staphylococcus aureus							✓								✓[5]										*Staphylococcus aureus*	
	Staphylococcus epidermidis							✓			‡				‡	‡[6]										*Staphylococcus epidermidis*	
	Staphylococcus saprophyticus										‡				✓											*Staphylococcus saprophyticus*	
	Streptococci, beta-hemolytic	✓	✓	✓	✓	✓	✓	✓	✓	✓	✓	✓	✓	✓	✓		‡	✓	✓	✓	✓	✓		✓	✓	*Streptococci*, beta-hemolytic	
	Streptococcus agalactiae										‡				‡	‡										*Streptococcus agalactiae*	
	Streptococcus bovis														‡											*Streptococcus bovis*	
	Streptococcus pneumoniae	✓	✓	✓	✓	✓	✓	✓	✓	✓	✓	✓	✓	✓	✓	✓[7]	✓	✓	✓	✓	✓	✓	✓[7]	✓	✓	*Streptococcus pneumoniae*	
	Streptococcus pyogenes						✓		✓		✓	✓	✓	✓	✓	✓	✓[8]	✓	✓	✓	✓	✓	✓	✓	✓	*Streptococcus pyogenes*	
	Streptococcus viridans														‡	‡										*Streptococcus viridans*	

Organisms Generally Susceptible to Cephalosporins																											
Organisms		First Generation					Second Generation									Third Generation										Organisms	
✓ = generally susceptible ‡ = demonstrated in vitro activity		Cefadroxil	Cefazolin	Cephalexin	Cephapirin	Cephradine	Cefaclor	Cefamandole	Cefonicid	Cefoxitin	Cefuroxime	Cefmetazole	Cefotetan	Cefprozil	Loracarbef	Cefdinir	Cefepime[1]	Cefixime	Cefoperazone	Cefotaxime	Cefpodoxime[2]	Ceftazidime	Ceftibuten	Ceftizoxime	Ceftriaxone	✓ = generally susceptible ‡ = demonstrated in vitro activity	
Gram-negative	*Acinetobacter* sp.																‡		✓[4]	✓		‡		✓	‡	*Acinetobacter* sp	Gram-negative
	Citrobacter sp.								‡		✓[4]	‡	‡	‡	‡	‡	‡	‡	✓	✓	‡	✓		‡	‡	*Citrobacter* sp	
	Enterobacter sp.		✓[4]						‡		✓[4]	‡	✓				✓		✓	✓		✓		✓	✓	*Enterobacter* sp	
	Escherichia coli	✓	✓	✓	✓	✓	✓	✓	✓	✓	✓	✓	✓	‡	✓	‡	✓	✓	✓	✓	✓	✓		✓	✓	*Escherichia coli*	
	Haemophilus influenzae		✓	✓	✓	✓	✓[5]	✓	✓[5]	✓[5]	✓[5]	✓[5]	✓[5]	✓[5]	✓[5]	✓[5]	‡[5]	✓[5]	✓[5]	✓[5]	✓[5]	✓[5]	✓[5]	✓[5]	✓[5]	*Haemophilus influenzae*	
	Haemophilus parainfluenzae						‡				‡				‡	✓[5]		‡[5]		✓	‡	‡			✓	*Haemophilus parainfluenzae*	
	Hafnia alvei																‡									*Hafnia alvei*	
	Klebsiella sp.	✓	✓	✓	✓	✓	✓	✓[4]	✓	✓	✓	✓	✓	‡	‡	‡	✓	‡	✓	✓	✓	✓		✓	✓	*Klebsiella* sp	
	Klebsiella pneumoniae						‡																			*Klebsiella pneumoniae*	
	Moraxella (Branhamella) catarrhalis	‡		‡			✓[5]				‡	‡	‡	✓[5]	✓[5]	✓[5]	‡[5]	✓[5]			✓	✓	✓[5]	‡		*Moraxella (Branhamella) catarrhalis*	
	Morganella (Proteus) morganii							✓	✓	✓	✓[4]	✓	✓				‡		✓	✓		‡		✓	✓	*Morganella (Proteus) morganii*	

Organisms Generally Susceptible to Cephalosporins																										
Organisms		First Generation					Second Generation									Third Generation										Organisms
✓ = generally susceptible ‡ = demonstrated in vitro activity		Cefadroxil	Cefazolin	Cephalexin	Cephapirin	Cephradine	Cefaclor	Cefamandole	Cefonicid	Cefoxitin	Cefuroxime	Cefmetazole	Cefotetan	Cefprozil	Loracarbef	Cefdinir	Cefepime[1]	Cefixime	Cefoperazone	Cefotaxime	Cefpodoxime[2]	Ceftazidime	Ceftibuten	Ceftizoxime	Ceftriaxone	✓ = generally susceptible ‡ = demonstrated in vitro activity
Gram-negative (cont'd.)	*Neisseria catarrhalis*			✓																						*Neisseria catarrhalis*
	Neisseria gonorrhoeae						‡		‡	✓	✓	‡	‡	‡	‡[3]			‡	✓[5]	✓	✓[4]	‡		✓	✓	*Neisseria gonorrhoeae*
	Neisseria meningitidis										✓								‡	✓		✓		‡	✓	*Neisseria meningitidis*
	Pasteurella multocida														‡											*Pasteurella multocida*
	Proteus inconstans										‡															*Proteus inconstans*
	Proteus mirabilis	✓	✓	✓	✓	✓	✓	✓	✓	✓	✓	✓	✓	‡	‡	‡	✓	✓	✓	✓	✓	✓		✓	✓	*Proteus mirabilis*
	Proteus vulgaris							✓[4]	✓	✓		✓	✓				‡	‡	✓	✓	‡	✓		✓	✓	*Proteus vulgaris*
	Providencia sp.									✓	✓	✓	✓				‡	‡		‡		‡		‡	‡	*Providencia* sp
	Providencia rettgeri							✓	✓	✓	✓	‡	✓				‡	‡	✓	✓	‡	‡		✓	‡	*Providencia rettgeri*
	Pseudomonas aeruginosa																✓		✓	✓[4]		✓		✓[4]	✓[4]	*Pseudomonas aeruginosa*
	Salmonella sp.										✓	‡	‡	‡	‡			‡	‡	‡		‡		‡	‡	*Salmonella* sp
	Salmonella typhi																			‡				‡	‡	*Salmonella typhi*
	Serratia sp.												‡				‡	‡	✓	✓		✓		✓	✓	*Serratia* sp
	Shigella sp.										✓	‡	‡	‡	‡			‡	‡	‡		‡		‡	‡	*Shigella* sp
	Yersinia enterocolitica												✓		‡											*Yersinia enterocolitica* (Gram-negative (con't))

Organisms Generally Susceptible to Cephalosporins																											
Organisms		First Generation					Second Generation									Third Generation										Organisms	
✓ = generally susceptible; ‡ = demonstrated in vitro activity		Cefadroxil	Cefazolin	Cephalexin	Cephapirin	Cephradine	Cefaclor	Cefamandole	Cefonicid	Cefoxitin	Cefuroxime	Cefmetazole	Cefotetan	Cefprozil	Loracarbef	Cefdinir	Cefepime[1]	Cefixime	Cefoperazone	Cefotaxime	Cefpodoxime[2]	Ceftazidime	Ceftibuten	Ceftizoxime	Ceftriaxone	✓ = generally susceptible; ‡ = demonstrated in vitro activity	
Anaerobes	*Bacteroides* sp.						✓	✓		✓	✓	✓	✓[4]	‡					✓	✓		✓[4]		‡	✓	*Bacteroides* sp	Anaerobes
	Bacteroides fragilis									✓		✓	✓						✓	✓				✓	‡	*Bacteroides fragilis*	
	Clostridium sp.							✓	‡	✓	✓	✓	✓	‡	‡				✓	✓		‡		‡	‡	*Clostridium* sp	
	Clostridium difficile												‡	‡					‡							*Clostridium difficile*	
	Eubacterium sp.																		‡						‡	*Eubacterium* sp	
	Fusobacterium sp.							✓	‡		✓	✓	✓	‡	‡				‡	✓				‡	‡	*Fusobacterium* sp	
	Peptococcus sp.						‡	✓	‡	✓	✓	‡	✓		‡				✓	✓		‡		✓	‡	*Peptococcus* sp	
	Peptococcus niger						‡								‡											*Peptococcus niger*	
	Peptostreptococcus sp.						‡	✓	‡	✓	✓	‡	✓	‡	‡				✓	✓	‡	‡		✓	‡	*Peptostreptococcus* sp	
	Porphyromonas asaccharolytica												‡													*Porphyromonas asaccharolytica*	
	Prevotella bivia												✓													*Prevotella bivia*	
	Prevotella digiens												✓													*Prevotella digiens*	
	Prevotella melaninogenica												‡													*Prevotella melaninogenica*	
	Prevotella oralis												‡													*Prevotella oralis*	
	Propionibacterium acnes						‡								‡											*Propionibacterium acnes*	
	Propionibacterium sp.												‡													*Propionibacterium* sp	
	Veillonella sp.												‡													*Veillonella* sp	
Other	*Borrelia burgdorferi*										✓															*Borrelia burgdorferi*	Other

[1] Extended spectrum agent.
[2] Some other references consider this fourth generation.
[3] Coagulase-positive, coagulase-negative and penicillinase-producing.
[4] Some strains are resistant.
[5] Including some β-lactamase-producing strains.
[6] Methicillin-susceptible strains only.
[7] Penicillin-susceptible strains only.
[8] Lancefield's Group A streptococci.

Contraindications

Hypersensitivity to cephalosporins or related antibiotics.

Cefditoren: Cefditoren is contraindicated in patients with carnitine deficiency or inborn errors of metabolism that may result in clinically significant carnitine deficiency because use of cefditoren causes renal excretion of carnitine.

Cefditoren contains sodium caseinate, a milk protein. Do not administer cefditoren to patients with milk protein hypersensitivity (not lactose intolerance).

Warnings

Hypersensitivity: Reactions range from mild to life-threatening. Before therapy is instituted, inquire about previous hypersensitivity reactions to cephalosporins and penicillins.

Cross-allergenicity with penicillin: Administer cautiously to penicillin-sensitive patients. There is evidence of partial cross-allergenicity; cephalosporins cannot be assumed to be an absolutely safe alternative to penicillin in the penicillin-allergic patient. The estimated incidence of cross-sensitivity is 5% to 16%; however, it is possibly as low as 3% to 7%.

Serum sickness-like reactions: (erythema multiforme or skin rashes accompanied by polyarthritis, arthralgia and, frequently, fever) have been reported; these reactions usually occurred following a second course of therapy. Signs and symptoms occur after a few days of therapy and resolve a few days after drug discontinuation with no serious sequelae.

Seizures: Several cephalosporins have been implicated in triggering seizures, particularly in patients with renal impairment when the dosage was not reduced.

Coagulation abnormalities: **Cefamandole**, **cefmetazole**, **cefoperazone**, **cefotetan**, and **ceftriaxone** may be associated with a fall in prothrombin activity. Those at risk include patients with renal impairment, cancer, impaired vitamin K synthesis, or low vitamin K stores (eg, chronic hepatic disease or malnutrition), as well as patients receiving a protracted course of antimicrobial therapy. Monitor prothrombin time for patients at risk and administer exogenous vitamin K as indicated. Vitamin K administration may be necessary if the prothrombin time is prolonged before therapy.

Predisposing factors – Predisposing factors to cephalosporin bleeding abnormalities include hepatic and renal dysfunction, thrombocytopenia and the concomitant use of "high dose" heparin (> 20,000 units/day), oral anticoagulants, or other drugs that affect hemostasis (eg, aspirin). Elderly, malnourished or debilitated patients are more likely to experience bleeding abnormalities than other patients.

Pseudomembranous colitis: Pseudomembranous colitis occurs with the use of cephalosporins (and other broad spectrum antibiotics); therefore, consider its diagnosis in patients who develop diarrhea with antibiotic use.

Immune hemolytic anemia: Immune hemolytic anemia has been observed in patients receiving cephalosporin class antibiotics.

Renal function impairment: Cephalosporins may be nephrotoxic; use with caution in the presence of markedly impaired renal function (Ccr < 50 mL/min/1.73 m^2).

Hepatic function impairment: Cefoperazone is extensively excreted in bile. Serum half-life increases 2-fold to 4-fold in patients with hepatic disease or biliary obstruction.

Pregnancy: Category B. These agents cross the placenta.

Lactation: Most of these agents are excreted in breast milk in small quantities.

Children: When using cephalosporins in infants, consider the relative benefit to risk. In neonates, accumulation of cephalosporin antibiotics (with resulting prolongation of drug half-life) has occurred.

Safety and efficacy in children < 1 month (**cefazolin** and **cefaclor** capsule and suspension), < 3 months (**cefuroxime**, **cephapirin**, and **cefoxitin**), < 5 months (**cefpodoxime**), < 6 months (**cefdinir**, **loracarbef**, **cefixime**, **ceftozoxime**, and **cefprozil**), < 9 months (**oral cephradine**) and < 1 year of age (**cefepime** and **parenteral cephradine**) have not been established.

Safety and efficacy of **cefaclor** extended-release tablets in children < 16 years of age have not been established.

Safety and efficacy of **cefonicid, cefmetazole, cefoperazone, cephalexin,** and **cefotetan** in children have not been established.

Precautions

Parenteral use: Inject IM preparations deep into musculature; properly dilute IV preparations and administer over an appropriate time interval.

Gonorrhea: In the treatment of gonorrhea, all patients should have a serologic test for syphilis. Patients with incubating syphilis (seronegative without clinical signs of syphilis) are likely to be cured by the regimens used for gonorrhea.

Superinfection: Use of antibiotics (especially prolonged or repeated therapy) may result in bacterial or fungal overgrowth of nonsusceptible organisms.

Drug Interactions

Agents that may interact with cephalosporins include ethanol, aminoglycosides, anticoagulants, polypeptide antibiotics, probenecid, antacids, H_2 antagonists, iron supplements, and loop diuretics.

Drug/Lab test interactions: A false-positive reaction for **urine glucose** may occur with *Benedict's* solution, *Fehling's* solution, or with *Clinitest* tablets, but not with enzyme-based tests such as *Clinistix* and *Tes-Tape.*

Cephradine may cause false-positive reactions in urinary protein tests that use sulfosalicylic acid.

Cefuroxime may cause a false-negative reaction in the ferricyanide test for blood glucose.

Cefdinir may cause a false-positive reaction for ketones in urine when measured using nitroprusside but not nitroferricynide.

A false-positive direct *Coombs' test* has occurred in some patients receiving cephalosporins.

Cephalosporins may falsely elevate *urinary 17-ketosteroid* values.

High concentrations of **cefoxitin** (> 100 mcg/mL) may interfere with measurement of *creatinine levels* by the Jaffe reaction and produce false results. **Cefotetan** may also affect these measurements.

Drug/Food interactions: Food increases absorption of **cefpodoxime** and oral **cefuroxime.**

Adverse Reactions

Most common – GI disturbances (nausea, vomiting, diarrhea); hypersensitivity phenomena (most common); hypotension; fever; dyspnea; candidal overgrowth consisting of oral candidiasis, vaginitis, genital moniliasis, vaginal discharge and genitoanal pruritus; nervousness; insomnia; confusion; hypertonia; dizziness; somnolence.

CNS: Headache; dizziness; lethargy; fatigue; paresthesia; confusion; diaphoresis; flushing.

Hematologic: Eosinophilia; transient neutropenia; leukocytosis; leukopenia; thrombocythemia; thrombocytopenia; agranulocytosis; granulocytopenia; hemolytic anemia; bone marrow depression; pancytopenia; decreased platelet function; anemia; aplastic anemia; hemorrhage.

Hepatic: Elevated AST, ALT, GGTP, total bilirubin, alkaline phosphatase, LDH; hepatitis.

Local: IM administration commonly results in pain, induration, temperature elevation, and tenderness.

Renal: Transitory elevations in BUN with and without elevated serum creatinine (frequency increases in patients > 50 years of age and in children < 3 years of age).

FLUCYTOSINE

Capsules: 250 and 500 mg | *Ancobon* (ICN)

> **Warning:**
> Use with extreme caution in patients with renal impairment. Close monitoring of hematologic, renal, and hepatic status of all patients is essential.

Indications

Serious infections caused by susceptible strains of *Candida* or *Cryptococcus*.

Administration and Dosage

The usual dosage is 50 to 150 mg/kg/day in divided doses at 6-hour intervals. To reduce or avoid nausea or vomiting, take capsules a few at a time over 15 minutes. Use a lower initial dose if BUN or serum creatinine is elevated or if there are other signs of renal impairment.

Actions

Pharmacology: Flucytosine has in vitro and in vivo activity against *Candida* and *Cryptococcus*. Although the exact mechanism is unknown, it has been reported that flucytosine acts directly on fungal organisms by competitive inhibition of purine and pyrimidine uptake and indirectly by intracellular metabolism to 5-fluorouracil.

Pharmacokinetics:

Absorption/Distribution – Flucytosine is well absorbed after oral use with peak blood levels within 2 hours. It is well distributed into aqueous humor, joints, peritoneal fluid, and other body fluids and tissues; CSF concentrations are ≈ 65% to 90% of serum levels. Bioavailability is 78% to 89%. Plasma protein binding is minimal. Toxicity occurs at blood levels > 100 mcg/mL.

Metabolism/Excretion – More than 90% of the dose is excreted unchanged in the urine by glomerular filtration; < 10% is found unchanged in the feces. Serum half-life is 2.4 and 4.8 hours in patients with normal renal function; half-life increases significantly in renal failure. The drug is removed easily by hemodialysis or peritoneal dialysis.

Contraindications

Hypersensitivity to flucytosine.

Warnings

Bone marrow depression: Give with extreme caution to patients with bone marrow depression. Frequently monitor hepatic function and the hematopoietic system during therapy.

Renal function impairment: Give with extreme caution; drug accumulation may occur. Monitor blood levels to determine the adequacy of renal excretion in such patients. Adjust dosage or dosing interval to maintain blood levels at < 100 mcg/mL.

Pregnancy: *Category* C. Flucytosine is teratogenic in rats and mice at 40 mg/kg/day. There are no adequate and well-controlled studies in pregnant women. Use only if the potential benefit justifies the potential risk to the fetus.

Lactation: It is not known whether this drug is excreted in breast milk. Because of potential serious adverse reactions in nursing infants, decide whether to discontinue nursing or the drug, taking into account the importance of the drug to mother.

Children: Safety and efficacy in children have not been established.

Precautions

Before therapy is initiated, determine electrolytes and hematological and renal status of the patient. Monitor hematologic status (WBC and platelet count) and liver function (alkaline phosphatase, ALT, and AST) at frequent intervals during treatment.

Drug Interactions

Drugs that impair glomerular filtration may prolong the half-life of flucytosine.

Amphotericin B: Amphotericin B may increase the therapeutic action and toxicity of flucytosine.

Cytosine: Cytosine may inactivate the antifungal activity of flucytosine.

Drug/Lab test interactions: Flucytosine interferes with creatinine value determinations with the dry-slide enzymatic method (Kodak Ektachem analyzer). Use Jaffe method.

Adverse Reactions

Cardiovascular: Cardiac arrest; myocardial toxicity; ventricular dysfunction.

CNS: Ataxia; hearing loss; headache; paresthesia; parkinsonism; peripheral neuropathy; pyrexia; vertigo; sedation; confusion; hallucinations; psychosis; convulsions.

Dermatologic: Rash; pruritus; urticaria; photosensitivity.

GI: Nausea; emesis; abdominal pain; diarrhea; anorexia; dry mouth; duodenal ulcer; GI hemorrhage; acute hepatic injury with possible fatal outcome in debilitated patients; hepatic dysfunction; jaundice; ulcerative colitis; bilirubin elevation; elevation of hepatic enzymes.

GU: Azotemia; creatinine and BUN elevation; crystalluria; renal failure.

Hematologic: Anemia; agranulocytosis; aplastic anemia; eosinophilia; leukopenia; pancytopenia; thrombocytopenia.

Respiratory: Respiratory arrest; chest pain; dyspnea.

Miscellaneous: Fatigue; hypoglycemia; hypokalemia; weakness; allergic reactions; Lyell's syndrome.

FLUOROQUINOLONES

CIPROFLOXACIN	
Tablets: 250, 500, and 750 mg (*Rx*)	*Cipro* (Bayer)
Suspension, oral: 5 g/100 mL (5%) and 10 g/100 mL (10%)	*Cipro* (Bayer)
Injection: 200 and 400 mg (*Rx*)	*Cipro IV* (Bayer)
ENOXACIN	
Tablets: 200 and 400 mg (*Rx*)	*Penetrex* (Aventis)
GATIFLOXACIN	
Tablets: 200 and 400 mg (*Rx*)	*Tequin* (Bristol-Myers Squibb)
Solution for Injection (single-use vials): 200 and 400 mg (*Rx*)	*Tequin* (Bristol-Myers Squibb)
Solution for Injection (premix): 200 and 400 mg (*Rx*)	*Tequin* (Bristol-Myers Squibb)
LEVOFLOXACIN	
Tablets: 250, 500, and 750 mg (*Rx*)	*Levaquin* (Ortho-McNeil)
Injection (single-use vials): 500 mg (25 mg/mL) and 750 mg (25 mg/mL) (*Rx*)	*Levaquin* (Ortho-McNeil)
Injection (premix): 250 (5 mg/mL), 500 mg (5 mg/mL), and 750 mg (5 mg/mL) (*Rx*)	*Levaquin* (Ortho-McNeil)
LOMEFLOXACIN HCl	
Tablets: 400 mg (*Rx*)	*Maxaquin* (Unimed)
MOXIFLOXACIN HCl	
Tablets: 400 mg (*Rx*)	*Avelox* (Bayer)
Injection (premix): 400 mg (*Rx*)	*Avelox* (Bayer)
NORFLOXACIN	
Tablets: 400 mg (*Rx*)	*Noroxin* (Merck)
OFLOXACIN	
Tablets: 200, 300, and 400 mg (*Rx*)	*Floxin* (Ortho-McNeil)
Injection: 200 and 400 mg (*Rx*)	*Floxin* (Ortho-McNeil)
SPARFLOXACIN	
Tablets: 200 mg (*Rx*)	*Zagam* (Bertek)
TROVAFLOXACIN MESYLATE/ALATROFLOXACIN MESYLATE	
Tablets: 100 and 200 mg trovafloxacin mesylate (*Rx*)	*Trovan* (Pfizer)
Solution for injection: 5 mg/mL alatrofloxacin mesylate (*Rx*)	*Trovan* (Pfizer)

Warning:

Trovafloxacin: Trovafloxacin has been associated with serious liver injury leading to liver transplantation or death. Trovafloxacin-associated liver injury has been reported with short-term and long-term drug exposure. Trovafloxacin use exceeding 2 weeks in duration is associated with a significantly increased risk of serious liver injury. Liver injury also has been reported following trovafloxacin re-exposure. Reserve trovafloxacin for use in patients with serious, life- or limb-threatening infections who receive their initial therapy in an inpatient health care facility (eg, hospital, long-term nursing care facility). Do not use trovafloxacin when safer, alternative antimicrobial therapy will be effective.

Indications

For specific approved indications, refer to the Administration and Dosage section.

Administration and Dosage

CIPROFLOXACIN:

Ciprofloxacin Dosage Guidelines

Location of infection	Type or severity	Unit dose	Frequency	Daily dose	Usual durations[1] (oral doseforms only)
Urinary tract	acute uncomplicated	100 or 250 mg	q 12 h	200 or 500 mg	3 days
	mild/moderate	250 mg (200 mg IV)	q 12 h	500 mg (400 mg IV)	7 to 14 days
	severe/complicated[2]	500 mg (400 mg IV)	q 12 h	1000 mg (800 mg IV)	7 to 14 days
Lower respiratory tract Bone and joint Skin and skin structure	mild/moderate	500 mg (400 mg IV)	q 12 h	1000 mg (800 mg IV)	7 to 14 days ≥ 4 to 6 weeks (bone and joint only)
	severe/complicated	750 mg (400 mg IV)	q 12 h (q 8 h)	1500 mg (1200 mg)	7 to 14 days ≥ 4 to 6 weeks (bone and joint only)
Nosocomial pneumonia	mild/moderate/severe	400 mg IV	q 8 h	1200 mg IV	
Intra-abdominal[3]	complicated	500 mg (400 mg IV)	q 12 h	1000 mg (800 mg IV)	7 to 14 days
Acute sinusitis	mild/moderate	500 mg (400 mg IV)	q 12 h	1000 mg (800 mg IV)	10 days
Chronic bacterial prostatitis	mild/moderate	500 mg (400 mg IV)	q 12 h	1000 mg (800 mg IV)	28 days
Empirical therapy in febrile neutropenic patients	severe: ciprofloxacin	400 mg IV	q 8 h	1200 mg IV	
	+ piperacillin	50 mg/kg IV	q 4 h	not to exceed 24 g/day	
Infectious diarrhea	mild/moderate/severe	500 mg	q 12 h	1000 mg	5 to 7 days
Typhoid fever	mild/moderate	500 mg	q 12 h	1000 mg	10 days
Urethral/Cervical gonococcal infections	uncomplicated	250 mg	single dose	250 mg	single dose

Ciprofloxacin Dosage Guidelines

Location of infection	Type or severity	Unit dose	Frequency	Daily dose	Usual durations[1] (oral doseforms only)
Inhalational anthrax (postexposure)[4]	adult	500 mg (400 mg IV)	q 12 h	1000 mg (800 mg IV)	60 days
	pediatric	15 mg/kg/dose, not to exceed 500 mg/dose (10 mg/kg/IV dose, not to exceed 400 mg/IV dose)	q 12 h	not to exceed 1000 mg (not to exceed 800 mg IV)	60 days

[1] Generally, ciprofloxacin should be continued for ≥ 2 days after the signs and symptoms of infection have disappeared, except for inhalational anthrax (postexposure).
[2] Including secondary bacteremia from *Escherichia coli* (IV only).
[3] Used in conjunction with metronidazole.
[4] Begin drug administration as soon as possible after suspected or confirmed exposure. This indication is based on a surrogate endpoint, ciprofloxacin serum concentrations achieved in humans, reasonably likely to predict clinical benefit. Total duration of ciprofloxacin administration (IV or oral) for inhalational anthrax (postexposure) is 60 days.

The duration of treatment depends upon the severity of infection. Generally, continue ciprofloxacin for ≥ 2 days after the signs and symptoms of infection have disappeared. The usual duration is 7 to 14 days; however, for severe and complicated infections, more prolonged therapy may be required. Bone and joint infections may require treatment for 4 to 6 weeks or longer. Infectious diarrhea may be treated for 5 to 7 days. Typhoid fever should be treated for 10 days. Treat chronic prostatitis for 28 days.

Administer sucralfate or divalent and trivalent cations such as antacids or iron containing magnesium, aluminum, or calcium 6 hours before or 2 hours after ciprofloxacin dosing.

Renal function impairment –

Ciprofloxacin Dosage in Impaired Renal Function	
Ccr (mL/min)	Dose
> 50 (oral); > 30 (IV)	See usual dosage
30 to 50	250 to 500 mg q 12 h
5 to 29	250 to 500 mg q 18 h (oral); 200 to 400 mg q 18 to 24 h (IV)
Hemodialysis or peritoneal dialysis	250 to 500 mg q 24 h (after dialysis)

In patients with severe infections and severe renal impairment, 750 mg may be administered orally at the intervals noted in the table.

CDC-recommended treatment schedules for chancroid and gonorrhea –

Chancroid (H. ducreyi infection): 500 mg orally 2 times/day for 3 days.

Gonococcal infections:

Disseminated (alternative initial regimen) – 500 mg IV every 12 hours for 24 to 48 hours after improvement begins, then 500 mg orally twice daily for 7 days.

Uncomplicated – 500 mg orally in a single dose plus azithromycin 1 g orally in a single dose or doxycycline 100 mg orally twice a day for 7 days.

IV: Administer by IV infusion over 60 minutes. Slow infusion of a dilute solution into a large vein will minimize patient discomfort and reduce the risk of venous irritation.

IV admixture compatibility/stability – Stable for ≤ 14 days at refrigerated or room temperature when diluted with 0.9% NaCl Injection, 5% Dextrose Injection, Sterile Water for Injection, 10% Dextrose for Injection, 5% Dextrose and 0.225% NaCl for Injection, 5% Dextrose and 0.45% NaCl for Injection, or Lactated Ringer's for Injection. Protect from light and freezing. If a Y-type IV infusion set or a piggyback method is used, temporarily discontinue the administration of any other solutions during the ciprofloxacin infusion.

NORFLOXACIN: Take 1 hour before or 2 hours after meals or dairy products and with a glass of water. Patients should be well hydrated.

Recommended Norfloxacin Dosage					
Infection	Description	Dose	Frequency	Duration	Daily dose
Urinary tract infections (UTI)	Uncomplicated (cystitis) caused by *E. coli*, *Klebsiella pneumoniae*, or *Proteus mirabilis*	400 mg	q 12 h	3 days	800 mg
	Uncomplicated caused by other organisms	400 mg	q 12 h	7 to 10 days	800 mg
	Complicated	400 mg	q 12 h	10 to 21 days	800 mg
Sexually transmitted diseases	Uncomplicated gonorrhea	800 mg	single dose	1 day	800 mg
Prostatitis	Acute or chronic	400 mg	q 12 h	28 days	800 mg

Renal function impairment – In patients with Ccr ≤ 30 mL/min/1.73 m^2, administer 400 mg once daily for the duration given above.

Elderly – Dose based on normal or impaired renal function.

CDC-recommended treatment schedules for gonorrhea –

Gonococcal infections, uncomplicated: 800 mg as a single dose (alternative regimen to **ciprofloxacin** or **ofloxacin**).

OFLOXACIN: Usual daily dose is 200 to 400 mg every 12 hours as described in the following table:

Ofloxacin Dosage Guidelines (Oral and IV)[1]					
Infection	Description	Dose	Frequency	Duration	Daily dose
Lower respiratory tract	Exacerbation of chronic bronchitis	400 mg	q 12 h	10 days	800 mg
	Community acquired pneumonia	400 mg	q 12 h	10 days	800 mg
Sexually transmitted diseases	Acute, uncomplicated urethral and cervical gonorrhea	400 mg	single dose	1 day	400 mg
	Cervicitis/Urethritis caused by *Chlamydia trachomatis*	300 mg	q 12 h	7 days	600 mg
	Cervicitis/Urethritis caused by *C. trachomatis* and *Neisseria gonorrhoeae*	300 mg	q 12 h	7 days	600 mg
	Acute pelvic inflammatory disease	400 mg	q 12 h	10 to 14 days	800 mg
Skin and skin structure	Uncomplicated	400 mg	q 12 h	10 days	800 mg
Urinary tract	Uncomplicated cystitis caused by *E. coli* or *K. pneumoniae*	200 mg	q 12 h	3 days	400 mg
	Uncomplicated cystitis caused by other organisms	200 mg	q 12 h	7 days	400 mg
	Complicated UTIs	200 mg	q 12 h	10 days	400 mg
Prostatitis	Caused by *E. coli*	300 mg	q 12 h	6 weeks[2]	600 mg

[1] Caused by the designated pathogens (see Indications).
[2] Because there are no safety data presently available to support the use of the IV formulation for > 10 days, switch to oral or other appropriate therapy after 10 days.

Do not take antacids containing calcium, magnesium, or aluminum; sucralfate; divalent or trivalent cations such as iron; multivitamins containing zinc; or didanosine (chewable/buffered tablets or pediatric powder for oral solution) 2 hours before or 2 hours after taking ofloxacin.

Renal function impairment – Adjust dosage in patients with Ccr ≤ 50 mL/min. After a normal initial dose, adjust the dosing interval as follows:

Ofloxacin Dosage in Impaired Renal Function		
Ccr (mL/min)	Maintenance dose	Frequency
20 to 50	usual recommended unit dose	q 24 hr
< 20	½ usual recommended unit dose	q 24 hr

Chronic hepatic impairment (cirrhosis) – The excretion of ofloxacin may be reduced in patients with severe liver function disorders (eg, cirrhosis with or without ascites). Do not exceed a maximum dose of 400 mg/day.

CDC-recommended treatment schedules for chlamydia, epididymitis, pelvic inflammatory disease (PID), and gonorrhea – †

Chlamydia: 300 mg orally 2 times/day for 7 days (alternative regimen).

Epididymitis: 300 mg orally 2 times/day for 10 days.

PID, outpatient: 400 mg orally 2 times/day for 14 days plus metronidazole.

Gonococcal infections, uncomplicated: 400 mg orally in a single dose plus doxycycline or azithromycin.

IV – Administer by IV infusion only. Do not give IM, intrathecally, intraperitoneally, or SC. Avoid rapid or bolus IV infusion; administer slowly over a period of ≥ 60 minutes.

Compatible IV solutions: 0.9% Sodium Chloride; 5% Dextrose; 5% Dextrose/0.9% Sodium Chloride; 5% Dextrose in Lactated Ringer's; 5% Sodium Bicarbonate; *Plasma-Lyte* 56 in 5% Dextrose; 5% Dextrose, 0.45% Sodium Chloride and 0.15% Potassium Chloride; Sodium Lactate (M/6); Water for Injection.

† CDC 1998 Sexually Transmitted Diseases Treatment Guidelines. *MMWR*. 1998;47(RR-1):1-118.

ENOXACIN: Take ≥ 1 hour before or 2 hours after a meal.

Enoxacin Dosage Guidelines					
Infection	Description	Dose	Frequency	Duration	Daily dose
Urinary tract infections	Uncomplicated (cystitis)	200 mg	q 12 h	7 days	400 mg
	Complicated	400 mg	q 12 h	14 days	800 mg
Sexually transmitted diseases	Uncomplicated urethral or cervical gonorrhea	400 mg	single dose	1 day	400 mg

Renal function impariment – Adjust dosage in patients with Ccr ≤ 30 mL/min/1.73 m^2. After a normal initial dose, use a 12-hour interval and ½ the recommended dose.

Elderly – Dosage adjustment is not necessary with normal renal function.

CDC recommended treatment schedules for gonorrhea –

Gonococcal infections, uncomplicated: 400 mg as a single dose (alternative regimen to ciprofloxacin or ofloxacin).

LOMEFLOXACIN HCl: Risk of reaction to solar UVA light may be reduced by taking lomefloxacin ≥ 12 hours before exposure to the sun (eg, in the evening). Lomefloxacin may be taken without regard to meals (see Actions).

Recommended Daily Dose of Lomefloxacin					
Body system	Infection	Dose	Frequency	Duration	Daily dose
Lower respiratory tract	Acute bacterial exacerbation of chronic bronchitis	400 mg	once daily	10 days	400 mg
Urinary tract	Uncomplicated cystitis caused by *K. pneumoniae, P. mirabilis*, or *Staphylococcus saprophyticus*	400 mg	once daily	10 days	400 mg
	Uncomplicated cystitis in females caused by *E. coli*	400 mg	once daily	3 days	400 mg
	Complicated UTI	400 mg	once daily	14 days	400 mg

Elderly – No dosage adjustment needed for elderly patients with normal renal function (Ccr ≥ 40 mL/min/1.73 m^2).

Renal function impairment – Lomefloxacin primarily is eliminated by renal excretion. Modification of dosage is recommended in patients with renal dysfunction. In patients with a Ccr > 10 but < 40 mL/min/1.73 m^2, the recommended dosage is an initial loading dose of 400 mg followed by daily maintenance doses of 200 mg once daily for the duration of the treatment.

Dialysis patients – Hemodialysis removes only a negligable amount of lomefloxacin (3% in 4 hours). Give hemodialysis patients an initial loading dose of 400 mg followed by maintenance dose of 200 mg once daily for duration of treatment.

Preoperative prevention –

Transrectal prostate biopsy: The recommended dose for transrectal prostate biopsy is a single 400 mg dose 1 to 6 hours prior to the procedure.

Transurethral surgical procedures: A single 400 mg dose 2 to 6 hours prior to surgery when oral preoperative prophylaxis for transurethral surgical procedures is considered appropriate.

CDC-recommended treatment schedules for gonorrhea –

Gonococcal infections, uncomplicated: 400 mg as a single dose (alternative regimen to ciprofloxacin or ofloxacin).

SPARFLOXACIN: Sparfloxacin may be taken with or without food.

Community-acquired pneumonia; acute bacterial exacerbations of chronic bronchitis – The recommended daily dose of sparfloxacin in patients with normal renal function is two 200 mg tablets taken on the first day as a loading dose. Thereafter, take one 200 mg tablet every 24 hours for a total of 10 days of therapy (11 tablets).

Renal function impairment – The recommended daily dose of sparfloxacin in patients with renal impairment (Ccr < 50 mL/min) is two 200 mg tablets taken on the first

† CDC 1998 Guidelines for the Treatment of Sexually Transmitted Diseases. MMWR. 1998;47(RR-1):1-118.

day as a loading dose. Thereafter, take one 200 mg tablet every 48 hours for a total of 9 days of therapy (6 tablets).

LEVOFLOXACIN: The usual dose of levofloxacin tablets/injection is 250 or 500 mg administered orally or by slow infusion over 60 minutes every 24 hours or 750 mg administered by slow infusion over 90 minutes every 24 hours, as indicated by infection and described in the following dosing chart. These recommendations apply to patients with normal renal function (ie, Ccr > 80 mL/min). For patients with altered renal function, see Levofloxacin Dosing with Renal Function Impairment table. Administer oral doses ≥ 2 hours before or 2 hours after antacids containing magnesium or aluminum, as well as sucralfate, metal cations such as iron and multivitamin preparations with zinc, or didanosine (chewable/buffered tablets or pediatric powder for oral solution).

Levofloxacin Dosing with Normal Renal Function

Infection[1]	Unit dose	Frequency	Duration[2]	Daily dose
Acute bacterial exacerbation of chronic bronchitis	500 mg	q 24 hr	7 days	500 mg
Community-acquired pneumonia	500 mg	q 24 hr	7 to 14 days	500 mg
Acute maxillary sinusitis	500 mg	q 24 hr	10 to 14 days	500 mg
Complicated SSSI[3]	750 mg	q 24 hr	7 to 14 days	750 mg
Uncomplicated SSSI[3]	500 mg	q 24 hr	7 to 10 days	500 mg
Complicated UTI	250 mg	q 24 hr	10 days	250 mg
Uncomplicated UTI	250 mg	q 24 hr	3 days	250 mg
Acute pyelonephritis	250 mg	q 24 hr	10 days	250 mg

[1] Caused by the designated pathogens (see Indications).
[2] Sequential therapy (IV to oral) may be instituted at the discretion of the physician.
[3] Skin and skin structure infection.

Levofloxacin Dosing with Renal Function Impairment

Renal status	Initial dose	Subsequent dose
Acute bacterial exacerbation of chronic bronchitis/community-acquired pneumonia/acute maxillary sinusitis/uncomplicated SSSI		
Ccr from 50 to 80 mL/min	No dosage adjustment required	
Ccr from 20 to 49 mL/min	500 mg	250 mg q 24 hr
Ccr from 10 to 19 mL/min	500 mg	250 mg q 48 hr
Hemodialysis	500 mg	250 mg q 48 hr
CAPD[1]	500 mg	250 mg q 48 hr
Complicated SSSI		
Ccr from 50 to 80 mL/min	No dosage adjustment required	
Ccr from 20 to 49 mL/min	750 mg	750 mg q 48 hr
Ccr from 10 to 19 mL/min	750 mg	500 mg q 48 hr
Hemodialysis	750 mg	500 mg q 48 hr
CAPD[1]	750 mg	500 mg q 48 hr
Complicated UTI/acute pyelonephritis		
Ccr ≥ 20 mL/min	No dosage adjustment required	
Ccr from 10 to 19 mL/min	250 mg	250 mg q 48 hr
Uncomplicated UTI	No dosage adjustment required	

[1] CAPD = chronic ambulatory peritoneal dialysis.

IV administration – Administer by IV infusion only, slowly over a period of ≥ 60 minutes. Avoid rapid or bolus IV infusion. Do not administer by IM, intrathecal, intraperitoneal, or SC routes.

TROVAFLOXACIN MESYLATE/ALATROFLOXACIN MESYLATE: Administer oral doses ≥ 2 hours before or 2 hours after antacids containing magnesium or aluminum, as well as sucralfate, citric acid buffered with sodium citrate, metal cations (eg, ferrous sulfate), and didanosine (chewable/buffered tablets or pediatric powder for oral solution).

If trovafloxacin is taken on an empty stomach, administer IV morphine ≥ 2 hours later. If trovafloxacin is taken with food, administer IV morphine ≥ 4 hours later.

Administer alatrofloxacin only by IV infusion. Do not administer by IM, intrathecal, intraperitoneal, or SC routes.

Single-use vials require dilution prior to administration.

Trovafloxacin/Alatrofloxacin Dosage Guidelines

Infection[1]/ Location and type	Daily unit dose and route of administration	Frequency	Total duration
Nosocomial pneumonia[2]	300 mg IV[3] followed by 200 mg oral	q 24 hr	10 to 14 days
Community-acquired pneumonia	200 mg oral or 200 mg IV followed by 200 mg oral	q 24 hr	7 to 14 days
Complicated intra-abdominal infections, including post-surgical infections	300 mg IV[3] followed by 200 mg oral	q 24 hr	7 to 14 days
Gynecologic and pelvic infections	300 mg IV[3] followed by 200 mg oral	q 24 hr	7 to 14 days
Skin and skin structure infections, complicated, including diabetic foot infections	200 mg oral or 200 mg IV followed by 200 mg oral	q 24 hr	10 to 14 days

[1] Caused by the designated pathogens (see Indications).
[2] As with other antimicrobials, where *Pseudomonas aeruginosa* is a documented or presumptive pathogen, combination therapy with either an aminoglycoside or aztreonam may be clinically indicated.
[3] Where the 300 mg IV dose is indicated, decrease therapy to 200 mg as soon as clinically indicated.

Do not administer trovafloxacin for > 2 weeks unless the treating physician believes the benefits to the individual patient clearly outweigh the risks of longer-term treatment.

Renal function impairment – No dosage adjustment is necessary in patients with impaired renal function.

Chronic hepatic disease (cirrhosis) – The following table provides dosing guidelines for patients with mild or moderate cirrhosis (Child-Pugh Class A and B). There are no data in patients with severe cirrhosis (Child-Pugh Class C).

Trovafloxacin/Alatrofloxacin Dosage in Chronic Hepatic Disease

Indicated dose (normal hepatic function)	Chronic hepatic disease dose
300 mg IV	200 mg IV
200 mg IV or oral	100 mg IV or oral

IV administration – After dilution with an appropriate diluent, administer by IV infusion over a period of 60 minutes.

Admixture incompatibility – Do not dilute alatrofloxacin with 0.9% Sodium Chloride Injection (normal saline), alone or in combination with other diluents. A precipitate may form under these conditions. In addition, do not dilute alatrofloxacin with Lactated Ringer's.

Compatible IV solutions: 5% Dextrose Injection; 0.45% Sodium Chloride Injection; 5% Dextrose and 0.45% Sodium Chloride Injection; 5% Dextrose and 0.2% Sodium Chloride Injection; Lactated Ringer's and 5% Dextrose Injection.

Normal saline, 0.9% Sodium Chloride Injection, can be used for flushing IV lines prior to or after administration of alatrofloxacin.

MOXIFLOXACIN HCl: The dose of moxifloxacin is 400 mg (orally or as an IV infusion) once every 24 hours.

Administer IV moxifloxacin by IV infusion only. It is not intended for IM, intrathecal, intraperitoneal, or SC administration.

Administer by IV infusion over a period of 60 minutes by direct infusion or through a Y-type IV infusion set that may already be in place. Caution: Rapid or bolus IV infusion must be avoided.

Moxifloxacin Dosage Guidelines (IV and Oral)

Infection[1]	Daily dose (mg)	Frequency	Duration (days)
Acute bacterial sinusitis	400	q 24 hr	10
Acute bacterial exacerbation of chronic bronchitis	400	q 24 hr	5
Community-acquired pneumonia	400	q 24 hr	10
Uncomplicated skin and skin structure infections	400	q 24 hr	7

[1] Caused by the designated pathogens (see Indications).

Impaired renal function: No dosage adjustment is required in renally impaired patients. Moxifloxacin has not been studied in patients on hemodialysis or continuous ambulatory peritoneal dialysis (CAPD).

Impaired hepatic function: No dosage adjustment is required in patients with mild hepatic insufficiency. The use of moxifloxacin is not recommended in patients with moderate and severe hepatic insufficiency.

Switching from IV to oral dosing: When switching from IV to oral dosage administration, no dosage adjustment is necessary.

GATIFLOXACIN: Gatifloxacin may be administered without regard to food, including milk and dietary supplements containing calcium, and without regard to age (≥ 18 years) or gender.

Oral: Administer oral gatifloxacin ≥ 4 hours before the administration of ferrous sulfate; dietary supplements containing zinc, magnesium, or iron (such as multivitamins); aluminum/magnesium-containing antacids; or didanosine (buffered tablets, buffered solution, or buffered powder for oral suspension).

When switching from IV to oral dosage administration, no dosage adjustment is necessary. Patients whose therapy is started with the injection may be switched to tablets when clinically indicated at the discretion of the physician.

IV: Administer injection by IV infusion only. It is not intended for IM, intrathecal, intraperitoneal, or SC administration.

Gatifloxacin Dosage Guidelines

Infection[1]	Daily dose (mg)[2]	Frequency	Duration
Acute bacterial exacerbation of chronic bronchitis	400	q 24 hr	5 days
Acute sinusitis	400	q 24 hr	10 days
Community-acquired pneumonia	400	q 24 hr	7 to 14 days
Uncomplicated UTIs (cystitis)	400	q 24 hr	Single dose
	or 200		3 days
Complicated UTIs	400	q 24 hr	7 to 10 days
Acute pyelonephritis	400	q 24 hr	7 to 10 days
Uncomplicated urethal gonorrhea in men; endocervical and rectal gonorrhea in women	400	q 24 hr	Single dose

[1] Caused by the designated pathogens (see Indications).
[2] For either the oral and IV routes of administration.

Renal function impairment: Because gatifloxacin is eliminated primarily by renal excretion, a dosage modification of gatifloxacin is recommended for patients with Ccr < 40 mL/min, including patients on hemodialysis and on continuous ambulatory peritoneal dialysis (CAPD). The recommended dosage of gatifloxacin follows:

Recommended Dosage of Gatifloxacin in Adult Patients with Renal Impairment		
Ccr	Initial dose (mg)	Subsequent dose[1]
≥ 40 mL/min	400	400 mg daily
< 40 mL/min	400	200 mg daily
Hemodialysis	400	200 mg daily
Continuous peritoneal dialysis	400	200 mg daily

[1] Start of subsequent dose on day 2 of dosing.

Administer gatifloxacin after a dialysis session for patients on hemodialysis.

Uncomplicated UTIs and gonorrhea – Single 400 mg dose regimen (for the treatment of uncomplicated UTIs and gonorrhea) and 200 mg once daily for 3 days regimen (for the treatment of uncomplicated UTIs) require no dosage adjustment in patients with impaired renal function.

Actions

Pharmacology: The fluoroquinolones are synthetic, broad-spectrum antibacterial agents that inhibit DNA gyrase and topoisomerase IV. DNA gyrase is an essential enzyme that is involved in the replication, transcription, and repair of bacterial DNA. Topoisomerase IV is an enzyme known to play a key role in the partitioning of the chromosomal DNA during bacterial cell division.

Pharmacokinetics:

Pharmacokinetics of Fluoroquinolones

Fluoroquinolone	Bioavailability (%)	Max urine concentration (mcg/mL) (dose)	Mean peak plasma concentration (mcg/mL) (dose)	Area under curve (AUC) (mcg • hr/mL) (dose)	Protein binding (%)	t½ (hr)	Urine recovery unchanged (%)
Ciprofloxacin Oral	≈ 70-80	> 200 (250 mg)	1.2 (250 mg) 2.4 (500 mg) 4.3 (750 mg) 5.4 (1000 mg)	4.8 (250 mg) 11.6 (500 mg) 20.2 (750 mg) 30.8 (1000 mg)	20 to 40	≈ 4	≈ 40 to 50
IV		> 200 (200 mg) > 400 (400 mg)	4.4 (400 mg)	4.8 (200 mg) 11.6 (400 mg)		≈ 5 to 6	≈ 50 to 70
Enoxacin	≈ 90	nd[1]	0.93 (200 mg) 2 (400 mg)		≈ 40	3 to 6	> 40
Gatifloxacin[2] Oral	≈ 96		≈ 2 (200 mg single dose) ≈ 3.8 (400 mg single dose) ≈ 4.2 (400 mg multiple dose)	≈ 14.2 (200 mg single dose) ≈ 33 (400 mg single dose) ≈ 34.4 (400 mg multiple dose)	≈ 20	≈ 7.8 (400 mg single dose) ≈7.1 (400 mg multiple dose)	≈ 73.8 (200 mg single dose) ≈72.4 (400 mg single dose) ≈ 80.2 (400 mg multiple dose)
IV			≈ 2.2 (200 mg single dose) ≈ 2.4 (200 mg multiple dose) ≈ 5.5 (400 mg single dose) ≈ 4.6 (400 mg multiple dose)	≈ 15.9 (200 mg single dose) ≈ 16.8 (200 mg multiple dose) ≈ 35.1 (400 mg single dose) ≈ 35.4 (400 mg multiple dose)		≈ 11.1 (200 mg single dose) ≈ 12.3 (200 mg multiple dose) ≈ 7.4 (400 mg single dose) ≈ 13.9 (400 mg multiple dose)	≈ 71.7 (200 mg single dose) ≈ 72.4 (200 mg multiple dose) ≈ 62.3 (400 mg single dose) ≈ 83.5 (400 mg multiple dose)
Levofloxacin	≈ 99		≈ 2.8 to 11.5 (single dose oral or IV) ≈ 5.7 to 12.1 (multiple dose oral or IV)	≈ 27.2 to 110 (single dose oral or IV) ≈ 47.5 to 108 (multiple dose oral or IV)	≈ 24-38	≈ 6.3 to 7.5 (single dose oral or IV) ≈ 7 to 8.8 (multiple dose oral or IV)	≈ 87 (oral)
Lomefloxacin	≈ 95-98	> 300 (400 mg)	0.8 (100 mg) 1.4 (200 mg) 3.2 (400 mg)	5.6 (100 mg) 10.9 (200 mg) 26.1 (400 mg)	≈ 10	≈ 8	≈ 65
Moxifloxacin	≈ 90		4.5 (400 mg)	≈ 48 (400 mg)	≈ 50	≈ 12	≈ 20
Norfloxacin	30 to 40	≥ 200 (400 mg)	0.8 (200 mg) 1.5 (400 mg) 2.4 (800 mg)		10 to 15	3 to 4	26 to 32

Pharmacokinetics of Fluoroquinolones

Fluoroquinolone	Bioavail-ability (%)	Max urine concentration (mcg/mL) (dose)	Mean peak plasma concentration (mcg/mL) (dose)	Area under curve (AUC) (mcg • hr/mL) (dose)	Protein binding (%)	t½ (hr)	Urine recovery unchanged (%)
Ofloxacin Oral	≈ 98	≈ 220 (200 mg)	1.5 (200 mg) 2.4 (300 mg) 2.9 (400 mg) 4.6 (400 mg steady-state)	14.1 (200 mg) 21.2 (300 mg) 31.4 (400 mg) 61 (400 mg steady-state)	≈ 32	≈ 9	65 to 80
IV		nd[1]	2.7 (200 mg) 4 (400 mg)	43.5 (400 mg)	≈ 32	5 to 10	≈ 65
Sparfloxacin	92		≈ 1.3 (400 mg)	≈ 34 (400 mg)	≈ 45	≈ 20	≈ 10
Trovafloxacin/ Alatrofloxacin[2] Trovafloxacin Single-dose	≈ 88 (oral)	> 12 (400 mg)[3] ≈ 12.1 (200 mg)	≈ 1 (100 mg) ≈ 2.1 (200 mg)	≈ 11.2 (100 mg) ≈ 26.7 (200 mg)	≈ 76	9.1 (100 mg) 9.6 (200 mg)	≈ 6 (oral)
Multiple dose			≈ 1.1 (100 mg) ≈ 3.1 (200 mg)	≈ 11.8 (100 mg) ≈ 34.4 (200 mg)		10.5 (100 mg) 12.2 (200 mg)	
Alatrofloxacin[4] Single-dose			≈ 2.7 (200 mg) ≈ 3.6 (300 mg)	≈ 28.1 (200 mg) ≈ 46.1 (300 mg)		9.4 (200 mg) 11.2 (300 mg)	
Multiple dose			≈ 3.1 (200 mg) ≈ 4.4 (300 mg)	≈ 32.2 (200 mg) ≈ 46.3 (300 mg)		11.7 (200 mg) 12.7 (300 mg)	

[1] nd = no data.
[2] Single dose: AUC (0-∞); Multiple dose: AUC (0-24).
[3] Following a 400 mg loading dose of sparfloxacin, the mean urine concentration 4 hours postdose was in excess of 12 mcg/mL.
[4] Trovafloxacin equivalents.

Microbiology:

	Organisms Generally Susceptible to Fluoroquinolones In Vitro										
	Organism	Ciprofloxacin	Enoxacin	Gatifloxacin	Levofloxacin	Lomefloxacin	Moxifloxacin	Norfloxacin	Ofloxacin	Sparfloxacin	Trovafloxacin/ Alatrofloxacin
Gram-negative	*Acinetobacter anitritus*									✓[1]	
	Acinetobacter iwoffi	✓[1]		✓[1]	✓[1]					✓[1]	
	Acinetobacter calcoaceticus								✓[1]		
	Aeromonas hydrophilia	✓[1]	✓[1]			✓[1]					
	Bacteroides distasonis										✓[1]
	Bacteroides ovatus										✓[1]
	Bordetella pertussis				✓[1]				✓[1]		
	Campylobacter jejuni	✓[2]									
	Chlamydia trachamotis								✓		
	Citrobacter diversus	✓	✓[1]	✓[1]	✓[1]	✓		✓[1]	✓	✓[1]	
	Citrobacter freundii	✓		✓[1]		✓[1]	✓[1]	✓	✓[1]		✓[1]
	Citrobacter koseri		✓[1]	✓[1]							
	Enterobacter cloacae	✓	✓	✓[1]	✓	✓	✓[1]	✓	✓[1]	✓	
	Enterobacter aerogenes	✓[1]	✓[1]	✓[1]	✓[1]	✓[1]		✓	✓	✓[1]	✓[1]
	Enterobacter agglomerans				✓[1]	✓[1]		✓[1]			
	Enterobacter sakazakii				✓[1]						
	Escherichia coli	✓	✓	✓	✓	✓	✓[1]	✓	✓	✓	✓
	Edwardsiella tarda	✓[1]						✓[1]			
	Fusobacterium sp.						✓[1]				
	Gardenella vaginalis								✓		✓
	Haemophilus ducreyi		✓[1]					✓[1]	✓[1]		
	Haemophilus influenzae	✓		✓	✓	✓	✓		✓	✓	✓
	Haemophilus parainfluenzae	✓		✓	✓	✓[1]	✓			✓	
	Hafnia alvei					✓[1]					
	Klebsiella pneumoniae	✓	✓	✓	✓	✓	✓	✓	✓	✓	✓

Organisms Generally Susceptible to Fluoroquinolones In Vitro

	Organism	Ciprofloxacin	Enoxacin	Gatifloxacin	Levofloxacin	Lomefloxacin	Moxifloxacin	Norfloxacin	Ofloxacin	Sparfloxacin	Trovafloxacin/ Alatrofloxacin
Gram-negative (cont'd.)	*Klebsiella oxytoca*	✔[1]	✔[1]	✔[1]	✔[1]	✔[1]	✔[1]	✔[1]	✔[1]	✔[1]	
	Klebsiella ozaenae		✔[1]			✔[1]					
	Moraxella-catarrhalis	✔[2]		✔	✔	✔	✔		✔[1]	✔	✔
	Morganella morganii	✔	✔[1]	✔[1]	✔[1]	✔[1]	✔	✔[1]	✔[1]	✔[1]	✔[1]
	Mycoplasma hominis								✔[1]		✔[1]
	Neisseria gonorrhoeae	✔[2]	✔	✔				✔	✔		
	Pasteurella multocida	✔[1]									
	Prevotella sp.						✔[1]				✔
	Proteus mirabilis	✔	✔	✔	✔	✔	✔[1]	✔	✔	✔[1]	✔
	Proteus vulgaris	✔	✔[1]	✔[1]	✔[1]	✔[1]		✔	✔[1]	✔[1]	✔[1]
	Providencia alcalifaciens		✔[1]			✔[1]		✔[1]			
	Providencia rettgeri	✔			✔[1]	✔[1]		✔[1]	✔[1]		
	Providencia stuartii	✔	✔[1]		✔[1]			✔[1]	✔[1]		
	Pseudomonas aeruginosa	✔	✔		✔[3]	✔[4]		✔	✔[3]		✔
	Pseudomonas fluorescens				✔[1]			✔[1]			
	Pseudomonas stutzeri							✔[1]			
	Salmonella sp.	✔[5]		✔	✔		✔		✔	✔	✔
	Salmonella typhi	✔									
	Salmonella enteritidis	✔[1]									
	Serratia marcescens	✔	✔[1]		✔[1]	✔[1]		✔	✔[1]		
	Serratia proteomaculans		✔[1]			✔[1]					
	Shigella sp.	✔[5]		✔	✔		✔		✔	✔	✔
	Shigella boydii	✔[2]									
	Shigella dysenteriae	✔[2]									
	Shigella flexneri	✔[2]									
	Shigella sonnei	✔[2]									

Organisms Generally Susceptible to Fluoroquinolones In Vitro

	Organism	Ciprofloxacin	Enoxacin	Gatifloxacin	Levofloxacin	Lomefloxacin	Moxifloxacin	Norfloxacin	Ofloxacin	Sparfloxacin	Trovafloxacin/ Alatrofloxacin
Gram-negative (cont'd.)	*Ureoplasma urealtycium*							✓[1]	✓[1]		✓[1]
	Vibrio parahemolyticus	✓[1]									
	Vibrio vulnificus	✓[1]									
	Vibrio cholerae	✓[1]									
	Yersinia enterocolitica	✓[1]									
Gram-positive	*Staphylococcus aureus* methicillin susceptible	✓		✓	✓	✓[1]	✓	✓[6]	✓	✓[6]	✓
	Staphylococcus aureus methicillin resistant					✓[1]					
	Staphylococcus epidermidis methicillin susceptible	✓[6]	✓[6]	✓	✓[1]	✓[1]	✓	✓[6]	✓[1]	✓	✓
	Staphylococcus epidermidis methicillin resistant			✓		✓[1]	✓				
	Staphylococcus hemolyticus	✓									
	Staphylococcus hominis	✓									
	Staphylococcus saprophyticus	✓	✓	✓[1]	✓	✓		✓	✓[1]		
	Streptococci pyogenes	✓		✓[1]	✓		✓[1]		✓	✓[1]	✓
	Streptococcus viridans				✓[1]					✓[1]	✓
	Streptococcus group c/f, g				✓[1]						
	Streptococcus milleri				✓[1]						
	Streptococcus agalactiae				✓[1]		✓	✓		✓[1]	✓
	Enteroccus faecalis	✓[7]			✓[7]			✓			✓[7]
	Penicillin susceptible			✓	✓		✓		✓	✓	✓
	Penicillin resistant			✓[1]	✓		✓[1]		✓[1]	✓[1]	✓[1]

Organisms Generally Susceptible to Fluoroquinolones In Vitro											
	Organism	Ciprofloxacin	Enoxacin	Gatifloxacin	Levofloxacin	Lomefloxacin	Moxifloxacin	Norfloxacin	Ofloxacin	Sparfloxacin	Trovafloxacin/ Alatrofloxacin
Atypical bacteria	*Legionella pneumophilia*	✓[1]		✓	✓	✓[1]	✓[1]		✓[1]	✓[1]	✓
	Mycoplasma pneumoniae			✓	✓		✓		✓[1]	✓	✓
	Chlamydia pneumoniae			✓	✓	✓	✓		✓[1]	✓	✓
Anaerobe bacteria	*Bacteroides fragilis*										✓
	Peptostreptococcus sp.			✓[1]			✓[1]				✓
	Clostridium perfringes				✓[1]			✓	✓[1]		✓[1]

[1] Exhibits in vitro MIC of ≤ 1 mcg/mL (ciprofloxacin, sparfloxacin); ≤ 2 mcg/mL (enoxacin, gatifloxacin, levofloxacin, lomefloxacin, moxifloxacin, ofloxacin, and trovafloxacin); ≤ 4 mcg/mL norfloxacin against most (≥ 90%) strains of microorganisms; however, the safety and effectiveness in treating clinical infections caused by these microorganisms have not been established in adequate and well-controlled clinical trials.
[2] Oral ciprofloxacin.
[3] As with other drugs in this class, some strains of *P. aeruginosa* may develop resistance fairly rapidly during treatment.
[4] Urinary tract only.
[5] See following text for individual microorganisms.
[6] Does not specify susceptible or resistant.
[7] Many strains are moderately susceptible.

Contraindications

Hypersensitivity to fluoroquinolones or the quinolone group; tendinitis or tendon rupture associated with quinolone use; patients receiving disopyramide and amiodarone as well as other QT_c-prolonging antiarrhythmic drugs reported to cause torsade de pointes, such as class IA antiarrhythmic agents (eg, quinidine, procainamide), class III antiarrhythmic agents (eg, sotalol), and bepridil (**sparfloxacin**); patients with known QT_c prolongation or in patients being treated concomitantly with medications known to produce an increase in the QT_c interval or torsades de pointes (**sparfloxacin**); patients whose lifestyle or employment will not permit compliance with required safety precautions concerning phototoxicity (**sparfloxacin**).

Warnings

Phototoxicity: Moderate-to-severe phototoxic reactions have occurred in patients exposed to direct or indirect sunlight or to artificial ultraviolet light (eg, sunlamps) during or following treatment with **lomefloxacin**, **sparfloxacin**, **ofloxacin**, or **trovafloxacin/alatrofloxacin**.

Avoid direct exposure to direct or indirect sunlight (even when using sunscreens or sunblocks) while taking lomefloxacin and other fluoroquinolones for several days following therapy. Discontinue therapy at first signs or symptoms of phototoxicity.

Hepatic failure: **Trovafloxacin/alatrofloxacin**-associated liver enzyme abnormalities, symptomatic hepatitis, jaundice, and liver failure (including rare reports of acute hepatic necrosis with eosinophilic infiltration, liver transplantation, or death) have been reported with short- and long-term drug exposure in men and women. Use exceeding 2 weeks in duration is associated with a significantly increased risk of serious liver injury. Liver injury also has been reported following trovafloxacin/alatrofloxacin re-exposure. Monitor liver function tests (eg, AST, ALT, bilirubin) in recipients who develop signs or symptoms consistent with hepatitis. Consider discontinuing the drug in those patients who develop liver function test abnormalities (see Warning Box).

Cardiac toxicity: **Moxifloxacin** and **gatifloxacin** have been shown to prolong the QT interval of the electrocardiogram in some patients. Avoid in patients with known prolongation of the QT interval, patients with uncorrected hypokalemia, and patients receiving class IA (eg, quinidine, procainamide) or class III (eg, amiodarone, sotalol) antiarrhythmic agents, because of the lack of clinical experience with these drugs in these patient populations.

Increases in the QT_c interval have been observed in healthy volunteers treated with **sparfloxacin**.

Avoid the concomitant prescription of medications known to prolong the QT_c interval (eg, erythromycin, terfenadine, astemizole, cisapride, pentamidine, tricyclic antidepressants, some antipsychotics including phenothiazines). **Sparfloxacin** is not recommended for use in patients with proarrhythmic conditions (eg, hypokalemia, significant bradycardia, CHF, myocardial ischemia, atrial fibrillation).

Hypotension: Life-threatening hypotension has been reported with **alatrofloxacin** administration. This has occurred in patients receiving alatrofloxacin either at the recommended rate of infusion or if given more rapidly. Hypotension may be potentiated with the concomitant administration of anesthetic agents. Alatrofloxacin should be only administered by slow IV infusion over a period of 60 minutes. Monitor blood pressure closely during infusion.

Tendon rupture/Tendinitis: Ruptures of the shoulder, hand, and Achilles tendons that required surgical repair or resulted in prolonged disability have been reported with fluoroquinolone antimicrobials. Discontinue therapy if the patient experiences pain, inflammation, or rupture of a tendon. Patients should rest and refrain from exercise until the diagnosis of tendinitis or tendon rupture has been confidently excluded. Tendon rupture can occur at any time during or after therapy.

Convulsions: Increased intracranial pressure, convulsions, and toxic psychosis have occurred. CNS stimulation also may occur and may lead to tremor, restlessness, lightheadedness, confusion, dizziness, depression, hallucinations, and rarely, suicidal thoughts or acts. Use with caution in patients with known or suspected CNS disorders (eg, severe cerebral arteriosclerosis, epilepsy) or other factors that predispose to seizures or lower the seizure threshold, or in the presence of other risk factors that may predispose to seizures or lower the seizure threshold (eg, certain drug therapy, renal dysfunction). If these reactions occur, stop the drug, and institute appropriate measures.

Syphilis: **Ciprofloxacin, enoxacin, gatifloxacin, norfloxacin, ofloxacin**, and **trovafloxacin** are not effective for syphilis. High doses of antimicrobial agents for short periods of time to treat gonorrhea may mask or delay symptoms of incubating syphilis. All patients should have a serologic test for syphilis at the time of gonorrhea diagnosis. Patients treated with ciprofloxacin, enoxacin, gatifloxacin, norfloxacin, ofloxacin, and trovafloxacin should have a follow-up serologic test after 3 months.

Chronic bronchitis due to Streptococcus pneumoniae: **Lomefloxacin** is not indicated for the empiric treatment of acute bacterial exacerbation of chronic bronchitis when it is probable that *S. pneumoniae* is a causative pathogen because it exhibits in vitro resistance to lomefloxacin.

P. aeruginosa: In clinical trials of complicated UTIs due to *P. aeruginosa*, 12 of 16 patients had the microorganism eradicated from the urine after therapy with **lomefloxacin**. No patients had concomitant bacteremia. Serum levels of lomefloxacin do not reliably exceed the MIC of *Pseudomonas* isolates. The safety and efficacy of lomefloxacin in treating patients with *Pseudomonas* bacteremia have not been established.

Hypersensitivity reactions: Hypersensitivity reactions, serious and occasionally fatal, have occurred in patients receiving quinolone therapy, some following the first dose. Refer to Management of Acute Hypersensitivity Reactions.

Pseudomembranous colitis: Pseudomembranous colitis has been reported with nearly all antibacterial agents, including fluoroquinolones, and may range from mild to life-threatening in severity.

Renal function impairment: Alteration in dosage regimen is necessary. See Administration and Dosage.

Hepatic function impairment: The oral clearance of **trovafloxacin** in mild and moderate cirrhosis is reduced ≈ 30%, which corresponds to prolongation of half-life by 2 to 2.5 hours (25% to 30%) increase. There are no data in patients with severe cirrhosis. Dosage adjustment is recommended in patients with mild-to-moderate cirrhosis.

Elderly: **Norfloxacin** is eliminated more slowly because of decreased renal function; absorption appears unaffected. The apparent half-life of **ofloxacin** is 6 to 8 hours, compared to ≈ 5 hours in younger adults; absorption is unaffected. **Lomefloxacin** plasma clearance was reduced by ≈ 25% and the AUC was increased by ≈ 33% in the elderly, which may be caused by decreased renal function in this population. **Enoxacin** plasma concentrations are 50% higher in the elderly than in young adults.

Pregnancy: Category C.

Lactation: **Norfloxacin** was not detected in breast milk following the administration of 200 mg to nursing mothers; however, this was a low dose. **Ciprofloxacin** is excreted in breast milk. **Ofloxacin**, as a single 200 mg dose, resulted in breast milk concentrations in nursing females that were similar to those found in plasma. **Levofloxacin** has not been measured in breast milk. Based upon data from ofloxacin, it can be presumed that levofloxacin will be excreted in breast milk. **Sparfloxacin** is excreted in breast milk. **Gatifloxacin** and **moxifloxacin** are excreted in the breast milk of rats. **Trovafloxacin** is excreted in breast milk and was found in measurable concentrations in the breast milk of lactating subjects. It is not known whether

lomefloxacin, **gatifloxacin**, or **enoxacin** are excreted in breast milk. Because of the potential for serious adverse reactions in nursing infants, decide whether to discontinue nursing or to discontinue the drug, taking into account the importance of the drug to the mother.

Children: Safety and efficacy of **enoxacin**, **gatifloxacin**, **levofloxacin**, **lomefloxacin**, **moxifloxacin**, **norfloxacin**, **ofloxacin**, **sparfloxacin**, and **trovafloxacin** in children < 18 years of age have not been established. **Ciprofloxacin**, **enoxacin**, **gatifloxacin**, **levofloxacin**, **lomefloxacin**, **moxifloxacin**, **ofloxacin**, **sparfloxacin**, and **trovafloxacin** cause arthropathy and osteochondrosis in immature animals. Administration of **ciprofloxacin**, **moxifloxacin**, and **norfloxacin** caused lameness in immature dogs because of permanent cartilage lesions.

Precautions

Monitoring: Periodic assessment of organ system functions, including renal, hepatic, and hematopoietic, is advisable during prolonged therapy.

Symptomatic pancreatitis has been reported with **trovafloxacin/alatrofloxacin** therapy. Monitor pancreatic tests in patients who develop symptoms consistent with pancreatitis.

Crystalluria: Needle-shaped crystals were found in the urine of some volunteers who received either placebo or 800 or 1600 mg **norfloxacin**. While crystalluria is not expected to occur under usual conditions with 400 mg twice daily, do not exceed the daily recommended dosage. Crystalluria related to **ciprofloxacin** has occurred only rarely in humans because human urine is usually acidic. The patient should drink sufficient fluids to ensure proper hydration and adequate urinary output.

Hemolytic reactions: Rarely, hemolytic reactions have been reported in patients with latent or actual defects in glucose-6-phosphate dehydrogenase activity who take quinolone antibacterial agents, including **norfloxacin**.

Myasthenia gravis: Quinolones may exacerbate the signs of myasthenia gravis and lead to life-threatening weakness of the respiratory muscles. Exercise caution when using quinolones in patients with myasthenia gravis.

Blood glucose abnormalities: As with other quinolones, disturbances of blood glucose, including symptomatic hyper- and hypoglycemia, have been reported, usually in diabetic patients receiving concomitant treatment with an oral hypoglycemic agent (eg, glyburide/glibenclamide) or with insulin. In these patients, careful monitoring of blood glucose is recommended. If a hypoglycemic reaction occurs, initiate appropriate therapy immediately.

Drug Interactions

Drugs that may affect fluoroquinolones include antacids, didanosine, iron salts, sucralfate, azlocillin, bismuth subsalicylate, cimetidine, nitrofurantoin, cisapride, nonsteroidal anti-inflammatory drugs (NSAIDs), morphine, and probenecid.

Drugs that may be affected by fluoroquinolones include caffeine, cyclosporine, digoxin, antiarrhythmic agents, bepridil, erythromycin, phenothiazine, tricyclic antidepressants, procainamide, anticoagulants, cyclosporine, and theophylline.

Drug/Food interactions: Food may decrease the absorption of **norfloxacin**. Food delays the absorption of **ciprofloxacin**, resulting in peak concentrations that are closer to 2 hours after dosing rather than 1 hour; however, overall absorption is not substantially affected. Dairy products such as milk and yogurt reduce the absorption of ciprofloxacin; avoid concurrent use. The bioavailability of ciprofloxacin may also be decreased by enteral feedings. Food delays the rate of absorption of **lomefloxacin** and decreases the extent of absorption (AUC) by 12%.

Adverse Reactions

Fluoroquinolone Adverse Reactions (%)											
	Adverse reaction	Ciprofloxacin[1]	Enoxacin[2]	Gatifloxacin	Levofloxacin	Lomefloxacin	Moxifloxacin	Norfloxacin[2]	Ofloxacin[1]	Sparfloxacin	Trovafloxacin/ Alatrofloxacin[1]
CNS	Headache	1.2	≤ 2	3	0.1-6.4	3.6	2	2-2.8	1-9	4.2-8.1	1-5
	Dizziness	< 1	≤ 3	3	0.3-2.7	2.1	3	1.7-2.6	1-5	2-3.8	2-11
	Fatigue/Lethargy/Malaise	< 1	< 1		< 1-1.2	< 1	> 0.05-< 1	0.3-1	1-3	< 1	< 1
	Somnolence/Drowsiness	< 1	< 1	< 0.1	< 1	< 1	> 0.05-< 1	0.3-1	1-3	< 1-1.5	< 1
	Depression	< 1	< 1	< 0.1	< 1	< 1		0.1-0.2	< 1	< 1	< 1
	Insomnia	< 1	1	≥ 0.1-< 3	0.5-4.6	< 1	> 0.05-< 1	0.3-1	3-7	1.9	< 1
	Seizures/Convulsions[3]	< 1	< 1	< 0.1	< 1	< 1		✓[4]	< 1		< 1
	Confusion	≤ 1	< 1	< 0.1	< 1	< 1	> 0.05-< 1	✓[4]	< 1	< 1	< 1
	Psychotic reactions	< 1	< 0.1					✓[4]			
	Paresthesia	< 1	< 1	≥ 0.1-< 3	< 1	< 1		✓[4]	< 1	< 1	
	Hallucinations	< 1	< 0.1	< 0.1	< 1		> 0.05-< 1		< 1	< 1	< 1
Dermatologic	Photosensitivity[3]	< 1	< 1			2.3		✓[4]	✓[4]		
	Rash	1.1	≤ 1	≥ 0.1-< 3	0.3-1.2	< 1	> 0.05-< 1	0.3-1	1-3	1.1	< 1-2
	Pruritus	< 1	1	< 0.1	0.4-1.3	< 1	> 0.05-< 1	0.3-1	1-3	1.8-3.3	< 1-2
	Toxic epidermal necrolysis	< 1	< 1					✓[4]			
	Stevens-Johnson syndrome	< 1	< 1					✓[4]			
	Exfoliative dermatitis	< 1						✓[4]			
	Hypersensitivity[3]	< 1				< 1		✓[4]	✓[3]		

	Fluoroquinolone Adverse Reactions (%)										
	Adverse reaction	Ciprofloxacin[1]	Enoxacin[2]	Gatifloxacin	Levofloxacin	Lomefloxacin	Moxifloxacin	Norfloxacin[2]	Ofloxacin[1]	Sparfloxacin	Trovafloxacin/ Alatrofloxacin[1]
GI	Nausea	5.2	2-8	8	1.3-7.2	3.5	8	2.6-4.2	3-10	4.3-7.6	4-8
	Abdominal pain/discomfort/ cramping	≤ 1-1.7	≤ 2	≥ 0.1-< 3	0.4-2.5	1.2	> 0.05-≤ 2	0.3-1.6	1-3	1.8-2.4	1
	Diarrhea	2.3	1-2	4	1-5.6	1.4	6	0.3-1	1-4	3.2-4.6	2
	Vomiting	≤ 1-2	2-9	≥ 0.1-< 3	0.2-2.3	< 1	2	0.3-1	1-4	< 1-1.3	1-3
	Dry/Painful mouth	< 1	< 1		< 1	< 1	> 0.05-< 1	0.3-1	1-3	< 1-1.4	
	Dyspepsia/Heartburn	< 1	1	≥ 0.1-< 3	0.3-2.4	< 1	1	0.3-1	< 1	1.6-2.3	
	Constipation	< 1	< 1	≥ 0.1-< 3	0.1-3.2	< 1	> 0.05-< 1	0.3-1	1-3	< 1	
	Flatulence	< 1	< 1	< 0.1	0.4-1.5	< 1		0.3-1	1-3	< 1-1.1	< 1
	Pseudomembranous colitis[3]	< 1	< 0.1	< 0.1	< 1	✓[4]		✓[4]	✓[3]		< 1
Miscellaneous	Visual disturbances	< 1	< 1			< 1		0.1-0.2	1-3		
	Hearing loss	< 1						✓[4]	< 1		
	Vaginitis	< 1	< 1	6	0.7-1.8	< 1	> 0.05-< 1		1-5	< 1	< 1-2
	Hypertensio	< 1		< 0.1	< 1	< 1	> 0.05-< 1		< 1	< 1	< 1
	Palpitations	< 1	< 1	≥ 0.1-< 3	< 1		> 0.05-< 1		< 1	< 1	
	Syncope	< 1	< 1		< 1	< 1			< 1		< 1
	Chills	< 1	< 1	≥ 0.1-< 3		< 1	> 0.05-< 1	0.1-0.2	< 1	< 1	
	Edema	< 1	< 1	< 0.1	< 1	< 1		0.1-0.2	< 1		< 1
	Fever	< 1	< 1	≥ 0.1-< 3	< 1			0.3-1	1-3	< 1	< 1

Fluoroquinolone Adverse Reactions (%)

	Adverse reaction	Ciprofloxacin[1]	Enoxacin[2]	Gatifloxacin	Levofloxacin	Lomefloxacin	Moxifloxacin	Norfloxacin[2]	Ofloxacin[1]	Sparfloxacin	Trovafloxacin/ Alatrofloxacin[1]
Abnormal laboratory values	↑ ALT/↑ AST	1.9/1.7	≥ 1	< 1		≤ 0.4		1.4/1.4-1.6	≥ 1	2-2.3	≥ 1
	↑ Alkaline phosphatase	0.8	< 1	< 1		0.1		1.1	≥ 1	< 1	≥ 1
	↑ LDH	0.4			< 1			✓[4]			
	↑ or ↓ Bilirubin	0.3	< 1	< 1		0.1	≥ 2			< 1	
	Eosinophilia	0.6	< 1			0.1	> 0.05-< 1	0.6-1.5	≥ 1		≥ 1
	Leukopenin	0.4	< 1		< 1	0.1	> 0.05-< 1	1.4	≥ 1		
	↑ or ↓ Platelets	0.1	< 1			< 1		1		< 1	≥ 1
	Pancytopenia	0.1									
	↑ ESR/Lymphocytopenia					< 0.1			≥ 1		
	Neutropenia			< 1				1.4	≥ 1		
	↑ Serum creatinine	1.1				0.1		✓[4]	≥ 1		
	↑ BUN	0.9				0.1		✓[4]	≥ 1		≥ 1
	Crystalluria/Cylinduria/Candi-duria	✓[4]						✓[4]			
	Hematuria	✓[4]							≥ 1		
	Glucosuria/Pyuria							✓[4]	≥ 1		
	Proteinuria/Albuminuria		< 1			< 0.1		1	≥ 1		

Fluoroquinolone Adverse Reactions (%)

	Adverse reaction	Ciprofloxacin[1]	Enoxacin[2]	Gatifloxacin	Levofloxacin	Lomefloxacin	Moxifloxacin	Norfloxacin[2]	Ofloxacin[1]	Sparfloxacin	Trovafloxacin/ Alatrofloxacin[1]
Abnormal laboratory values con't	↑ γ-glutamyltransferase	< 0.1				< 0.1					
	↑ Serum amylase	< 0.1		< 1						< 1	
	↑ Uric acid	< 0.1									
	↑ or ↓ Blood glucose	< 0.1			2.2	< 0.1			≥ 1	< 1	
	↓ Hemoglobin/Hematocrit	< 0.1	< 1			< 0.1	≥ 2	0.6			≥ 1
	↑ or ↓ Potassium	✓[4]	< 1			0.1				< 1	
	Anemia	< 0.1				< 0.1			≥ 1		
	Bleeding/↑ PT	< 0.1				< 0.1					
	↑ Monocytes	< 0.1				0.2				< 1	
	Leukocytosis	< 0.1	< 1		< 1	0.1			≥ 1		
	↑ Triglycerides/Cholesterol	✓[4]									

[1] Includes data for oral and IV formulations.
[2] From single- and multiple-dose studies.
[3] See Warnings or Precautions.
[4] ✓ = Adverse reaction observed; incidence not reported.

GASTROINTESTINAL ANTICHOLINERGICS/ANTISPASMODICS

ANISOTROPINE METHYLBROMIDE	
Tablets: 50 mg (*Rx*)	Various
ATROPINE SULFATE	
Injection: 0.05, 0.1, 0.3, 0.4, 0.5, 0.8, andl mg/mL (*Rx*)	Various
Tablets: 0.4 mg (*Rx*)	*Atropine Sulfate* (Lilly), *Sal-Tropine* (Hope)
Tablets, soluble: 0.4 and 0.6 mg (*Rx*)	*Atropine Sulfate* (Lilly)
BELLADONNA	
Liquids: 27 to 33 mg belladonna alkaloids/100 mL (*Rx*)	Various
CLIDINIUM BROMIDE	
Capsules: 2.5 and 5 mg (*Rx*)	*Quarzan* (Roche)
DICYCLOMINE HCl	
Capsules: 10 and 20 mg (*Rx*)	Various, *Bentyl* (Lakeside Pharm.)
Tablets: 20 mg (*Rx*)	Various, *Bentyl* (Lakeside Pharm.)
Syrup: 10 mg/5 mL (*Rx*)	Various, *Bentyl* (Lakeside Pharm.)
Injection: 10 mg/mL (*Rx*)	Various, *Bentyl* (Lakeside Pharm.)
GLYCOPYRROLATE	
Tablets: 1 and 2 mg (*Rx*)	*Robinul* (Robins)
Injection: 0.2 mg/mL (*Rx*)	Various, *Robinul* (Robins)
LEVOROTATORY ALKALOIDS OF BELLADONNA	
Tablets: 0.25 mg (*Rx*)	*Bellafoline* (Sandoz)
L-HYOSCYAMINE SULFATE	
Tablets: 0.125 and 0.15 mg (*Rx*)	*Levsin* (Schwarz Pharma), *Gastrosed* (Roberts/ Hauck), *Cystospaz* (PolyMedica), *Donnamar* (Marnel), *ED-SPAZ* (Edwards)
Tablets, sublingual: 0.125 mg (*Rx*)	*Levsin/SL* (Schwarz Pharma), *A-Spas S/L* (Hyrex)
Tablets, extended release: 0.375 mg (*Rx*)	*Levbid* (Schwarz Pharma)
Capsules, timed release: 0.375 mg (*Rx*)	Various, *Cystospaz-M* (PolyMedica), *Levsinex Timecaps* (Schwarz Pharma)
Solution: 0.125 mg/mL (*Rx*)	*Levsin Drops* (Schwarz Pharma), *Gastrosed* (Roberts Hauck)
Elixir: 0.125 mg/5 mL (*Rx*)	*Levsin* (Schwarz Pharma)
Injection: 0.5 mg/mL (*Rx*)	*Levsin* (Schwarz Pharma)
METHSCOPOLAMINE BROMIDE	
Tablets: 2.5 mg (*Rx*)	*Pamine* (Kenwood/Bradley)
MEPENZOLATE BROMIDE	
Tablets: 25 mg (*Rx*)	*Cantil* (Aventis)
METHANTHELINE BROMIDE	
Tablets: 50 mg (*Rx*)	*Banthine* (Schiapparelli Searle)
OXYPHENCYCLIMINE HCl	
Tablets: 10 mg (*Rx*)	*Daricon* (GlaxoSmithKline)
PROPANTHELINE BROMIDE	
Tablets: 7.5 and 15 mg (*Rx*)	Various, *Pro-Banthine* (Schiapparelli Searle)
SCOPOLAMINE HBr (Hyoscine HBr)	
Injection: 0.3, 0.4, 0.86, and 1 mg/mL (*Rx*)	Various
TRIDIHEXETHYL CHLORIDE	
Tablets: 25 mg (*Rx*)	*Pathilon* (Lederle)

Indications

Peptic ulcer: Adjunctive therapy for peptic ulcer. These agents suppress gastric acid secretion.

Other GI conditions: Functional GI disorders (diarrhea, pylorospasm, hypermotility, neurogenic colon), irritable bowel syndrome (spastic colon, mucous colitis), acute enterocolitis, ulcerative colitis, diverticulitis, mild dysenteries, pancreatitis, splenic flexure syndrome, and infant colic.

Biliary tract: For spastic disorders of the biliary tract. Given in conjunction with a narcotic analgesic.

Urogenital tract: Uninhibited hypertonic neurogenic bladder.

Bradycardia: **Atropine** is used in the suppression of vagally mediated bradycardias.

Preoperative medication: **Atropine**, **scopolamine**, **hyoscyamine**, and **glycopyrrolate** are used as preanesthetic medication to control bronchial, nasal, pharyngeal, and salivary secretions and to block cardiac vagal inhibitory reflexes during induction of anesthesia and intubation. Scopolamine is used for preanesthetic sedation and for obstetric amnesia.

Antidotes for poisoning by cholinergic drugs: Atropine is used for poisoning by organophosphorous insecticides, chemical warfare nerve gases, and as an antidote for mushroom poisoning caused by muscarine in certain species, such as *Amanita muscaria.*

Miscellaneous uses: Calming delirium; motion sickness (**scopolamine**); parkinsonism.

Unlabeled uses:

Bronchial asthma – Atropine and related agents are effective in some patients with cholinergic-mediated bronchospasm.

Glycopyrrolate may be effective in the treatment of bronchial asthma.

Administration and Dosage

ANISOTROPINE METHYLBROMIDE: 50 mg 3 times daily.

ATROPINE SULFATE:

Adults – 0.4 to 0.6 mg.

Children –

Atropine Dosage Recommendations in Children

Weight		Dose
lb	kg	mg
7 to 16	3.2 to 7.3	0.1
16 to 24	7.3 to 10.9	0.15
24 to 40	10.9 to 18.1	0.2
40 to 65	18.1 to 29.5	0.3
65 to 90	29.5 to 40.8	0.4
> 90	40.8	0.4 to 0.6

Hypotonic radiography – 1 mg IM.

Surgery – Give SC, IM, or IV. The average adult dose is 0.5 mg (range, 0.4 to 0.6 mg). In children, it has been suggested to use a dose of 0.01 mg/kg to a maximum of 0.4 mg, repeated every 4 to 6 hours as needed. A recommended infant dose is 0.04 mg/kg (infants < 5 kg) or 0.03 mg/kg (infants > 5 kg), repeated every 4 to 6 hours as needed.

Bradyarrhythmias – The usual IV adult dosage ranges from 0.4 to 1 mg every 1 to 2 hours as needed; larger doses, up to a maximum of 2 mg, may be required. In children, IV dosage ranges from 0.01 to 0.03 mg/kg.

Poisoning – In anticholinesterase poisoning from exposure to insecticides, give large doses of at least 2 to 3 mg parenterally; repeat until signs of atropine intoxication appear.

BELLADONNA:

Belladonna tincture –

Adults: 0.6 to 1 mL 3 to 4 times daily.

Children: 0.03 mL/kg (0.8 mL/m^2) 3 times daily.

CLIDINIUM BROMIDE:

Adults – 2.5 to 5 mg 3 or 4 times daily before meals and at bedtime.

Geriatric or debilitated patients – 2.5 mg 3 times daily before meals.

DICYCLOMINE HCl:

Oral –

Adults: The only oral dose shown to be effective is 160 mg/day in 4 equally divided doses. However, because of side effects, begin with 80 mg/day (in 4 equally divided doses). Increase dose to 160 mg/day unless side effects limit dosage.

Parenteral – IM only. Not for IV use.

Adults: 80 mg/day in 4 divided doses.

GLYCOPYRROLATE: Not recommended for children < 12 years of age for the management of peptic ulcer.

Oral – 1 mg 3 times daily or 2 mg 2 to 3 times daily.

Maintenance: 1 mg 2 times daily.

Parenteral –

Peptic ulcer: 0.1 to 0.2 mg IM or IV 3 or 4 times daily.

Preanesthetic medication: 0.002 mg/lb (0.004 mg/kg) IM, 30 minutes to 1 hour prior to anesthesia. Children < 2 years of age may require up to 0.004 mg/lb. Children < 12 years of age, give 0.002 to 0.004 mg/lb IM.

Intraoperative medication: Adults, 0.1 mg IV. Repeat as needed at 2- to 3-minute intervals. Children, give 0.002 mg/lb (0.004 mg/kg) IV, not to exceed 0.1 mg in a single dose; may be repeated at 2- to 3-minute intervals.

Reversal of neuromuscular blockade: Adults and children, 0.2 mg for each 1 mg neostigmine or 5 mg pyridostigmine. Administer IV simultaneously.

L-HYOSCYAMINE SULFATE:

Oral –

Adults: 0.125 to 0.25 mg 3 or 4 times/day orally or sublingually; or 0.375 to 0.75 mg in sustained release form every 12 hours.

Children: Individualize dosage according to weight.

Parenteral – 0.25 to 0.5 mg SC, IM or IV, 2 to 4 times daily, as needed.

LEVOROTATORY ALKALOIDS OF BELLADONNA:

Oral –

Adults: 0.25 to 0.5 mg 3 times daily.

Children (> 6 years of age): 0.125 to 0.25 mg 3 times daily.

METHSCOPOLAMINE BROMIDE: 2.5 mg 30 minutes before meals and 2.5 to 5 mg at bedtime.

MEPENZOLATE BROMIDE:

Adults – 25 to 50 mg 4 times daily with meals and at bedtime.

Children – Safety and efficacy have not been established.

METHANTHELINE BROMIDE:

Adults – 50 to 100 mg every 6 hours.

Pediatric –

Newborns: 12.5 mg 2 times daily, then 12.5 mg 3 times daily.

Infants (1 to 12 months of age): 12.5 mg 4 times daily, increased to 25 mg 4 times daily.

Children (> 1 year of age): 12.5 to 50 mg 4 times daily.

OXPHENCYCLIMINE HCl:

Adults – 5 to 10 mg 2 or 3 times daily, preferably in the morning and at bedtime. Some respond to 5 mg 2 times/day, while some may require higher dosage 3 times/day.

Children – Not for use in children < 12 years of age.

PROPANTHELINE BROMIDE:

Adults – 15 mg 30 minutes before meals and 30 mg at bedtime. For patients with mild manifestations, geriatric patients, or those of small stature, take 7.5 mg 3 times daily.

Children –

Peptic ulcer: Safety and efficacy have not been established.

Antisecretory: 1.5 mg/kg/day divided 3 to 4 times daily.

Antispasmodic: 2 to 3 mg/kg/day divided every 4 to 6 hours and at bedtime.

SCOPOLAMINE HBr (Hyoscine HBr): Give SC or IM; may give IV after dilution with Sterile Water for Injection.

Adults – 0.32 to 0.65 mg.

Children – 0.006 mg/kg. Maximum dosage, 0.3 mg.

TRIDIHEXETHYL CHLORIDE: 25 to 50 mg 3 or 4 times daily before meals and at bedtime. Bedtime dose, 50 mg.

Actions

Pharmacology: GI anticholinergics are used primarily to decrease motility (smooth muscle tone) in GI, biliary, and urinary tracts and for antisecretory effects. Antispasmodics, related compounds, decrease GI motility by acting on smooth muscle.

These agents inhibit the muscarinic actions of acetylcholine at postganglionic parasympathetic neuroeffector sites including smooth muscle, secretory glands, and CNS sites. Large doses may block nicotinic receptors at the autonomic ganglia and at the neuromuscular junction.

Pharmacokinetics:

Belladonna alkaloids – Belladonna alkaloids are rapidly absorbed after oral use. They readily cross the blood-brain barrier and affect the CNS.

Atropine – Atropine has a half-life of ≈ 2.5 hours; 94% of a dose is eliminated through the urine in 24 hours.

Quaternary anticholinergics – Synthetic or semisynthetic derivatives structurally related to the belladonna alkaloids, they are poorly and unreliably absorbed orally. Because they do not cross the blood-brain barrier, CNS effects are negligible. Duration of action is more prolonged than alkaloids.

Contraindications

Hypersensitivity: Hypersensitivity to anticholinergic drugs. Patients hypersensitive to belladonna or to barbiturates may be hypersensitive to **scopolamine.**

Ocular: Narrow-angle glaucoma; adhesions (synechiae) between the iris and lens.

Cardiovascular: Tachycardia; unstable cardiovascular status in acute hemorrhage; myocardial ischemia.

GI: Obstructive disease (eg, achalasia, pyloroduodenal stenosis or pyloric obstruction, cardiospasm); paralytic ileus; intestinal atony of the elderly or debilitated; severe ulcerative colitis; toxic megacolon complicating ulcerative colitis; hepatic disease.

GU: Obstructive uropathy (eg, bladder neck obstruction caused by prostatic hypertrophy); renal disease.

Musculoskeletal: Myasthenia gravis.

Atropine: Atropine is contraindicated in asthma patients.

Dicyclomine: Dicyclomine is contraindicated in infants < 6 months of age.

Warnings

Heat prostration: Heat prostration can occur with anticholinergic drug use (fever and heat stroke caused by decreased sweating) in the presence of a high environmental temperature.

Diarrhea: Diarrhea may be an early symptom of incomplete intestinal obstruction, especially in patients with ileostomy or colostomy. Treatment of diarrhea with these drugs is inappropriate and possibly harmful.

Anticholinergic psychosis: Anticholinergic psychosis has been reported in sensitive individuals given anticholinergic drugs.

Gastric ulcer: Gastric ulcer may produce a delay in gastric emptying time and may complicate therapy (antral stasis).

Elderly: Elderly patients may react with excitement, agitation, drowsiness, and other untoward manifestations to even small doses of anticholinergic drugs.

Pregnancy: *Category B* (glycopyrrolate, parenteral); *Category C* (hyoscyamine, atropine, scopolamine, propantheline, methantheline).

Lactation: **Hyoscyamine** is excreted in breast milk; other anticholinergics (especially **atropine**) may be excreted in milk, causing infant toxicity, and may reduce milk production.

Children: Safety and efficacy are not established. **Hyoscyamine** has been used in infant colic. Safety and efficacy of **glycopyrrolate** in children < 12 years of age are not established for peptic ulcer. **Dicyclomine** is contraindicated in infants < 6 months of age.

Precautions

Use with caution in:

Ocular – Glaucoma; light irides. Use caution in the elderly because of increased incidence of glaucoma.

GI – Hepatic disease; early evidence of ileus, as in peritonitis; ulcerative colitis; hiatal hernia associated with reflux esophagitis.

GU – Renal disease; prostatic hypertrophy.

Cardiovascular – Coronary heart disease; CHF; cardiac arrhythmias; tachycardia; hypertension.

Pulmonary – Debilitated patients with chronic lung disease; reduction in bronchial secretions can lead to inspissation and formation of bronchial plugs.

Miscellaneous: Autonomic neuropathy; hyperthyroidism.

Special risk: Use cautiously in infants, small children, and people with Down's syndrome, brain damage, or spastic paralysis.

Hazardous tasks: May produce drowsiness, dizziness, or blurred vision; observe caution while driving or performing other tasks requiring alertness.

Drug Interactions

Drugs that may interact with GI anticholinergics include amantadine, atenolol, digoxin, phenothiazines, and tricyclic antidepressants.

Adverse Reactions

Xerostomia; altered taste perception; nausea; vomiting; dysphagia; heartburn; constipation; bloated feeling; paralytic ileus; urinary hesitancy and retention; impotence; blurred vision; mydriasis; photophobia; cycloplegia; increased intraocular pressure; dilated pupils; palpitations; tachycardia (after higher doses); headache; flushing; nervousness; drowsiness; weakness; dizziness; confusion; insomnia; fever (especially in children); mental confusion or excitement; CNS stimulation (restlessness, tremor with large doses); severe allergic reactions including anaphylaxis, urticaria and other dermal manifestations; nasal congestion; decreased sweating.

GLUCOCORTICOIDS

BETAMETHASONE	
BETAMETHASONE, ORAL	
Tablets: 0.6 mg (*Rx*)	*Celestone* (Schering)
Syrup: 0.6 mg/5 mL (*Rx*)	
BETAMETHASONE SODIUM PHOSPHATE	
Injection: 4 mg sodium phosphate/mL (*Rx*)	*Celestone Phosphate* (Schering)
BETAMETHASONE SODIUM PHOSPHATE AND ACETATE	
Injection: 3 mg acetate and 3 mg sodium phosphate/mL (*Rx*)	*Celestone Soluspan* (Schering)
BUDESONIDE	
Capsules: 3 mg micronized budesonide	*Entocort EC* (AstraZeneca)
CORTISONE	
Tablets: 5, 10, and 25 mg (*Rx*)	Various, *Cortisone Acetate* (Merck)
Injection: 50 mg/mL (*Rx*)	*Cortone Acetate* (Merck)
DEXAMETHASONE	
DEXAMETHASONE, ORAL	
Tablets: 0.25, 0.5, 0.75, 1, 1.5, 2, 4, and 6 mg (*Rx*)	Various, *Decadron* (Merck), *Dexone* (Solvay), *Hexadrol* (Organon)
Elixir: 0.5 mg/5 mL (*Rx*)	Various, *Decadron* (Merck), *Hexadrol* (Organon)
Oral Solution: 0.5 mg/5 mL (*Rx*)	Various
DEXAMETHASONE ACETATE	
Injection: 8 and 16 mg/mL (*Rx*)	Various, *Dalalone L.A.* (Forest), *Dalalone D.P.* (Forest) *Decadron-LA* (Merck)
DEXAMETHASONE SODIUM PHOSPHATE	
Injection: 4, 10, 20, and 24 mg/mL (*Rx*)	Various, *Dalalone* (Forest), *Decadron Phosphate* (Merck), *Hexadrol Phosphate* (Organon)
HYDROCORTISONE (CORTISOL)	
HYDROCORTISONE	
Tablets: 5, 10, and 20 mg (*Rx*)	Various, *Cortef* (Upjohn), *Hydrocortone* (Merck)
HYDROCORTISONE CYPIONATE	
Oral Suspension: 10 mg/5 mL (*Rx*)	*Cortef* (Upjohn)
HYDROCORTISONE SODIUM PHOSPHATE	
Injection: 50 mg/mL (*Rx*)	*Hydrocortone Phosphate* (Merck)
HYDROCORTISONE SODIUM SUCCINATE	
Injection: 100, 250, 500, and 1000 mg per vial (*Rx*)	*A-Hydrocort* (Abbott), *Solu-Cortef* (Upjohn)
HYDROCORTISONE ACETATE	
Injection: 25 and 50 mg/mL (*Rx*)	Various, *Hydrocortone Acetate* (Merck)
METHYLPREDNISOLONE	
METHYLPREDNISOLONE, ORAL	
Tablets: 2, 4, 8, 16, 24, and 32 mg (*Rx*)	Various, *Medrol* (Upjohn)
METHYLPREDNISOLONE SODIUM SUCCINATE	
Powder for Injection: 40, 125, and 500 mg and 1 and 2 g per vial (*Rx*)	Various, *A-Methapred* (Abbott), *Solu-Medrol* (Upjohn)
METHYLPREDNISOLONE ACETATE	
Injection: 20, 40, and 80 mg/mL (*Rx*)	Various, *Depo-Medrol* (Upjohn), *depMedalone* (Forest), *Adlone* (UAD)
PREDNISOLONE	
PREDNISOLONE, ORAL	
Tablets: 5 mg (*Rx*)	Various, *Delta-Cortef* (Upjohn)
Syrup: 15 mg/5 mL (*Rx*)	*Prelone* (Muro)
PREDNISOLONE ACETATE	
Injection: 25 and 50 mg/mL (*Rx*)	Various, *Key-Pred 25* (Hyrex), *Key-Pred 50* (Hyrex)
PREDNISOLONE TEBUTATE	
Injection: 20 mg/mL (*Rx*)	Various, *Hydeltra-T.B.A.*(Merck)
PREDNISOLONE SODIUM PHOSPHATE	
Injection: 20 mg/mL (*Rx*)	*Hydeltrasol* (Merck)
Oral Liquid: 5 mg/5 mL (*Rx*)	*Pediapred* (Fisons)

PREDNISONE	
Tablets: 1, 2.5, 5, 10, 20, and 50 mg (*Rx*)	Various, *Meticorten* (Schering), *Orasone* (Solvay), *Deltasone* (Upjohn)
Oral Solution: 5 mg/5 mL (*Rx*)	Various
Syrup: 5 mg/5 mL (*Rx*)	*Liquid Pred* (Muro)
TRIAMCINOLONE	
TRIAMCINOLONE, ORAL	
Tablets: 1, 2, 4, and 8 mg (*Rx*)	Various, *Aristocort* (Fujisawa)
TRIAMCINOLONE DIACETATE	
Injection: 25 and 40 mg/mL (*Rx*)	Various, *Aristocort Intralesional* (Fujisawa), *Aristocort Forte* (Fujisawa), *Triamolone 40* (Forest)
TRIAMCINOLONE HEXACETONIDE	
Injection: 5 mg/mL (*Rx*)	*Aristospan Intralesional* (Fujisawa)
20 mg/mL (*Rx*)	*Aristospan Intra-articular* (Fujisawa)
TRIAMCINOLONE ACETONIDE	
Injection: 3, 10, and 40 mg/mL (*Rx*)	Various, *Tac-3* (Herbert), *Kenalog-10* (Westwood-Squibb), *Kenalog-40* (Westwood-Squibb), *Triamonide 40* (Forest)

Indications

Endocrine disorders: Primary or secondary adrenal cortical insufficiency (hydrocortisone or cortisone is the drug of choice; synthetic analogs may be used in conjunction with mineralocorticoids; in infancy, mineralocorticoid supplementation is important); congenital adrenal hyperplasia; nonsuppurative thyroiditis; hypercalcemia associated with cancer.

Parenteral – Acute adrenal cortical insufficiency (hydrocortisone or cortisone is drug of choice); preoperatively or in serious trauma or illness with known adrenal insufficiency or when adrenal cortical reserve is doubtful; shock unresponsive to conventional therapy if adrenal cortical insufficiency exists or is suspected.

Various rheumatic disorders.

Collagen diseases.

Dermatologic diseases.

Allergic states: Control of severe or incapacitating allergic conditions intractable to conventional treatment in serum sickness and drug hypersensitivity reactions. Parenteral therapy is indicated for urticarial transfusion reactions and acute noninfectious laryngeal edema (epinephrine is the drug of first choice).

Ophthalmic: Severe acute and chronic allergic and inflammatory processes involving the eye and its adnexa.

Respiratory diseases.

Hematologic disorders.

Neoplastic diseases.

Edematous states: To induce diuresis or remission of proteinuria in the nephrotic syndrome (without uremia) of the idiopathic type or that due to lupus erythematosus.

GI diseases: Crohn's disease and intractable sprue.

Multiple sclerosis.

Miscellaneous: Tuberculous meningitis with subarachnoid block or impending block when accompanied by appropriate antituberculous chemotherapy; in trichinosis with neurologic or myocardial involvement.

Intralesional administration: Keloids; localized hypertrophic, infiltrated, inflammatory lesions of lichen planus, psoriatic plaques, granuloma annulare, lichen simplex chronicus (neurodermatitis); discoid lupus erythematosus; necrobiosis lipoidica diabeticorum; alopecia areata. May be useful in cystic tumors of an aponeurosis or tendon (ganglia).

Triamcinolone: Treatment of pulmonary emphysema where bronchospasm or bronchial edema plays a significant role, and diffuse interstitial pulmonary fibrosis (Hamman-

Rich syndrome); in conjunction with diuretic agents to induce a diuresis in refractory CHF and in cirrhosis of the liver with refractory ascites; and for postoperative dental inflammatory reactions.

Unlabeled uses:

Glucocorticoid Unlabeled Uses	
Use	Drug/Comment
Acute mountain sickness	Dexamethasone 4 mg q 6 h; prevention or treatment
Antiemetic	Dexamethasone most common, 16 to 20 mg
Bacterial meningitis	Dexamethasone 0.15 mg/kg q 6 h; to decrease incidence of hearing loss
Bronchopulmonary dysplasia in preterm infants	Dexamethasone 0.5 mg/kg, then taper.
COPD	Prednisone 30 to 60 mg/day for 1 to 2 weeks, then taper
Depression, diagnosis of	Dexamethasone 1 mg
Duchenne's muscular dystrophy	Prednisone 0.75 to 1.5 mg/kg/day; to improve strength and function
Graves' ophthalmopathy	Prednisone 60 mg/day, taper to 20 mg/day
Hepatitis, severe alcoholic	Methylprednisolone 32 mg/day
Hirsutism	Dexamethasone 0.5 to 1 mg/day
Respiratory distress syndrome	Prevention in premature neonates (betamethasone most common); adults, methylprednisolone 30 mg/kg (controversial)
Septic shock	Methylprednisolone 30 mg/kg IV most common (very controversial)
Spinal cord injury, acute	Methylprednisolone IV within 8 hrs of injury; to improve neurologic function
Tuberculous pleurisy	Prednisolone 0.75 mg/kg/day, then taper; concurrently w/antituberculous therapy

Administration and Dosage

The maximal activity of the adrenal cortex is between 2 and 8 am, and it is minimal between 4 pm and midnight. Exogenous corticosteroids suppress adrenocortical activity the least when given at the time of maximal activity (am). Therefore, administer glucocorticoids in the morning prior to 9 am.

Initiation of therapy: The initial dosage depends on the specific disease entity being treated. Maintain or adjust the initial dosage until a satisfactory response is noted. If after a reasonable period of time there is a lack of satisfactory clinical response, discontinue the drug and transfer the patient to other appropriate therapy. For infants and children, the recommended dosage should be governed by the same considerations rather than by strict adherence to the ratio indicated by age or body weight. It should be emphasized that dosage requirements are variable and must be individualized.

Maintenance therapy: After a favorable response is observed, determine the maintenance dosage by decreasing the initial dosage in small amounts at intervals until the lowest dosage that will maintain an adequate clinical response is reached.

Withdrawal of therapy: If, after long-term therapy, the drug is to be stopped, it must be withdrawn gradually. If spontaneous remission occurs in a chronic condition, discontinue treatment gradually.

Alternate day therapy: Alternate day therapy is a dosing regimen in which twice the usual daily dose is administered every other morning. The purpose is to provide the patient requiring long-term treatment with the beneficial effects of corticosteroids while minimizing pituitary-adrenal suppression, the cushingoid state, withdrawal symptoms and growth suppression in children. The benefits of alternate day therapy are only achieved by using the intermediate-acting agents.

Intra-articular injection: Dose depends on the joint size and varies with the severity of the condition. In chronic cases, injections may be repeated at intervals of ≥ 1 to 5 weeks depending upon the degree of relief obtained from the initial injection. Injection must be made into the synovial space.

Miscellaneous (tendinitis, epicondylitis, ganglion): In the treatment of conditions such as tendinitis or tenosynovitis, inject into the tendon sheath rather than into the substance of the tendon. When treating conditions such as epicondylitis, outline the area of greatest tenderness and infiltrate the drug into the area.

Injections for local effect in dermatologic conditions: Avoid injection of sufficient material to cause blanching, since this may be followed by a small slough. One to four injections are usually employed.

BETAMETHASONE:

Betamethasone, oral –

Initial dosage: 0.6 to 7.2 mg/day.

Betamethasone sodium phosphate –

Systemic and local: The initial dosage may vary up to 9 mg/day.

Betamethasone sodium phosphate and acetate – Betamethasone sodium phosphate provides prompt activity, while betamethasone acetate is only slightly soluble and affords sustained activity.

Systemic: Not for IV use.

Initial dose – 0.5 to 9 mg/day. Dosage ranges are 33% to 50% of the oral dose given every 12 hours. In certain acute, life-threatening situations, dosages exceeding the usual may be justified and may be in multiples of oral dosages.

Bursitis, tenosynovitis, peritendinitis: 1 mL given intrabursally.

Rheumatoid arthritis and osteoarthritis: 0.5 to 2 mL given intra-articularly.

Very large joints – 1 to 2 mL.

Large joints – 1 mL.

Medium joints – 0.5 to 1 mL.

Small joints – 0.25 to 0.5 mL.

Dermatologic conditions: 0.2 mL/cm^2 intradermally.

Maximum dose – 1 mL/week.

Foot disorders – The following doses are recommended at 3- to 7-day intervals:

Bursitis:

Under heloma durum or heloma molle – 0.25 to 0.5 mL.

Under calcaneal spur – 0.5 mL.

Over hallux rigidus or digiti quinti varus – 0.5 mL.

Tenosynovitis, periostitis of cuboid: 0.5 mL.

Acute gouty arthritis: 0.5 to 1 mL.

BUDESONIDE:

Adults – Take 9 mg once daily in the morning for up to 8 weeks. Swallow capsules whole; do not chew or break. Safety and efficacy of budesonide in the treatment of active Crohn's disease have not been established beyond 8 weeks. For recurring episodes of active Crohn's disease, a repeat 8-week course of budesonide can be given. Treatment with budesonide capsules can be tapered to 6 mg/day for 2 weeks prior to complete cessation.

Patients with mild-to-moderately active Crohn's disease involving the ileum or ascending colon have been switched from oral prednisolone to budesonide with no reported episodes of adrenal insufficiency. Because prednisolone should not be stopped abruptly, tapering should begin concomitantly with initiating budesonide treatment.

Hepatic insufficiency: Consider reducing the dose of budesonide capsules in patients with hepatic insufficiency.

CORTISONE:

Initial dosage – 25 to 300 mg/day. In less severe diseases, lower doses may suffice.

DEXAMETHASONE:

Dexamethasone, oral –

Initial dosage: 0.75 to 9 mg/day.

In acute, self-limited allergic disorders or acute exacerbations of chronic allergic disorders: In acute, self-limited allergic disorders or acute exacerbations of chronic allergic disorders, the following dosage schedule combining parenteral (dexamethasone sodium phosphate injection, 4 mg/mL) and oral therapy (0.75 mg tablets) is suggested: First day, 1 or 2 mL IM; second day, 4 tablets in 2 divided doses; third day, 4 tablets in 2 divided doses; fourth day, 2 tablets in 2 divided doses; fifth day, 1 tablet; sixth day, 1 tablet; seventh day, no treatment; eighth day, follow-up visit.

Suppression tests: For Cushing's syndrome – Give 1 mg at 11 pm. Draw blood for plasma cortisol determination the following day at 8 am. For greater accuracy, give 0.5 mg every 6 hours for 48 hours. Collect 24 hour urine to determine 17-hydroxycorticosteroid excretion.

Test to distinguish Cushing's syndrome due to pituitary ACTH excess from Cushing's syndrome due to other causes – Give 2 mg every 6 hours for 48 hours. Collect 24 hour urine to determine 17-hydroxycorticosteroid excretion.

Dexamethasone acetate – Not for IV use.

Systemic: 8 to 16 mg IM, may repeat in 1 to 3 weeks.

Intralesional: 0.8 to 1.6 mg.

Intra-articular and soft tissue: 4 to 16 mg; may repeat at 1 to 3 week intervals.

Dexamethasone sodium phosphate –

Systemic:

Initial dosage – 0.5 to 9 mg daily. Usual dose ranges are 33% to 50% of the oral dose given every 12 hours. However, in certain acute, life-threatening situations, dosages exceeding the usual may be justified and may be in multiples of the oral dosages.

Cerebral edema: In adults, administer an initial IV dose of 10 mg, followed by 4 mg IM every 6 hours until maximum response has been noted. Response is usually noted within 12 to 24 hours. Dosage may be reduced after 2 to 4 days and gradually discontinued over 5 to 7 days. For palliative management of patients with recurrent or inoperable brain tumors, maintenance therapy with either the injection or tablets in a dosage of 2 mg 2 or 3 times daily may be effective.

Unresponsive shock – Reported regimens range from 1 to 6 mg/kg as a single IV injection, to 40 mg initially followed by repeated IV injections every 2 to 6 hours while shock persists.

HYDROCORTISONE (Cortisol):

Hydrocortisone, oral –

Initial dosage: 20 to 240 mg/day.

Hydrocortisone sodium phosphate – Administer by IV, IM or SC injection. Initial dose is 15 to 240 mg/day. Usually, 33% to 50% of the oral dose every 12 hours. For acute diseases, doses > 240 mg may be required.

Hydrocortisone sodium succinate – May be administered IV or IM. The initial dose is 100 to 500 mg, and may be repeated at 2, 4 or 6 hour intervals depending on patient response and clinical condition.

Hydrocortisone acetate – For intralesional, intra-articular or soft tissue injection only. Not for IV use. Dosage range is 5 to 37.5 mg. If desired, a local anesthetic may be injected before hydrocortisone acetate or mixed in a syringe and given simultaneously.

METHYLPREDNISOLONE:

Methylprednisolone, oral –

Initial dose: 4 to 48 mg/day; adjust until a satisfactory response is noted. Determine maintenance dose by decreasing initial dose in small decrements at appropriate intervals until reaching the lowest effective dose.

Dosepak 21 therapy: Follow manufacturer's directions.

Methylprednisolone sodium succinate –

Initial dose: 10 to 40 mg IV, administered over 1 to several minutes. Give subsequent doses IV or IM.

Infants and children: Not less than 0.5 mg/kg/24 hours.

For high dose therapy, give 30 mg/kg IV, infused over 10 to 20 minutes. May repeat every 4 to 6 hours, not beyond 48 to 72 hours.

Methylprednisolone acetate – Not for IV use. As a temporary substitute for oral therapy, administer the total daily dose as a single IM injection. For prolonged effect, give a single weekly dose.

Adrenogenital syndrome: A single 40 mg injection IM every 2 weeks.

Rheumatoid arthritis: Weekly IM maintenance dose varies from 40 to 120 mg.

Dermatologic lesions: 40 to 120 mg IM weekly for 1 to 4 weeks. In severe dermatitis (eg, poison ivy), relief may result within 8 to 12 hours of a single dose of 80 to 120 mg IM. In chronic contact dermatitis, repeated injections every 5 to 10 days may be necessary. In seborrheic dermatitis, a weekly dose of 80 mg IM may be adequate.

Asthma and allergic rhinitis: 80 to 120 mg IM.

Intra-articular and soft tissue: 4 to 80 mg.

Intralesional: 20 to 60 mg.

PREDNISOLONE:

Prednisolone –

Initial dosage: 5 to 60 mg/day.

Multiple sclerosis: In treatment of acute exacerbations of multiple sclerosis, 200 mg daily for a week followed by 80 mg every other day for 1 month.

Prednisolone acetate – Not for IV use.

Initial dosage: 4 to 60 mg/day, IM.

Intralesional, intra-articular or soft tissue injection: 4 mg, up to 100 mg.

Multiple sclerosis: 200 mg daily for a week, followed by 80 mg every other day or 4 to 8 mg dexamethasone every other day for 1 month.

Prednisolone tebutate –

Intra-articular, intralesional or soft tissue administration: 8 to 30 mg. Doses > 40 mg are not recommended.

Prednisolone sodium phosphate –

Parenteral: For IV or IM use.

Initial dosage – 4 to 60 mg/day.

Intra-articular, intralesional or soft tissue administration: 2 to 30 mg.

Oral:

Initial dosage – 5 to 60 mL (5 to 60 mg base) per day.

Multiple sclerosis (acute exacerbations) – 200 mg daily for a week, followed by 80 mg every other day or 4 to 8 mg dexamethasone every other day for 1 month.

PREDNISONE: Initial dosage varies from 5 to 60 mg/day. Prednisone is inactive and must be metabolized to prednisolone. This may be impaired in patients with liver disease.

TRIAMCINOLONE:

Triamcinolone, oral –

Adrenocortical insufficiency: 4 to 12 mg, in addition to mineralocorticoid therapy.

Rheumatic and dermatological disorders and bronchial asthma: 8 to 16 mg.

Allergic states: 8 to 12 mg.

Ophthalmological diseases: 12 to 40 mg.

Respiratory diseases: 16 to 48 mg.

Hematologic disorders: 16 to 60 mg.

Tuberculous meningitis: 32 to 48 mg.

Acute rheumatic carditis: 20 to 60 mg.

Acute leukemia and lymphoma (adults): 16 to 40 mg. It may be necessary to give as much as 100 mg/day in leukemia.

Acute leukemia (children): 1 to 2 mg/kg.

Edematous states: 16 to 20 mg (up to 48 mg) until diuresis occurs.

Systemic lupus erythematosus: 20 to 32 mg.

Triamcinolone diacetate –

Systemic: Not for IV use. May be administered IM for initial therapy; however, most clinicians prefer to adjust the dose orally until adequate control is attained.

The average dose is 40 mg IM per week. In general, a single parenteral dose 4 to 7 times the oral daily dose controls the patient from 4 to 7 days, up to 3 to 4 weeks.

Intra-articular and intrasynovial: 5 to 40 mg.

Intralesional or sublesional: 5 to 48 mg. Do not use > 12.5 mg/injection site. The usual average dose is 25 mg per lesion.

Triamcinolone hexacetonide – Not for IV use.

Intra-articular: 2 to 20 mg average.

Intralesional or sublesional: Up to 0.5 mg per square inch of affected area.

Triamcinolone acetonide –

Systemic:

Initial IM dose – 2.5 to 60 mg/day. Not for IV use.

Intra-articular or intrabursal administration and for injection into tendon sheaths:

Initial dose – 2.5 to 5 mg for smaller joints and 5 to 15 mg for larger joints. For adults, doses up to 10 mg for smaller areas and up to 40 mg for larger areas are usually sufficient.

Intradermal: Use only 3 or 10 mg/mL. Initial dose varies; limit to 1 mg per site.

Actions

Pharmacology: The naturally occurring adrenal cortical steroids have both anti-inflammatory (glucocorticoid) and salt-retaining (mineralocorticoid) properties. Glucocorticoids cause profound and varied metabolic effects. In addition, they modify the body's immune responses to diverse stimuli. These compounds are used as replacement therapy in adrenocortical deficiency states and may be used for their anti-inflammatory effects.

Pharmacokinetics: Hydrocortisone and most of its congeners are readily absorbed from the GI tract; greatly altered onsets and durations are usually achieved with injections of suspensions and esters. Hydrocortisone is metabolized by the liver, which is the rate-limiting step in its clearance. The metabolism and excretion of the synthetic glucocorticoids generally parallel hydrocortisone. Induction of hepatic enzymes will increase the metabolic clearance of hydrocortisone and the synthetic glucocorticoids.

The half-life values refer to the intrinsic activity of each agent; insoluble salts of these drugs are used as repository injections and have sustained effects due to delayed absorption from the injection site.

Glucocorticoid Equivalencies, Potencies and Half-Life

Glucocorticoid	Approximate equivalent dose (mg)	Relative anti-inflammatory (glucocorticoid) potency	Relative mineralocorticoid potency	Plasma (min)	Biologic (hrs)
Short-acting					
Cortisone	25	0.8	2	30	8-12
Hydrocortisone	20	1	2	80-118	8-12
Intermediate-acting					
Prednisone	5	4	1	60	18-36
Prednisolone	5	4	1	115-212	18-36
Triamcinolone	4	5	0	200+	18-36
Methylprednisolone	4	5	0	78-188	18-36
Long-acting					
Dexamethasone	0.75	20-30	0	110-210	36-54
Betamethasone	0.6-0.75	20-30	0	300+	36-54

Contraindications

Systemic fungal infections; hypersensitivity to the drug; IM use in idiopathic thrombocytopenic purpura; administration of live virus vaccines (eg, smallpox) in patients receiving immunosuppressive corticosteroid doses (see Warnings).

Warnings

Infections: Corticosteroids may mask signs of infection, and new infections may appear during their use. There may be decreased resistance and inability of the host defense mechanisms to prevent dissemination of the infection. Restrict use in active tuberculosis to cases of fulminating or disseminated disease in which the corticosteroid is used for disease management with appropriate chemotherapy. Corticosteroids may exacerbate systemic fungal infections and may activate latent amebiasis.

Hepatitis: Corticosteroids may be harmful in chronic active hepatitis positive for hepatitis B surface antigen.

Ocular effects: Prolonged use may produce posterior subcapsular cataracts, glaucoma with possible damage to the optic nerves, and may enhance the establishment of secondary ocular infections due to fungi or viruses.

Fluid and electrolyte balance: Average and large doses of hydrocortisone or cortisone can cause elevation of blood pressure, salt and water retention and increased excretion of potassium. These effects are less likely to occur with the synthetic derivatives except when used in large doses.

Immunosuppression: During therapy, do not use live virus vaccines (eg, smallpox). Do not immunize patients who are receiving corticosteroids, especially high doses, because of possible hazards of neurological complications and a lack of antibody response. This does not apply to patients receiving corticosteroids as replacement therapy.

Adrenal suppression: Prolonged therapy of pharmacologic doses may lead to hypothalamic-pituitary-adrenal suppression. The degree of adrenal suppression varies with the dosage, relative glucocorticoid activity, biological half-life, and duration of glucocorticoid therapy within each individual. Adrenal suppression may be minimized by the use of intermediate-acting glucocorticoids (prednisone, prednisolone, methylprednisolone) on an alternate day schedule.

Stress: In patients receiving or recently withdrawn from corticosteroid therapy subjected to unusual stress, increased dosage of rapidly acting corticosteroids is indicated before, during, and after stressful situations, except in patients on high-dose therapy.

Cardiovascular: Reports suggest an apparent association between corticosteroid use and left ventricular free wall rupture after a recent MI.

Hypersensitivity reactions: Anaphylactoid reactions have occurred rarely with corticosteroid therapy.

Renal function impairment: Edema may occur in the presence of renal disease with a fixed or decreased glomerular filtration rate.

Elderly: Consider the risk/benefit factors of steroid use. Consider lower doses because of body changes caused by aging (ie, diminution of muscle mass and plasma volume).

Pregnancy: Corticosteroids cross the placenta (prednisone has the poorest transport). Chronic maternal ingestion during the first trimester has shown a 1% incidence of cleft palate in humans. Hypoadrenalism has occurred.

Lactation: Corticosteroids appear in breast milk and could suppress growth, interfere with endogenous corticosteroid production or cause other unwanted effects in the nursing infant. However, large doses for short periods may not harm the infant. Alternatives to consider include waiting 3 to 4 hours after the dose before breastfeeding and using prednisolone rather than prednisone.

Children: Carefully observe growth and development of infants and children on prolonged corticosteroid therapy.

Precautions

Monitoring: Observe patients for weight increase, edema, hypertension, and excessive potassium excretion, as well as for less obvious signs of adrenocortical steroid-induced untoward effects. Monitor for a negative nitrogen balance due to protein catabolism. Evaluate blood pressure and body weight, and do routine laboratory studies, including 2 hour postprandial blood glucose and serum potassium and a chest x-ray at regular intervals during prolonged therapy. Upper GI x-rays are desirable in patients with known or suspected peptic ulcer disease or significant dyspepsia or in patients complaining of gastric distress.

Use the lowest possible dose: Make a benefit/risk decision in each individual case as to the size of the dose, duration of treatment and the use of daily or intermittent therapy, since complications of treatment are dependent on these factors.

Steroid psychosis: Steroid psychosis is characterized by a delirious or toxic psychosis with clouded sensorium. Other symptoms may include euphoria, insomnia, mood swings, personality changes and severe depression. The onset of symptoms usually occurs within 15 to 30 days. Predisposing factors include doses > 40 mg prednisone equivalent, female predominance, and, possibly, a family history of psychiatric illness.

Multiple sclerosis: Although corticosteroids are effective in speeding the resolution of acute exacerbations of multiple sclerosis, they do not affect the ultimate outcome or natural history of the disease.

Repository injections: To minimize the likelihood and severity of atrophy, do not inject SC, avoid injection into the deltoid and avoid repeated IM injections into the same site, if possible. Repository injections are not recommended as initial therapy in acute situations.

Local injections: Intra-articular injection may produce systemic and local effects. A marked increase in pain accompanied by local swelling, further restriction of joint motion, fever and malaise is suggestive of septic arthritis. Frequent intra-articular injection may damage joint tissues.

Special risk: Use with caution in the following situations: Nonspecific ulcerative colitis if there is a probability of impending perforation, abscess or other pyogenic infection; diverticulitis; fresh intestinal anastomoses; hypertension; CHF; thromboembolitic tendencies; thrombophlebitis; osteoporosis; exanthema; Cushing's syndrome; antibiotic-resistant infections; convulsive disorders; metastatic carcinoma; myasthenia gravis; vaccinia; varicella; diabetes mellitus.; hypothyroidism, cirrhosis (enhanced effect of corticosteroids).

Drug Interactions

Drugs that may be affected by glucocorticoids include anticholinesterases, anticoagulants, cyclosporine, digitalis glycosides, isoniazid, nondepolarizing neuromuscular blockers, potassium-depleting agents (eg, diuretics), salicylates, somatrem and theophyllines. Drugs that may affect corticosteroids include aminoglutethimide, barbiturates, cholestyramine, oral contraceptives, ephedrine, estrogens, hydantoins, ketoconazole, macrolide antibiotics, and rifampin.

CYP3A4 inhibitors: If concomitant administration with a CYP3A4 inhibitor is indicated, closely monitor patients for increased signs or symptoms of hypercorticism. Consider reduction in **budesonide** dose.

Drug/Lab test interactions: Urine glucose and serum cholesterol levels may increase. Decreased serum levels of potassium, triiodothyronine (T_3), and a minimal decrease of thyroxine (T_4) may occur. Thyroid I^{131} uptake may be decreased. False-negative results with the nitroblue-tetrazolium test for bacterial infection. Dexamethasone, given for cerebral edema, may alter the results of a brain scan (decreased uptake of radioactive material).

Adverse Reactions

Adverse reactions that may occur include hypertension, myocardial rupture following recent MI, anaphylactoid/hypersensitivity reactions; sodium and fluid retention; hypokalemia; metabolic alkalosis; hypocalcemia; hypotension or shock-like reactions; muscle weakness; muscle mass loss; tendon rupture; osteoporosis; spontaneous fractures; thromboembolism or fat embolism; thrombophlebitis; cardiac arrhythmias or ECG changes due to potassium deficiency; syncopal episodes; pancreatitis; abdominal distension; ulcerative esophagitis; nausea; vomiting; increased appetite and weight gain; impaired wound healing; thin fragile skin; petechiae/ecchymoses; erythema; purpura; hirsutism; acneiform eruptions; allergic dermatitis; urticaria; convulsions; vertigo; headache; neuritis/paresthesias; aggravation of pre-existing psychiatric conditions; steroid psychoses; menstrual irregularities; development of Cushingoid state (eg, moonface, buffalo hump, supraclavicular fat pad enlargement, central obesity); suppression of growth in children; increased sweating; hyperglycemia; glycosuria; increased IOP; glaucoma; malaise; fatigue; insomnia.

HELICOBACTER PYLORI AGENTS

Helicobacter pylori: H. *pylori* is found in ≈ 100% of chronic active antral gastritis cases, 90% to 95% of duodenal ulcer patients, and 50% to 80% of gastric ulcer patients. The treatment of documented *H. pylori* infection in patients with confirmed peptic ulcer on first presentation or recurrence has been recommended by the National Institutes for Health in a 1994 Consensus Conference. Once *H. pylori* eradication has been achieved, reinfection rates are < 0.5% per year, and ulcer recurrence rates are dramatically reduced.

Numerous clinical trials have been done to determine the optimal regimen for *H. pylori* eradication, but there remains no gold standard of therapy to date. When selecting a regimen, take into account efficacy, tolerability, compliance, and cost. *H. pylori* is easily suppressed but, to ensure successful eradication, requires the use of 2 antimicrobial agents with either a bismuth compound, an antisecretory agent, or both. These combinations have been shown to enhance *H. pylori* cure, shorten the duration of treatment and decrease treatment failure caused by antimicrobial resistance.

Double antimicrobial therapy plus an antisecretory drug:

Regimens Used in the Eradication of *H. pylori* [1]

Regimen	Dosing	Duration	Eradication
Metronidazole Omeprazole Clarithromycin	500 mg twice daily with meals 20 mg twice daily with meals 500 mg twice daily with meals	1 week	87% to 91%
Amoxicillin Omeprazole Clarithromycin	1 g twice daily with meals 20 mg twice daily before meals 500 mg twice daily with meals	1 to 2 weeks	77% to 83%
Metronidazole Omeprazole Amoxicillin	500 mg twice daily with meals 20 mg twice daily before meals 1 g twice daily with meals	1 to 2 weeks	77% to 83%

[1] Extending therapy to 10 to 14 days in the above regimens may provide additional benefit. H_2 blockers may be used with 2 antibiotics, but a longer treatment course (10 to 14 days), higher antibiotic doses, and 3 times daily administration are required.

Triple-therapy regimens: These regimens have proven to be very effective in eradicating *H. pylori*. The primary disadvantage of these regimens is compliance because of the variety and number of medications used. Likewise, adverse effects are more common in patients taking these regimens compared with alternatives.

Regimens Used in the Eradication of *H. pylori* [1]

Regimen	Dosing	Duration	Eradication
Bismuth subsalicylate Metronidazole Tetracycline	525 mg 4 times daily with meals and at bedtime 250 mg 4 times daily with meals and at bedtime 500 mg 4 times daily	2 weeks 1 week	88% to 90% 86% to 90%
Bismuth subsalicylate Metronidazole Tetracycline Omeprazole	525 mg 4 times daily with meals and at bedtime 250 mg 4 times daily with meals and at bedtime 500 mg 4 times daily 20 mg 2 times daily before meals	1 week	94% to 98%
Bismuth subsalicylate Metronidazole Amoxicillin	525 mg 4 times daily with meals and at bedtime 250 mg 4 times daily with meals and at bedtime 500 mg 4 times daily with meals and at bedtime	2 weeks 1 week	80% to 86% 75% to 81%

[1] One week of 4 times daily therapy may be sufficient in the absence of antibiotic resistance. Adding a proton pump inhibitor facilitates shorter treatment periods. Until more data is available, the use of H_2 antagonists or proton pump inhibitors with the above regimens is appropriate to enhance ulcer healing and provide symptomatic relief.

Quadruple therapy regimens (2 antibiotics, bismuth, antisecretory agent): Like triple therapy regimens, these have proven to be effective in *H. pylori* eradication. The primary disadvantage of these regimens is compliance. In addition, because of the variety and number of medications used, adverse effects are more common in patients taking these regimens compared with alternatives.

FDA-Approved Regimens for the Eradication of *H. pylori*			
Regimen	Dosing	Eradication	Comments
Omeprazole	40 mg once daily followed by a 2-week course of 20 mg once daily	64% to 74%	The American College of Gastroenterology recommends that either tetracycline or amoxicillin be added to this regimen.
Clarithromycin	500 mg 3 times daily for 2 weeks		
Ranitidine bismuth citrate	400 mg twice daily for 4 weeks	82%	The American College of Gastroenterology recommends that either tetracycline or amoxicillin be added to this regimen.
Clarithromycin	500 mg 3 times daily for 2 weeks		
Metronidazole	250 mg 4 times daily at meals and bedtime	82%	*Helidac* therapy combines bismuth subsalicylate, metronidazole, and tetracycline in a consumer-tested, patient-friendly kit.
Tetracycline HCl	500 mg 4 times daily at meals and bedtime		
Bismuth subsalicylate	525 mg 4 times daily at meals and bedtime		

Practice Guidelines from the American College of Gastroenterology: In the 1996 Consensus Statement on Medical Treatment of Peptic Ulcer Disease, the American College of Gastroenterology does not recommend single-antibiotic combinations of either clarithromycin or amoxicillin with proton pump inhibitors because efficacy is < 70% (cure), and a high-dose, 2-week treatment period is required. The Consensus Statement recommends a 2-antibiotic combination of clarithromycin, metronidazole, or amoxicillin in regimens that do not employ a bismuth compound. In addition, the American College of Gastroenterology suggests adding either tetracycline or amoxicillin to the recently approved ranitidine-bismuth citrate-clarithromycin combination to enhance successful *H. pylori* eradication. Combining a proton pump inhibitor, either omeprazole or lansoprazole, with 2 antibiotics is thought to enhance effectiveness and allow for a shorter duration of treatment.

There are a number of factors that limit the effectiveness of regimens designed to eradicate *H. pylori*. The first, antibiotic resistance, is seen with metronidazole and clarithromycin but has not been reported with bismuth, amoxicillin, or tetracycline.

Second, mild adverse effects (eg, diarrhea, metallic taste, black stools) do occur in ≈ 30% to 50% of patients. Therefore, shorter treatment periods in this group of patients may be better tolerated.

Finally, patient compliance is often a problem because of cumbersome regimens and adverse effects.

Maintenance therapy with antisecretory agents: Currently, it is advisable to continue maintenance until *H. pylori* cure has been confirmed in patients with a history of complications, frequent or troublesome recurrences or refractory ulcers.

Successful eradication: Confirming successful eradication is important in patients with a history of complicated or refractory ulcers but is controversial in those with uncomplicated ulcers who remain asymptomatic after therapy.

Refractory ulcers: Refractory ulcers in patients receiving antibiotic therapy for *H. pylori* eradication is often due to failure to successfully eradicate *H. pylori* infection. Resistance patterns, as well as noncompliance, and concurrent NSAID use may play a role in refractory cases.

HEPATITIS A VACCINE, INACTIVATED

Injection (pediatric formulation): 360 ELU/0.5 mL or 25 U/0.5 mL of viral antigen (*Rx*)	*Havrix* (GlaxoSmithKline), *Vaqta* (Merck)
Injection (adult formulation): 1440 ELU/1 mL or 50 U/1 mL of viral antigen (*Rx*)	

Indications

Hepatitis A virus (HAV): For active immunization of people ≥ 2 years of age against disease caused by HAV.

Primary immunization: Primary immunization should be completed at least 2 weeks prior to expected exposure to HAV. Immunization with hepatitis A vaccine is indicated for those people desiring protection against hepatitis A who are, or will be, at increased risk of infection by HAV:

Travelers – People traveling to areas of higher endemicity for hepatitis A.

Populations with high incidence of the disease – Native people of Alaska and the Americas.

People at increased risk because of their employment – Certain institutional workers (eg, caretakers for the developmentally challenged); employees of child day care centers; laboratory workers who handle live hepatitis A virus; handlers of primate animals that may be harboring HAV.

Others – People engaging in high-risk sexual activity (such as homosexually active males); users of illicit injectable drugs; residents of a community experiencing an outbreak of hepatitis A; military personnel; people living in or relocating to areas of high endemicity.

Administration and Dosage

Route and site: For IM use. Do not inject IV, ID, or SC. In adults, give the injection in the deltoid region. It should not be administered in the gluteal region; such injections may result in suboptimal response.

Primary immunization regimen:

Adults – A single dose of 1440 EL.U.

Children (2 to 18 years of age) – 2 doses, each containing 360 EL.U. given 1 month apart.

Booster dose – A booster dose is recommended anytime between 6 and 12 months after the initiation of the primary course in order to ensure the highest antibody titers.

In those with an impaired immune system, adequate anti-HAV response may not be obtained after the primary immunization course. Such patients may therefore require administration of additional doses of vaccine.

Contraindications

Hypersensitivity to any component of the vaccine.

Warnings

Hepatitis: Hepatitis A vaccine will not prevent hepatitis caused by other agents such as hepatitis B, C, or E virus or other pathogens known to infect the liver.

Hypersensitivity reactions: Epinephrine should be available for use in case of anaphylaxis or anaphylactoid reaction.

Pregnancy: Category C.

Lactation: It is not known whether the vaccine is excreted in breast milk.

Children: Hepatitis A vaccine is well tolerated and highly immunogenic and effective in children ≥ 2 years of age.

Precautions

Febrile illness: Febrile illness is reason to delay use of hepatitis A vaccine, except when withholding the vaccine entails a greater risk.

Bleeding disorders: Administer cautiously to people with thrombocytopenia or a bleeding disorder as bleeding may occur following IM use.

Immunosuppressed people: Immunosuppressed people or people receiving immunosuppressive therapy may not obtain the expected immune response.

Injection site: Do not inject into a blood vessel.

Drug Interactions

When concomitant administration of other vaccines or immune globulin is required, they should be given with different syringes and at different injection sites.

Adverse Reactions

Adverse reactions occurring in ≥ 3% of patients include injection site soreness/pain, tenderness, induration, redness, swelling, fatigue, fever, malaise, anorexia, nausea, and headache.

HISTAMINE H_2 ANTAGONISTS

CIMETIDINE	
Tablets: 100 mg (*otc*)	*Tagamet HB* (GlaxoSmithKline)
Tablets: 200, 300, 400, and 800 mg (*Rx*)	Various, *Tagamet* (GlaxoSmithKline)
Liquid: 300 mg (as HCl)/5 mL (*Rx*)	*Cimetidine Oral Solution* (Barre-National), *Tagamet* (GlaxoSmithKline)
Injection: 300 mg (as HCl)/2 mL (*Rx*)	*Cimetidine* (Endo), *Tagamet* (GlaxoSmithKline)
Injection, premixed: 300 mg (as HCl) in 50 mL 0.9% Sodium Chloride (*Rx*)	*Tagamet* (GlaxoSmithKline)
FAMOTIDINE	
Tablets: 10 mg (*otc*)	*Pepcid AC Acid Controller* (J & J Merck)
Tablets: 20 and 40 mg (*Rx*)	*Pepcid* (J & J Merck)
Gelcaps: 10 mg (*otc*)	*Pepcid AC* (J & J Merck)
Tablets, chewable: 10 mg (*otc*)	*Pepcid AC* (J & J Merck)
Tablets, orally disintegrating: 20 and 40 mg (*Rx*)	*Pepcid RPD* (J & J Merck)
Powder for oral suspension: 40 mg/5 mL when reconstituted (*Rx*)	
Injection: 10 mg/mL (*Rx*)	
Injection, premixed: 20 mg/50 mL in 0.9% HCl (*Rx*)	
NIZATIDINE	
Tablets: 75 mg (*otc*)	*Axid AR* (Whitehall-Robins)
Capsules: 150 and 300 mg (*Rx*)	*Axid Pulvules* (Lilly)
RANITIDINE	
Tablets: 75 mg (*otc*)	*Zantac 75* (GlaxoSmithKline)
Tablets: 150 and 300 mg (as HCl) (*Rx*)	*Zantac* (GlaxoSmithKline)
Tablets, effervescent: 150 mg (*Rx*)	*Zantac EFFERdose* (GlaxoSmithKline)
Capsules: 150 and 300 mg (*Rx*)	*Zantac GELdose* (GlaxoSmithKline)
Syrup: 15 mg (as HCl)/mL (*Rx*)	*Ranitidine HCl* (UDL), *Zantac* (GlaxoSmithKline)
Granules, effervescent: 150 mg (*Rx*)	*Zantac EFFERdose* (GlaxoSmithKline)
Injection: 0.5 and 25 mg (as HCl)/mL (*Rx*)	*Zantac* (GlaxoSmithKline)
HISTAMINE H_2 ANTAGONIST COMBINATIONS	
Tablets, chewable: 10 mg famotidine, 800 mg calcium carbonate, 165 mg magnesium hydroxide (*otc*)	*Pepcid Complete* (J & J Merck)

Indications

Histamine H_2 Antagonists: Summary of Indications

✔ – Labeled x – Unlabeled	Cimetidine	Famotidine	Nizatidine	Ranitidine	Combinations
Duodenal ulcer					
Treatment	✔	✔	✔	✔	
Maintenance	✔	✔	✔	✔	
GERD (including erosive esophagitis)	✔	✔	✔	✔	
Gastric ulcer					
Treatment	✔	✔	✔	✔	
Maintenance				✔	
Pathological hypersecretory conditions	✔	✔		✔	
Heartburn/acid indigestion/ sour stomach	✔[1,2]	✔[1,3]			✔
Erosive esophagitis, maintenance				✔	
Prevent upper GI bleeding	✔	x		x	
Peptic ulcer [4]	x	x	x	x	
Prevent aspiration pneumonitis	x	x		x	
Prophylaxis of stress ulcers	x	x		x	
Prevent gastric NSAID damage				x	

Histamine H_2 Antagonists: Summary of Indications					
✓ – Labeled x – Unlabeled	Cimetidine	Famotidine	Nizatidine	Ranitidine	Combinations
Hyperparathyroidism	x				
Secondary hyperparathyroidism in hemodialysis	x				
Tinea capitis	x				
Herpes virus infection	x				
Hirsute women	x				
Chronic idiopathic urticaria	x				
Anaphylaxis (dermatological)	x				
Acetaminophen overdose	x				
Dyspepsia	x				
Warts	x				
Colorectal cancer	x				

[1] *otc* use only.
[2] Relief of symptoms only.
[3] Relief and prevention of symptoms.
[4] As part of a multi-drug regimen to eradicate *Helicobacter pylori*.

Administration and Dosage

CIMETIDINE:

Duodenal ulcer –

Short-term treatment of active duodenal ulcer: 800 mg at bedtime. Alternate regimens are 300 mg 4 times/day with meals and at bedtime, or 400 mg twice/day.

Maintenance therapy: 400 mg at bedtime.

Active benign gastric ulcer – For short-term treatment, 800 mg at bedtime or 300 mg 4 times/day with meals and at bedtime.

Erosive gastroesophageal reflux disease (GERD) –

Adults: 1600 mg daily in divided doses (800 mg twice daily or 400 mg 4 times/day) for 12 weeks. Use > 12 weeks has not been established.

Pathological hypersecretory conditions – 300 mg 4 times/day with meals and at bedtime. If necessary, give 300 mg doses more often. Do not exceed 2400 mg/day.

Prevention of upper GI bleeding – Continuous IV infusion of 50 mg/hour. Patients with Ccr < 30 mL/min should receive half the recommended dose. Treatment > 7 days has not been studied.

Severely impaired renal function – Accumulation may occur. Use the lowest dose; 300 mg every 12 hours orally or IV has been recommended. Dosage frequency may be increased to every 8 hours or even further with caution.

Parenteral – The usual dose is 300 mg IM or IV every 6 to 8 hours. If it is necessary to increase dosage, do so by more frequent administration of a 300 mg dose, not to exceed 2400 mg/day.

IM: Administer undiluted.

IV: Dilute to a total volume of 20 mL; inject over ≥ 2 minutes.

Intermittent IV infusion: Dilute 300 mg in at least 50 mL of compatible IV solution; infuse over 15 to 20 minutes.

Continuous IV infusion: 37.5 mg/hour (900 mg/day).

FAMOTIDINE:

Duodenal ulcer –

Acute therapy: 40 mg/day at bedtime. 20 mg twice/day is also effective.

Maintenance therapy: 20 mg once a day at bedtime.

Benign gastric ulcer –

Acute therapy: 40 mg orally once a day at bedtime.

Pathological hypersecretory conditions – The adult starting dose is 20 mg every 6 hours.

GERD – 20 mg twice daily for up to 6 weeks. For esophagitis including erosions and ulcerations and accompanying symptoms caused by GERD, 20 or 40 mg twice daily for up to 12 weeks.

Severe renal insufficiency –

Ccr < 10 mL/min: To avoid excess accumulation of the drug, the dose may be reduced to 20 mg at bedtime or the dosing interval may be prolonged to 36 to 48 hours, as indicated.

Parenteral –

IV: Give famotidine IV 20 mg every 12 hours.

Children – Studies suggest the following starting doses in pediatric patients 1 to 16 years of age.

Peptic ulcer: 0.5 mg/kg/day orally at bedtime or divided twice daily up to 40 mg/day.

GERD with or without esophagitis including erosions and ulcerations: 1 mg/kg/day orally divided twice daily up to 40 mg twice daily.

Heartburn, acid indigestion, and sour stomach (otc only) –

Acute therapy: 10 mg (1 tablet) with water.

Prevention: 10 mg 15 minutes before eating food or drinking a beverage that is expected to cause symptoms.

Use: Can be used up to twice daily (up to 2 tablets in 24 hours). Do not take maximum dose for > 2 weeks continuously unless otherwise directed by a physician.

Children: Do not give to children < 12 years of age unless otherwise directed.

Moderate (Ccr < 50 mL/min) or severe renal insufficiency (Ccr < 10 mL/min) – To avoid excess accumulation of the drug, the dose may be reduced to half the dose or the dosing interval may be prolonged to 36 to 48 hours, as indicated.

NIZATIDINE:

Active duodenal ulcer – 300 mg once daily at bedtime. An alternative dosage regimen is 150 mg twice daily.

Maintenance of healed duodenal ulcer – 150 mg once daily at bedtime.

GERD – 150 mg twice daily.

Benign gastric ulcer – 300 mg given either as 150 mg twice daily or 300 mg once daily at bedtime.

Heartburn, acid indigestion, and sour stomach (otc only) – Can be used up to twice daily (up to 2 tablets in 24 hours).

Relief: For relief of symptoms, take 1 tablet with a full glass of water.

Prevention: For prevention of symptoms, take 1 tablet with a full glass of water right before eating or up to 60 minutes before consuming food and beverages that cause heartburn.

Moderate to severe renal insufficiency –

Nizatidine Dosage in Renal Insufficiency

Ccr	Dosage	
	Active duodenal ulcer	Maintenance therapy
20 to 50 mL/min	150 mg/day	150 mg every other day
< 20 mL/min	150 mg every other day	150 mg every 3 days

RANITIDINE:

Duodenal ulcer –

Short-term treatment of active duodenal ulcer: 150 mg orally twice daily. An alternate dosage of 300 mg once daily at bedtime can be used for patients in whom dosing convenience is important.

Maintenance therapy: 150 mg at bedtime.

Pathological hypersecretory conditions – 150 mg orally twice a day. More frequent doses may be necessary. Doses up to 6 g/day have been used.

Benign gastric ulcer (oral doseforms only) and GERD – 150 mg twice daily.

Gastric ulcer –

Treatment: 150 mg twice daily.

Maintenance: 150 mg at bedtime.

Erosive esophagitis –

Treatment: 150 mg 4 times daily.

Maintenance: 150 mg twice daily.

Heartburn (otc only) –

Treatment: For relief of symptoms, swallow 1 tablet with a glass of water.

Prevention: To prevent symptoms, swallow 1 tablet with a glass of water 30 to 60 minutes before eating food or drinking beverages that cause heartburn.

Maintenance: Can be used up to twice daily (up to 2 tablets in 24 hours).

Children – The safety and effectiveness of ranitidine have been established in children from 1 month to 16 years of age. There is insufficient information about the pharmacokinetics of ranitidine in neonatal patients < 1 month of age to make dosing recommendations. Do not give *otc* ranitidine to children < 12 years of age unless directed by physician.

Active duodenal and gastric ulcers:

Treatment – 2 to 4 mg/kg/day twice daily to a maximum of 300 mg/day.

Maintenance – 2 to 4 mg/kg once daily to a maximum of 150 mg/day.

GERD and erosive esophagitis: Although limited data exist for these conditions in pediatric patients, published literature supports a dosage of 5 to 10 mg/kg/day, usually given as 2 divided doses.

EFFERdose (tablets and granules) – Dissolve each dose in ≈ 6 to 8 oz. of water before drinking.

Renal impairment – (Ccr < 50 mL/min): 150 mg orally every 24 hours or 50 mg parenterally every 18 to 24 hours. The frequency of dosing may be increased to every 12 hours or further with caution.

Parenteral –

IM: 50 mg (2 mL) every 6 to 8 hours (no dilution necessary).

IV injection: 50 mg (2 mL) every 6 to 8 hours. Dilute 50 mg to a total volume of 20 mL; inject over ≥ 5 minutes.

Intermittent IV infusion: 50 mg (2 mL) every 6 to 8 hours. Dilute 50 mg and infuse over 15 to 20 minutes; do not exceed 400 mg/day.

Continuous IV infusion: Add ranitidine injection to 5% Dextrose Injection or other compatible IV solution. Deliver at a rate of 6.25 mg/hr (eg, 150 mg [6 mL] ranitidine injection in 250 mL of 5% Dextrose Injection at 10.7 mL/hr).

Children – The recommended dose in pediatric patients is for a total daily dose of 2 to 4 mg/kg, to be divided and administered every 6 to 8 hours up to a maximum of 50 mg given every 6 to 8 hours. Limited data in neonatal patients (< 1 month of age) receiving ECMO have shown that a dose of 2 mg/kg is usually sufficient to increase gastric pH to > 4 for at least 15 hours. Therefore, consider doses of 2 mg/kg given every 12 to 24 hours or as a continuous infusion.

COMBINATIONS:

≥ 12 years of age – To relieve symptoms, chew 1 tablet before swallowing. Do not use > 2 tablets in 24 hours. Do not swallow tablet whole; chew completely.

Actions

Pharmacology: Histamine H_2 antagonists are reversible competitive blockers of histamine at the H_2 receptors, particularly those in the gastric parietal cells. They also inhibit fasting and nocturnal secretions, and secretions stimulated by food, insulin, caffeine, pentagastrin, and betazole. **Cimetidine**, **ranitidine**, and **famotidine** have no effect on gastric emptying, and cimetidine and famotidine have no effect on lower esophageal sphincter pressure. Ranitidine, **nizatidine**, and famotidine have little or no effect on fasting or postprandial serum gastrin.

Pharmacokinetics:

Pharmacokinetic Properties of Histamine H_2 Antagonists

H_2 receptor antagonist	Bioavailability (%)	Time to peak plasma concentration (hr)	Peak plasma concentration[1] (mcg/mL)	Half-life (hr)	Protein binding (%)	Volume of distribution (L/kg)	Elimination (%)		
							Urine, unchanged		
							Oral	IV	Metabolized
Cimetidine	60-70	0.75-1.5	0.7-3.2 (300 mg dose) (3.5-7.5 IV)	≈ 2[2]	13-25	0.8-1.2	48	75	30-40
Famotidine	40-45	1-3	0.076-0.1 (40 mg dose)	2.5-3.5[3]	15-20	1.1-1.4	25-30	65-70	30-35
Nizatidine	> 90	0.5-3	0.7-1.8/ 1.4-3.6 (150/ 300 mg dose)	1-2[3]	≈ 35	0.8-1.5	60	na[4]	< 18
Ranitidine	50-60 (90-100 IM)	1-3 (0.25 IM)	0.44-0.55 (0.58 IM)	2-3[3]	15	1.2-1.9	30-35	68-79	< 10

[1] Dose-dependent.
[2] Increased in renal and hepatic impairment and in the elderly.
[3] Increased in renal impairment.
[4] na = not applicable.

Contraindications

Hypersensitivity to individual agents or to other H_2-receptor antagonists.

Warnings

Benzyl alcohol: Benzyl alcohol, contained in some of these products as a preservative, has been associated with a fatal "gasping syndrome" in premature infants.

Hypersensitivity reactions: Rare cases of anaphylaxis have occurred as well as rare episodes of hypersensitivity (eg, bronchospasm, laryngeal edema, rash, eosinophilia).

Renal function impairment: Because these agents are excreted primarily via the kidneys, decreased clearance may occur; reduced dosage may be necessary.

Hepatic function impairment: Observe caution. Decreased clearance may occur; these agents are partly metabolized in the liver.

Elderly: Safety and efficacy appear similar to those of younger age; however, the elderly may have reduced renal function. Decreased **cimetidine** clearance may be more common.

Pregnancy: (*Category B* - cimetidine, famotidine, nizatidine, ranitidine.). Cimetidine crosses the placenta.

Lactation: **Cimetidine** is excreted in breast milk with milk:plasma ratios of ≈ 5:1 to 12:1. Potential daily infant ingestion is ≈ 6 mg.

Ranitidine is excreted in breast milk with milk:plasma ratios of 1:1 to 6.7:1.

Nizatidine is excreted in breast milk in a concentration of 0.1% of the oral dose in proportion to plasma concentrations.

Famotidine is excreted in the breast milk of rats. It is not known whether it is excreted in human breast milk.

Children: Safety and efficacy are not established. **Cimetidine** is not recommended for children < 16 years of age, unless anticipated benefits outweigh potential risks. In very limited experience, cimetidine 20 to 40 mg/kg/day has been used.

Precautions

Gastric malignancy: Symptomatic response to these agents does not preclude gastric malignancy.

CNS effects: Reversible CNS effects (eg, mental confusion, agitation, psychosis, depression, anxiety, hallucinations, disorientation) have occurred with **cimetidine,** predominantly in severely ill patients. Advancing age (≥ 50 years) and preexisting liver or renal disease appear to be contributing factors.

Hepatocellular injury: Hepatocellular injury may occur with **nizatidine** as evidenced by elevated liver enzymes (AST, ALT, or alkaline phosphatase).

Occasionally, reversible hepatitis, hepatocellular, or hepatocanalicular or mixed, with or without jaundice have occurred with oral **ranitidine.**

Monitoring – Laboratory test monitoring for liver abnormalities is appropriate.

Antiandrogenic effect: **Cimetidine** has a weak antiandrogenic effect in animals. Gynecomastia in patients treated for ≥ 1 month may occur.

Immunocompromised patients: Decreased gastric acidity, including that produced by acid-suppressing agents such as H_2 antagonists, may increase the possibility of strongyloidiasis.

Drug Interactions

Cimetidine reduces the hepatic metabolism of drugs metabolized via the cytochrome P-450 pathway, delaying elimination and increasing serum levels.

Cimetidine Drug Interactions (Decreased Hepatic Metabolism)	
Benzodiazepines[1]	Propafenone
Caffeine	Propranolol
Calcium channel blockers	Quinidine
Carbamazepine	Quinine
Chloroquine	Sulfonylureas
Labetalol	Tacrine
Lidocaine	Theophyllines[2]
Metoprolol	Triamterene
Metronidazole	Tricyclic antidepressants
Moricizine	Valproic acid
Pentoxifylline	Warfarin
Phenytoin	

[1] Does not include agents metabolized by glucuronidation (lorazepam, oxazepam, temazepam).
[2] Does not include dyphylline.

Ranitidine (which weakly binds to cytochrome P450 in vitro), **famotidine**, and **nizatidine** do not inhibit the cytochrome P450-linked oxygenase enzyme system in the liver. Drug interactions with these agents mediated by inhibition of hepatic metabolism are not expected.

Drugs that may affect histamine H_2 antagonists include antacids, anticholinergics, metoclopramide, and cigarette smoking. Drugs that may be affected by histamine H_2 antagonists include ferrous salts, indomethacin, ketoconazole, tetracyclines, carmustine, digoxin, flecainide, fluconazole, fluorouracil, narcotic analgesics, procainamide, succinylcholine, tocainide, salicylates, diazepam, sulfonylureas, theophyllines, warfarin, and ethanol.

Drug/Lab test interactions: False-positive tests for urobilinogen may occur during **nizatidine** therapy. False-positive tests for urine protein with *Multistix* may occur during **ranitidine** therapy; testing with sulfosalicylic acid is recommended.

Drug/Food interactions: Food may increase bioavailability of **famotidine** and **nizatidine**; this is of no clinical consequence. **Cimetidine** and **ranitidine** are not affected.

Adverse Reactions

Adverse reactions may include headache, somnolence/fatigue, dizziness, confusional states, hallucinations, insomnia, nausea, vomiting, abdominal discomfort, diarrhea, constipation, thrombocytopenia, alopecia, rash, gynecomastia, impotence, loss of libido, and arthralgia.

5-HT$_3$ RECEPTOR ANTAGONISTS

ONDANSETRON	
Tablets: 4, 8, 24 mg (as HCl dihydrate) (*Rx*)	*Zofran* (GlaxoSmithKline)
Solution, oral: 4 mg/5 mL (5 mg as HCl) (*Rx*)	
Injection: 2 mg/mL and 32 mg/50 mL (pre-mixed) (as HCl dihydrate) (*Rx*)	
Tablets, orally disintegrating: 4 and 8 mg (as base) (*Rx*)	*Zofran ODT* (GlaxoSmithKline)
GRANISETRON	
Tablets: 1 mg (1.12 mg as HCl) (*Rx*)	*Kytril* (GlaxoSmithKline)
Injection: 1 mg/mL (1.12 mg/mL as HCl) (*Rx*)	
DOLASETRON	
Tablets: 50 and 100 mg (*Rx*)	*Anzemet* (Aventis)
Injection: 20 mg/mL (*Rx*)	
ALOSETRON HCl	
Tablets: 1 mg (1.124 mg alosetron HCl equiv. to 1 mg alosetron) (*Rx*)	*Lotronex* (GlaxoSmithKline)

Warning:

Serious GI adverse events, some fatal, have been reported with the use of **alosetron**. These events, including ischemic colitis and serious complications of constipation, have resulted in hospitalization, blood transfusion, surgery, and death.

- Only physicians who have enrolled in GlaxoSmithKline's Prescribing Program for *Lotronex*, based on their attestation of qualifications and acceptance of responsibilities, should prescribe alosetron (see Administration and Dosage).
- Alosetron is indicated only for women with severe diarrhea-predominant irritable bowel syndrome (IBS) who have failed to respond to conventional therapy (see Indications). Less than 5% of IBS is considered severe. Before receiving the initial prescription for alosetron, the patient must read and sign the Patient-Physician Agreement.
- Alosetron should be discontinued immediately in patients who develop constipation or symptoms of ischemic colitis. Physicians should instruct patients to immediately report constipation or symptoms of ischemic colitis. Alosetron should not be resumed in patients who develop ischemic colitis. Physicians should instruct patients who report constipation to immediately contact them if the constipation does not resolve after discontinuation of alosetron. Patients with resolved constipation should resume alosetron only on the advice of their treating physician.

Indications

Antiemetic: Prevention of nausea and vomiting associated with initial and repeat courses of emetogenic cancer therapy, including high-dose cisplatin; prevention of postoperative nausea or vomiting (**ondansetron** and **dolasetron**); treatment of postoperative nausea or vomiting (**dolasetron** injection); prevention of nausea and vomiting associated with radiotherapy in patients receiving total body irradiation, single high-dose fraction, or daily fractions to the abdomen (oral **ondansetron** and **granisetron**).

IBS (alosetron): Because of serious GI adverse events, some fatal, alosetron is indicated only for women with severe diarrhea-predominant IBS who have:

- chronic IBS symptoms (generally lasting 6 months or longer),
- had anatomic or biochemical abnormalities of the GI tract excluded, and
- failed to respond to conventional therapy.

Diarrhea-predominant IBS is severe if it includes diarrhea and 1 or more of the following:

- frequent and severe abdominal pain/discomfort,

- frequent bowel urgency or fecal incontinence,
- disability or restriction of daily activities because of IBS.

Less than 5% of IBS is considered severe.

Unlabeled uses:

Granisetron – Acute nausea and vomiting following surgery (1 to 3 mg IV).

Dolasetron – Radiotherapy-induced nausea and vomiting (40 mg IV or 0.3 mg/kg IV).

Administration and Dosage

ONDANSETRON:

Prevention of nausea/vomiting associated with cancer chemotherapy –

Parenteral: The recommended IV dosage is three 0.15 mg/kg doses or a single 32 mg dose. With the 3 dose regimen, the first dose is infused over 15 minutes beginning 30 minutes before the start of emetogenic chemotherapy. Subsequent doses are administered 4 and 8 hours after the first dose. The single 32 mg dose is infused over 15 minutes beginning 30 minutes before the start of emetogenic chemotherapy.

Children – The dosage in children 4 to 18 years of age should be three 0.15 mg/kg doses (see above). Little information is available about dosage in children ≤ 3 years of age.

Oral (moderately emetogenic cancer chemotherapy): In patients greater than 12 years of age, the recommended dose is 8 mg twice/day. Administer the first dose 30 minutes before the start of emetogenic chemotherapy, with a subsequent dose 8 hours after the first dose. Administer 8 mg twice a day (every 12 hours) for 1 to 2 days after completion of chemotherapy.

Children – Dosage is same as adults; for children 4 to 11 years, use 4 mg 3 times a day. Give the first dose 30 minutes before chemotherapy, with subsequent doses 4 and 8 hours after the first dose. Give 4 mg 3 times a day (every 8 hours) for 1 to 2 days after completion of chemotherapy.

Prevention of nausea and vomiting associated with radiotherapy (oral) – 8 mg 3 times/day.

Total body irradiation: 8 mg 1 to 2 hours before each fraction of radiotherapy administered each day.

Single high-dose fraction radiotherapy to the abdomen: 8 mg 1 to 2 hours before radiotherapy, with subsequent doses every 8 hours after the first dose for 1 to 2 days after completion of radiotherapy.

Daily fractionated radiotherapy to the abdomen: 8 mg 1 to 2 hours before radiotherapy, with subsequent doses every 8 hours after the first dose for each day radiotherapy is given.

Prevention of postoperative nausea or vomiting –

Parenteral: Immediately before induction of anesthesia, or postoperatively if the patient experiences nausea or vomiting shortly after surgery, administer 4 mg undiluted IV in not less than 30 seconds, preferably over 2 to 5 minutes. Alternatively, 4 mg undiluted may be administered IM as a single injection in adults. In patients who do not achieve adequate control, administration of a second IV dose of 4 mg ondansetron postoperatively does not provide additional control of nausea and vomiting.

Children – Patients 2 to 12 years of age weighing ≤ 40 kg may receive 0.1 mg/kg IV; give a single 4 mg dose for those weighing > 40 kg. Administer over not less than 30 seconds, preferably over 2 to 5 minutes.

Oral: 16 mg given as a single dose 1 hour before induction of anesthesia.

Children: There is no experience in children.

Prevention of nausea and vomiting associated with highly emetogenic cancer chemotherapy (oral) – The recommended adult oral dosage is 24 mg administered 30 minutes before the start of single-day highly emetogenic chemotherapy, including cisplatin greater than 50 mg/m^2. Efficacy of the 32 mg single dose beyond 24 hours in these patients has not been established.

Hepatic function impairment – Do not exceed an 8 mg oral dose. For IV use, a single maximum daily dose of 8 mg infused over 15 minutes beginning 30 minutes before the start of emetogenic chemotherapy is recommended.

GRANISETRON:

IV – The recommended dosage is 10 mcg/kg infused IV over 5 minutes, beginning within 30 minutes before initiation of chemotherapy, and only on the day(s) chemotherapy is given.

Children: The recommended dose in children 2 to 16 years of age is 10 mcg/kg.

Elderly, renal, or hepatic function impairment: No dosage adjustment is recommended.

Oral – 2 mg once/day or 1 mg twice/day. In the 2 mg once/day regimen, two 1 mg tablets are given up to 1 hour before chemotherapy. In the 1 mg twice/day regimen, give the first dose up to 1 hour before chemotherapy and the second dose 12 hours after the first. Either regimen is administered only on the day(s) chemotherapy is given. Continued treatment while not on chemotherapy has not been found to be useful.

Radiation (either total body irradiation or fractionated abdominal radiation): 2 mg once/day. Two 1 mg tablets are taken within 1 hour of radiation.

Elderly, renal/hepatic function impairment: No dosage adjustment is recommended.

DOLASETRON:

Cardiac effects – Administer dolasetron with caution in patients who have or may develop prolongation of cardiac conduction intervals, particularly QT_c.

Infusion rate – Dolasetron injection can be safely infused IV as rapidly as 100 mg/30 seconds or diluted in a compatible IV solution to 50 mL and infused over a period of up to 15 minutes.

Chemotherapy-induced nausea and vomiting, prevention –

IV:

Adults – 1.8 mg/kg as a single dose ≈ 30 minutes before chemotherapy. Alternatively, a fixed dose of 100 mg can be administered over 30 seconds.

Children (2 to 16 years of age) – 1.8 mg/kg as a single dose ≈ 30 minutes before chemotherapy, up to a maximum of 100 mg.

Oral:

Adults – 100 mg within 1 hour before chemotherapy.

Children (2 to 16 years of age) – 1.8 mg/kg within 1 hour before chemotherapy, up to a maximum of 100 mg.

Postoperative nausea or vomiting, prevention/treatment –

IV:

Adults – 12.5 mg as a single dose ≈ 15 minutes before the cessation of anesthesia or as soon as nausea or vomiting presents.

Children (2 to 16 years of age) – 0.35 mg/kg as a single dose ≈ 15 minutes before the cessation of anesthesia or as soon as nausea or vomiting presents, up to a maximum of 12.5 mg.

Oral (prevention only) –

Adults: 100 mg 2 hours before surgery.

Children (2 to 16 years of age): 1.2 mg/kg within 2 hours before surgery, up to a maximum of 100 mg.

ALOSETRON: For safety reasons, alosetron is approved with marketing restrictions. Physicians must attest that they are able and willing to:

- diagnose and treat IBS,
- diagnose and manage ischemic colitis,
- diagnose and manage constipation and complications of constipation,
- understand the risks and benefits of treatment with alosetron for severe diarrhea-predominant IBS,
- educate patients on the risks and benefits of treatment with alosetron,
- report serious adverse events to GlaxoSmithKline at (888) 825-5249 or to the Food and Drug Administration's MedWatch Program at (800) FDA-1088.
- affix program stickers to all prescriptions for alosetron (ie, the original and all subsequent refill prescriptions). No telephone, facsimile, or computerized prescriptions are permitted with this program.

To enroll in the Prescribing Program for *Lotronex*, call (888) 825-5249 or visit www.LOTRONEX.com.

Usual adult dose – Start alosetron at a dosage of 1 mg orally once/day for 4 weeks. If, after 4 weeks, the 1 mg once daily dosage is well tolerated but does not adequately control IBS symptoms, then the dosage can be increased to 1 mg twice/day. Discontinue alosetron in patients who have not had adequate control of IBS symptoms after 4 weeks of treatment with 1 mg twice/day. Alosetron can be taken with or without food.

Discontinue alosetron immediately in patients who develop constipation or signs of ischemic colitis. Do not restart alosetron in patients who develop ischemic colitis.

Children – Safety and effectiveness have not been established in pediatric patients.

Elderly – Postmarketing experience suggests that elderly patients may be at greater risk for complications of constipation; therefore, exercise appropriate caution and follow-up if alosetron is prescribed for these patients.

Actions

Pharmacology: Selective 5-hydroxytryptamine$_3$ (5-HT$_3$) receptor antagonists are antinauseant and antiemetic agents with little or no affinity for other serotonin receptors, alpha- or beta-adrenergic, dopamine-D$_2$, histamine-H$_1$, benzodiazepine, picrotoxin, or opioid receptors. 5-HT$_3$ receptor antagonists such as **alosetron** inhibit activation of nonselective cation channels, which results in the modulation of the enteric nervous system.

Pharmacokinetics: The elimination half-lives of these drugs range from 4 to 8 hours. Elimination is primarily via hepatic metabosim. Plasma concentrations of **alosetron** are 30% to 50% lower and less variable in men compared with women given the same dose. Plasma protein binding is 82% for alosetron, 65% for **granisetron** and 70% to 76% for **ondansetron**. The terminal elimination half-life of alosetron is approximately 1.5 hours.

Contraindications

Dolasetron: Hypersensitivity to the drug or components of the product; markedly prolonged QTc or atrioventricular block II to III; patients receiving class I or III antiarrhythmic agents.

Alosetron: Do not initiate alosetron in patients with constipation. Alosetron is contraindicated in patients:

- with a history of chronic or severe constipation or with a history of sequelae from constipation,
- with a history of intestinal obstruction, stricture, toxic megacolon, GI perforation, or adhesions,
- with a history of ischemic colitis, impaired intestinal circulation, thrombophlebitis, or hypercoagulable state,
- with current or a history of Crohn's disease or ulcerative colitis,
- with active diverticulitis or a history of diverticulitis,
- who are unable to understand or comply with the Patient-Physician Agreement,
- with known hypersensitivity to any component of the product.

Warnings

Ischemic colitis: Ischemic colitis has been reported in patients receiving **alosetron**. Immediately discontinue alosetron in patients with signs of ischemic colitis, such as rectal bleeding, bloody diarrhea, or new or worsening abdominal pain. Do not resume alosetron in patients who develop ischemic colitis.

Constipation: Serious complications of constipation, including obstruction, perforation, impaction, toxic megacolon, secondary colonic ischemia, and death have been reported with use of **alosetron**. Immediately discontinue alosetron treatment in patients who develop constipation.

Postoperatively: Routine prophylaxis is not recommended for patients in whom there is little expectation that nausea or vomiting will occur postoperatively. In patients where nausea or vomiting must be avoided postoperatively, IV **ondansetron** is recommended even where the incidence of postoperative nausea or vomiting is low. For patients who have postoperative nausea or vomiting, ondansetron may be given to prevent further episodes.

Cardiac effects: Acute, usually reversible, ECG changes (PR and QTc prolongation; QRS widening) caused by **dolasetron** have been observed. Dolasetron appears to prolong depolarization and, to a lesser extent, repolarization time. The magnitude and frequency of the ECG changes increased with dose. These ECG interval prolongations usually returned to baseline within 6 to 8 hours but in some patients were present at 24-hour follow up.

Administer dolasetron with caution in patients who have or may develop prolongation of cardiac conduction intervals, particularly QTc. These include patients with hypokalemia or hypomagnesemia, patients taking diuretics with potential for inducing electrolyte abnormalities, patients with congential QT syndrome, patients taking antiarrhythmic drugs or other drugs that lead to QT prolongation and cumulative high dose anthracycline therapy.

Peristalsis: Ondansetron does not stimulate gastric or intestinal peristalsis. Do not use instead of nasogastric suction. Use in abdominal surgery may mask a progressive ileus or gastric distension.

Hypersensitivity reactions: Rare cases of hypersensitivity reactions, sometimes severe, have occurred.

Hepatic function impairment: Increased exposure to alosetron is likely to occur in patients with hepatic insufficiency.

Pregnancy: *Category B.*

Lactation: It is not known whether 5-HT$_3$ antagonists are excreted in breast milk.

Children:

Granisetron – Safety and efficacy of the injection in children < 2 years of age have not been established. Safety and efficacy of the oral doseform in children have not been established.

Ondansetron – Little information is available about dosage in children ≤ 3 years of age.

Dolasetron – Safety and efficacy in children < 2 years of age have not been established. See Adminstration and Dosage for use in children ≤ 2 years of age.

Alosetron – Safety and efficacy in pediatric patients have not been established.

Precautions

Benzyl alcohol: Some of these products contain benzyl alcohol, which has been associated with a fatal "gasping syndrome" in premature infants.

Drug Interactions

Inducers or inhibitors of P450 enzymes may change the clearance and, hence, the half-life of 5-HT$_3$ antagonists. No dosage adjustment is recommended for patients on these drugs. **Dolasetron** may be affected by atenolol, cimetidine, and rifampin. **Ondansetron** may be affected by rifampin.

Adverse Reactions

Adverse reactions occurring in ≥ 3% of patients:

Ondansetron: Anxiety/agitation; dizziness; drowsiness/sedation; malaise/fatigue; fever/pyrexia; gynecological disorder; hypoxia; injection site reaction; pruritus; urinary retention; hypotension; headache; chills/shivering; abdominal pain; constipation; diarrhea; increased AST and ALT; arrhythmias; wound problem; musculoskeletal pain; extrapyramidal syndrome.

Granisetron: Asthenia; headache; abdominal pain; constipation; diarrhea; nausea/vomiting; increased AST and ALT; somnolence; CNS stimulation; decreased appetite; leukopenia; shivers; anemia; alopecia; thrombocytopenia.

Dolasetron: Bradycardia/tachycardia; hypotension; dizziness; headache; malaise/fatigue; abdominal pain; dyspepsia; fever/pyrexia; pruritus; increased AST and ALT.

Alosetron: Abdominal pain; constipation; nausea; GI discomfort/pain.

INFLIXIMAB

Powder for injection, lyophilized: 100 mg (*Rx*)	*Remicade* (Centocor)

Warning:

Tuberculosis (frequently disseminated or extrapulmonary at clinical presentation), invasive fungal infections, and other opportunistic infections have been observed in patients receiving infliximab. Some of these infections have been fatal (see Warnings).

Evaluate patients for latent tuberculosis infection with a tuberculin skin test. Initiate treatment of latent tuberculosis infection prior to therapy with infliximab.

Indications

Rheumatoid arthritis (RA)

Crohn's disease, moderate to severe: For reducing signs and symptoms and inducing and maintaining clinical remission in patients with moderately to severely active Crohn's disease who have had an inadequate response to conventional therapy.

Crohn's disease, fistulizing: For reducing the number of draining enterocutaneous fistulas. The safety and efficacy of therapy continued beyond 3 doses have not been established.

Administration and Dosage

RA: 3 mg/kg given as an IV infusion followed with additional similar doses at 2 and 6 weeks after the first infusion, then every 8 weeks thereafter. Give infliximab in combination with methotrexate. For patients who have an incomplete response, consider adjusting the dose up to 10 mg/kg or treating as often as every 4 weeks.

Crohn's disease, moderate to severe: 5 mg/kg given as an induction regimen at 0, 2, and 6 weeks followed by a maintenance regimen of 5 mg/kg every 8 weeks thereafter. For patients who respond and then lose their response, consider treatment with 10 mg/kg. Patients who do not respond by week 14 are unlikely to respond with continued dosing; consider discontinuing infliximab in these patients.

Crohn's disease, fistulizing: Administer an initial 5 mg/kg dose followed with additional 5 mg/kg doses at 2 and 6 weeks after the first infusion.

There are insufficient safety and efficacy data for the use of infliximab for fistulizing Crohn's disease beyond the recommended duration.

Actions

Pharmacology: Infliximab is a chimeric IgG1κ monoclonal antibody that neutralizes the biological activity of tumor necrosis factor alpha (TNFα) by high-affinity binding to its soluble and transmembrane forms and inhibits TNFα receptor binding. Infliximab does not neutralize TNFβ (lymphotoxin α). Biological activities attributed to TNFα include the following: Induction of proinflammatory cytokines (eg, IL-1, IL-6), leukocyte migration enhancement by increasing endothelial layer permeability and expression of adhesion molecules by endothelial cells and leukocytes, activation of neutrophil and eosinophil functional activity, and induction of acute phase reactants and other liver proteins, as well as tissue-degrading enzymes produced by synoviocytes or chondrocytes.

Elevated concentrations of TNFα have been found in the joints of RA patients and the stools of Crohn's disease patients and correlate with elevated disease activity. In Crohn's disease, infliximab reduces infiltration of inflammatory cells and TNFα production in inflamed areas of the intestine and reduces the proportion of mononuclear cells from the lamina propria able to express TNFα and interferon. In RA, treatment with infliximab reduced infiltration of inflammatory cells into inflamed areas of the joint as well as expression of molecules mediating cellular adhesion and vascular cell adhesion molecule-1, chemoattraction, and tissue degradation. After treatment with infliximab, patients with Crohn's disease or RA have decreased levels of serum IL-6 and C-reactive protein compared with baseline.

However, peripheral blood lymphocytes from infliximab-treated patients showed no significant decrease in number or in proliferative responses to in vitro mitogenic stimulation when compared with cells from untreated patients.

Pharmacokinetics: A study of single IV infusions of 3 to 20 mg/kg showed a linear relationship between the dose and the maximum serum concentration. The volume of distribution at steady state was independent of dose and indicated that infliximab was distributed primarily within the vascular compartment. The median terminal half-life of infliximab ranged between 8 to 10 days.

No systemic accumulation of infliximab occurred. In Crohn's disease patients receiving maintenance treatment with 5 and 10 mg/kg infliximab, approximately 20% and 12%, respectively, had undetectable infliximab concentrations 8 weeks following their infusion.

With repeated dosing of infliximab, serum concentrations of infliximab were higher in RA patients who received concomitant methotrexate.

Contraindications

In patients with moderate or severe (NYHA Class III/IV) CHF (See Warnings).

Hypersensitivity to any murine proteins or other components of the product.

Warnings

CHF: Do not administer doses greater than 5 mg/kg to patients with CHF. Use infliximab with caution in patients with mild heart failure (NYHA Class I/II). Monitor patients closely; infliximab must not be continued in patients who develop new or worsening symptoms of heart failure.

Risk of infections: Serious infections, including sepsis, have been reported in patients receiving TNF-blocking agents. Some of these infections have been fatal. Many of the serious infections in patients treated with infliximab occurred in patients on concomitant immunosuppressive therapy that, in addition to their Crohn's disease or RA, could predispose them to infections. Do not give infliximab to patients with a clinically important active infection. Exercise caution when considering the use of infliximab in patients with a chronic infection or a history of recurrent infections. Monitor patients for signs and symptoms of infection while on or after treatment with infliximab. Closely monitor new infections. If a patient develops a serious infection, discontinue infliximab therapy (see Warning Box, Adverse Reactions).

Cases of histoplasmosis, listeriosis, pneumocystosis, and tuberculosis have been observed in patients receiving infliximab. For patients who have resided in regions where histoplasmosis is endemic, carefully consider the benefits and risks of infliximab treatment before initiation of infliximab therapy.

Autoimmunity: Treatment with infliximab therapy may result in the formation of autoantibodies and, rarely, in the development of a lupus-like syndrome. Discontinue treatment if a patient develops symptoms suggestive of a lupus-like syndrome following treatment with infliximab.

Neurologic events: Infliximab and other agents that inhibit TNF have been associated in rare cases with optic neuritis, seizure, and new onset or exacerbation of clinical symptoms or radiographic evidence of CNS demyelinating disorders, including multiple sclerosis. Exercise caution in considering the use of infliximab in patients with pre-existing or recent-onset CNS demyelinating or seizure disorders.

Hypersensitivity reactions: Infliximab has been associated with hypersensitivity reactions that vary in their time of onset. Urticaria, dyspnea, and hypotension have occurred during or within 2 hours of infliximab infusion. However, in some cases, serum sickness-like reactions have been observed in Crohn's disease patients 3 to 12 days after infliximab therapy was reinstituted following an extended period without infliximab treatment. Symptoms associated with these reactions include the following: Fever, rash, headache, sore throat, myalgias, polyarthralgias, hand and facial edema, dysphagia. These reactions were associated with a marked increase in antibodies to infliximab, loss of detectable serum concentrations of infliximab, and possible loss of drug efficacy. Discontinue infliximab for severe reactions. Have medications for the treatment of hypersensitivity reactions (eg, acetaminophen, antihistamines, corticosteroids, epinephrine) available for immediate use in the event of a reaction. Refer to Management of Acute Hypersensitivity Reactions.

Elderly: Because there is a higher incidence of infections in the elderly population in general, use caution when treating the elderly.

Pregnancy: *Category B*. Give to a pregnant woman only if clearly needed.

Lactation: Decide whether to discontinue nursing or discontinue the drug, taking into account the importance of the drug to the mother.

Children: Safety and efficacy have not been established.

Precautions

Malignancy: Patients with a long duration of Crohn's disease or RA and chronic exposure to immunosuppressant therapies are more prone to develop lymphomas (see Adverse Reactions). The impact of infliximab treatment on these phenomena is unknown.

Immunogenicity: Treatment with infliximab can be associated with the development of antibodies to infliximab. Approximately 10% of patients were antibody-positive. Patients who were antibody-positive were more likely to experience an infusion reaction. Antibody development was lower among Crohn's disease and RA patients receiving immunosuppressant therapies such as 6-mercaptopurine, azathioprine, and methotrexate.

Vaccinations: Do not administer live vaccines concurrently.

Adverse Reactions

The most common reasons for discontinuation of treatment were infusion-related reactions (dyspnea, flushing, headache, and rash). Adverse events have been reported in a higher proportion of RA patients receiving the 10 mg/kg dose than the 3 mg/kg dose; however, no differences were observed in the frequency of adverse events between the 5 and 10 mg/kg doses in patients with Crohn's disease.

Adverse reactions reported in 20% or more of patients include the following: Acute infusion reaction, serious infections, auto-antibody/lupus-like syndrome, increased ANA titers, headache, URI, nausea. Adverse reactions reported in 3% or more of patients include the following: Fatigue, insomnia, depression, rash, pruritus, arthralgia, back pain, myalgia, pharyngitis, sinusitis, cough, dyspnea, pain, fever, flu syndrome, chest pain, moniliasis, hypertension, abscess, diarrhea, vomiting, dyspepsia, abdominal pain.

INTERFERON ALFA-2b (IFN-alpha 2; rIFN-α2; α-2-interferon)

Powder for injection, lyophilized: 3, 5, 10, 18, 25, and 50 million IU/vial *(Rx)*	*Intron* A (Schering)
Solution for injection: 3, 5, 10, 18, and 25 million IU/vial (*Rx*)	
Injection: 3, 5, and 10 million IU/vial (*Rx*)	

Warning:

Alpha interferons, including interferon alfa-2b, recombinant, cause or aggravate fatal or life-threatening neuropsychiatric, autoimmune, ischemic, and infectious disorders. Closely monitor patients with periodic clinical and laboratory evaluations. Withdraw patients with persistently severe or worsening signs or symptoms of these conditions from therapy. In many, but not all, cases, these disorders resolve after stopping interferon alfa-2b, recombinant therapy. See Warnings and Adverse Reactions.

Indications

Hairy-cell leukemia: In patients 18 years of age and older with hairy-cell leukemia.

Malignant melanoma: Adjuvant to surgical treatment in patients 18 years of age and older with malignant melanoma who are free of disease but at high risk for systemic recurrence within 56 days of surgery.

Follicular lymphoma: Initial treatment of clinically aggressive follicular non-Hodgkin's lymphoma in conjunction with anthracycline-containing combination chemotherapy in patients 18 years of age and older.

Condylomata acuminata: Intralesional treatment of external genital or perianal warts in select patients 18 years of age and older.

AIDS-related Kaposi's sarcoma: In select patients 18 years of age and older with AIDS-related Kaposi's sarcoma.

Chronic hepatitis C: In patients 18 years of age and older with compensated liver disease and a history of blood or blood product exposure, or patients who are HCV-antibody-positive.

Chronic hepatitis B: In patients 1 year of age and older with compensated liver disease and HBV replication. Patients must be serum HBsAg-positive for at least 6 months and have HBV replication (serum HBeAg-positive) with elevated serum ALT.

Administration and Dosage

The patient may self-administer the dose at bedtime.

Hairy-cell leukemia: 2 million IU/m^2 IM or SC 3 times/week for up to 6 months. Do not use the 50 million IU strength of the powder for injection for the treatment of hairy-cell leukemia.

Malignant melanoma: 20 million IU/m^2 IV infusion on 5 consecutive days/week for 4 weeks. Maintenance dosage is 10 million IU/m^2 SC 3 times/week for 48 weeks.

Perform regular lab testing to monitor abnormalities for the purpose of dose modification. If adverse reactions develop during interferon alfa-2b treatment, particularly if granulocytes decrease to less than 500/mm^3 or ALT/AST rises to less than 5 times the upper limit of normal (ULN), temporarily discontinue treatment until adverse reactions abate. Restart interferon alfa-2b at 50% of the previous dose. If intolerance persists, or if granulocytes decrease to less than 250/mm^3, or ALT/AST rises to more than 10 times the ULN, discontinue interferon alfa-2b therapy.

Follicular lymphoma: 5 million IU SC 3 times/week for up to 18 months in conjunction with an anthracycline-containing chemotherapy regimen.

Discontinue interferon alfa-2b therapy if AST exceeds more than 5 times the upper limit of normal or serum creatinine more than 2 mg/dL.

Condylomata acuminata: Inject 1 million IU/lesion 3 times/week for 3 weeks on alternate days intralesionally. Use only 10 million IU vials because dilution of other strengths results in a hypertonic solution. Use a tuberculin or similar syringe and a 25- to 30-gauge needle.

The 10 million IU vial of interferon alfa-2b powder for injection must be reconstituted with 1 mL of diluent (Bacteriostatic Water for Injection).

Maximum response usually occurs 4 to 8 weeks after therapy initiation. If results are not satisfactory after 12 to 16 weeks, a second course may be instituted. Patients with 6 to 10 condylomata may receive a second (sequential) course. Patients with more than 10 condylomata may receive additional sequences.

Drug delivery – Do not go beneath the lesion too deeply or inject too superficially. As many as 5 lesions can be treated at one time. To reduce side effects, give in evening with acetaminophen.

Direct the needle at the center of the base of the wart and at an angle almost parallel to the plane of the skin. This will deliver the interferon to the dermal core of the lesion, infiltrating the lesion and causing a small wheal.

AIDS-related Kaposi's sarcoma: 30 million IU/m^2 3 times/week administered SC or IM. Do not use the 18 and 25 million IU multidose strengths of the interferon alfa-2b solution for injection for the treatment of AIDS-related Kaposi's sarcoma. Maintain the selected dosage regimen unless the disease progresses rapidly or severe intolerance occurs. If severe adverse reactions develop, modify dosage (50% reduction) or temporarily discontinue therapy until adverse reactions abate. When patients initiate therapy at 30 million IU/m^2 3 times/week, average dose tolerated at the end of 12 weeks of therapy is 110 million IU/week and 75 million IU/week at end of 24 weeks of therapy.

When disease stabilization or response to treatment occurs, continue treatment until there is no further evidence of tumor or until discontinuation is required by evidence of a severe opportunistic infection or adverse effect.

Chronic hepatitis C: 3 million IU 3 times/week SC or IM. At 16 weeks of treatment, extend therapy to 18 to 24 months at 3 million IU 3 times/week to improve the sustained response, normalization of ALT. Consider discontinuing therapy in nonresponders after 16 weeks. If severe adverse reactions develop, modify the dose (50% reduction) or temporarily discontinue therapy until reactions abate. If intolerance persists after dose adjustment, discontinue therapy.

Chronic hepatitis B:

Adults – 30 to 35 million IU/week SC or IM, either as 5 million IU daily or 10 million IU 3 times/week for 16 weeks.

Pediatrics – 3 million IU/m^2 3 times/week for the first week of therapy followed by dose escalation to 6 million IU/m^2 3 times/week (maximum of 10 million IU 3 times/week) administered SC for a total therapy duration of 16 to 24 weeks.

If serious adverse reactions or lab abnormalities develop during therapy, decrease the dose by 50% or discontinue if appropriate until adverse reactions abate. If intolerance persists after dose adjustment, discontinue the drug.

Decreased white blood cell, granulocyte, or platelet counts – Use the following guidelines:

Interferon Alfa-2b Dose with Decreased White Blood Cell, Granulocyte, or Platelet Counts

Granulocyte count	White blood cell count	Platelet count	Interferon alfa-2b dose
< 750/mm^3	< 1500/mm^3	< 50,000/mm^3	Reduce by 50%
< 500/mm^3	< 1000/mm^3	< 30,000/mm^3	Permanently discontinue

When platelet or granulocyte counts return to normal or baseline values, reinstitute therapy at up to 100% of initial dose.

Actions

Pharmacology: Interferon alfa-2b is a protein produced by recombinant DNA techniques. Interferons exert their cellular activities by binding to specific membrane receptors on the cell surface. Once bound to the cell membrane, interferon initiates a complex sequence of intracellular events that includes the induction of certain enzymes. These events include inhibition of virus replication in virus-infected cells, suppression of cell proliferation, and immunomodulating activities.

Pharmacokinetics:

Absorption/Distribution – Maximum serum concentrations obtained via SC and IM occurred 3 to 12 hours after administration. Serum concentrations were below the detection limit by 16 hours after the injections.

After IV use, serum concentrations peaked by the end of infusion, then declined at a slightly more rapid rate than after IM or SC administration, becoming undetectable 4 hours after infusion.

Metabolism/Excretion – Elimination half-lives were about 2 to 3 hours. Interferon could not be detected in urine; the kidney may be the main site of interferon catabolism.

Contraindications

Hypersensitivity to interferon alfa-2b or any components of the product. Interferon alfa-2b and ribavirin must not be used by women who are pregnant or by men whose female partners are pregnant. Extreme care must be taken to avoid pregnancy in female patients and in female partners of patients taking combination interferon alfa-2b/ribavirin therapy. Patients with autoimmune hepatitis must not be treated with combination interferon alfa-2b/ribavirin therapy.

Warnings

Benzyl alcohol: Some of these products contain benzyl alcohol, which has been associated with a fatal "gasping syndrome" in premature infants.

Interferon alfa-2b and ribavirin capsule combination: Therapy containing interferon alfa-2b and ribavirin capsules was associated with hemolytic anemia. Hemoglobin less than 10 g/dL was observed in about 10% of patients in clinical trials. Anemia occurred within 1 to 2 weeks of initiation of ribavirin therapy.

Thrombocytopenia: Do not give IM to patients with platelet counts less than 50,000/mm^3. Instead, give SC.

50 million IU vial size: This vial size is to be used *only* for treatment of patients with AIDS-related Kaposi's sarcoma or with malignant melanoma.

Condylomata acuminata:

Do not use – Do not use 3, 5, 18, 25, or 50 million IU vials of powder for injection or the 3 or 18 million IU multidose vials intralesionally to treat condylomata acuminata; concentrations are inappropriate.

Malignant melanoma: Interferon solution for injection is not recommended for the IV treatment of malignant melanoma.

Pre-existing psychiatric condition/history of severe psychiatric disorder: Depression and suicidal behavior including suicidal ideation, suicidal attempts, and completed suicides have been reported. Patients with a pre-existing psychiatric condition, especially depression, or a history of severe psychiatric disorder should not be treated with interferon alfa-2b.

Obtundation/Coma: Obtundation and coma also have been observed in some patients, usually elderly, treated at higher doses. These effects are usually rapidly reversible upon discontinuation of therapy; full resolution of symptoms has taken up to 3 weeks in a few severe episodes. Use concurrent narcotics, hypnotics, or sedatives with caution.

Bone marrow toxicity: Interferon alfa-2b therapy suppresses bone marrow function and may result in severe cytopenias, including very rare events of aplastic anemia. Obtain CBCs pretreatment and monitor routinely during therapy. Discontinue interferon alfa-2b therapy in patients who develop severe decreases in neutrophil (less than 0.5×10^9/L) or platelet counts (less than 25×10^9/L).

Thyroid abnormalities: Infrequently, patients receiving interferon alfa-2b therapy developed thyroid abnormalities, either hypothyroid or hyperthyroid. Patients developing symptoms consistent with possible thyroid dysfunction of therapy should have their thyroid function evaluated and appropriate treatment instituted. Discontinue therapy if thyroid function cannot be normalized by medication. Discontinuation of therapy has not always reversed thyroid dysfunction occurring during treatment.

Fever/"Flu-like" symptoms: Because of fever and other "flu-like" symptoms associated with this drug, use cautiously in patients with debilitating medical conditions, such as a history of pulmonary disease or diabetes mellitus prone to ketoacidosis. Observe caution in coagulation disorders or severe myelosuppression.

Pulmonary infiltrates: Pulmonary infiltrates, pneumonitis, and pneumonia, including fatality, have been observed.

Cardiovascular: Use therapy cautiously in patients with a history of cardiovascular disease. Cardiovascular adverse experiences include hypotension, arrhythmia, or tachycardia of at least 150 beats/min and, rarely, cardiomyopathy and MI. Hypotension may occur during administration, or up to 2 days posttherapy, and may require supportive therapy, including fluid replacement to maintain intravascular volume.

Retinal hemorrhages, cotton wool spots, and retinal artery or vein obstruction: Retinal hemorrhages, cotton wool spots, and retinal artery or vein obstruction have been observed rarely.

Hepatotoxicity: Hepatotoxicity, including fatality, has been observed.

Autoimmune disease: Rare cases of autoimmune diseases including thrombocytopenia, vasculitis, Raynaud's phenomenon, rheumatoid arthritis, lupus erythematosus, and rhabdomyolysis have been observed.

Hyperglycemia: Diabetes mellitus and hyperglycemia have been observed rarely in patients treated with interferon alfa-2b.

Hypersensitivity: Acute serious hypersensitivity reactions (eg, urticaria, angioedema, bronchoconstriction, anaphylaxis) have been observed rarely in treated patients.

Renal function impairment: Interferon alfa-2b/ribavirin capsule combination therapy is not recommended in patients with severe renal impairment; use with caution in patients with moderate renal impairment.

Hepatic function impairment: Do not treat patients with decompensated liver disease, autoimmune hepatitis, history of autoimmune disease, or immunocompromised transplant recipients.

Fertility impairment: Interferon may impair fertility. Fertile women should not receive interferon alfa-2b unless they are using effective contraception. Use with caution in fertile men.

Pregnancy: Category C.

Lactation: It is not known if this drug is excreted in breast milk.

Children: Safety and efficacy in children under 18 years of age have not been established.

Precautions

Monitoring: Prior to beginning treatment and periodically thereafter perform the following: Standard hematologic tests with complete blood counts and differential, platelet counts, blood chemistries, electrolytes, TSH, liver function tests. Patients with pre-existing cardiac abnormalities or those in advanced stages of cancer should have ECGs taken before and during treatment.

Baseline chest X-rays are suggested; repeat if clinically indicated.

For malignant melanoma patients, monitor differential, WBC count, and liver function tests weekly during the induction phase of therapy and monthly during the maintenance phase of therapy.

Chronic hepatitis B: Perform a liver biopsy to establish presence of chronic hepatitis and extent of liver damage.

ALT increase – A transient increase in ALT at least 2 times baseline (flare) can occur, generally 8 to 12 weeks after therapy initiation, and is more frequent in responders.

Chronic hepatitis C: Perform a liver biopsy to establish diagnosis. Test for presence of antibody to HCV. Exclude patients with other causes of chronic hepatitis, including autoimmune hepatitis.

Psoriasis: There have been reports of interferon exacerbating pre-existing psoriasis.

Photosensitivity: Photosensitivity may occur.

Drug Interactions

Drugs that may be affected by inteferon alfa-2b include theophylline and zidovudine.

Adverse Reactions

The most frequently reported reactions are "flu-like" symptoms, particularly fever, headache, chills, myalgia, and fatigue. Other adverse reactions occurring in more than 5% of patients include the following: Dizziness; paresthesia; depression; anxiety; confusion; hypesthesia; amnesia; impaired concentration; nervousness; irritability; somnolence; decreased libido; nausea; diarrhea; vomiting; anorexia; dyspnea; constipation; loose stools; abdominal pain; pharyngitis; nasal congestion; dyspnea; coughing; sinusitis; dry mouth; arthralgia; asthenia; rigors; back pain; muscle pain/weakness; rash; pruritus; dry skin; dermatitis; alopecia; moniliasis; edema/facial edema; chest pain; increased sweating; malaise; taste alteration; insomnia; weight loss; herpes simplex; gingivitis; thinning hair; nonproductive cough; asthenia; pain (unspecified); injection site inflammation; lab test abnormalities including hemoglobin, WBC count, platelet count, serum creatinine, alkaline phosphatase, AST, ALT, serum urea nitrogen, and granulocyte count.

LACTASE ENZYMES

Capsules: 250 mg standardized enzyme lactase	*Lactrase* (Schwarz Pharma)
Tablets, chewable: 3000 FCC lactase units	*Dairy Ease* (Blistex)

Indications

To digest lactose contained in milk for patients with lactose intolerance.

Administration and Dosage

Tablets: 1 to 3 tablets with the first bite of dairy food.

Capsules: 1 or 2 capsules taken with milk or dairy products. If the patient is severely intolerant to lactose, increase dosage until a satisfactory dose is achieved.

LAXATIVES

BISACODYL	
Tablets, enteric coated: 5 mg (*otc*)	Various, *Dulcolax* (Ciba Consumer), *Fleet Laxative* (Fleet), *Modane* (Savage), *Women's Gentle Laxative* (Goldline Consumer), *Bisac-Evac* (G & W), *Caroid* (Metholatum Co.), *Correctol* (Schering-Plough), *Feen-a-mint* (Schering-Plough)
Tablets, enteric coated, delayed-release: 5 mg	*Reliable Gentle Laxative* (Goldline Consumer)
Suppositories: 10 mg (*otc*)	Various, *Bisacodyl Uniserts* (Upsher-Smith), *Bisac-Evac* (G & W), *Dulcolax* (Novartis Consumer), *Reliable Gentle Laxative* (Goldline Consumer), *Fleet Laxative* (Fleet)
CASCARA SAGRADA	
Tablets: 325 mg (*otc*)	Various
Liquid: (*otc*)	*Aromatic Cascara Fluidextract* (Various), *Cascara Aromatic* (Humco)
CASTOR OIL	
Liquid: 95% castor oil (*otc*)	Various, *Purge* (Fleming)
Emulsion: 95% castor oil with emulsifying agents (*otc*)	*Emulsoil* (Paddock)
36.4% castor oil with 0.1% sodium benzoate, 0.2% potassium sorbate (*sf, otc*)	*Neoloid* (Kenwood)
CO_2 RELEASING SUPPOSITORIES	
Suppositories: Sodium bicarbonate and potassium bitartrate in a water soluble polyethylene glycol base (*otc*)	*Ceo-Two* (Beutlich)
DOCUSATE CALCIUM (DIOCTYL CALCIUM SULFOSUCCINATE)	
Capsules: 240 mg (*otc*)	Various, *DC Softgels* (Goldline), *Stool Softener* (Apothecary), *Stool Softener DC* (Rugby), *Surfak Liquigels* (Pharmacia)
DOCUSATE SODIUM (DIOCTYL SODIUM SULFOSUCCINATE; DSS)	
Tablets: 100 mg (*otc*)	*ex-lax Stool Softener* (Novartis Consumer)
Capsules: 50 and 100 mg (*otc*)	Various, *Colace* (Roberts), *D-S-S* (Magno-Humphries), *Modane Soft* (Savage), *Non-Habit Forming Stool Softener*, *Stool Softener* (Rugby), *Regulax SS* (Republic)
Capsules: 250 mg (*otc*)	Various, *Stool Softener* (Rugby)
Capsules, soft gel: 50, 100, and 250 mg (*otc*)	Various, *D.O.S.*, *Genasoft* (Goldline Consumer), *Phillip's Liqui-Gels* (Bayer Consumer), *Stool Softener* (Rugby)
Syrup: 50, 60, 150 mg/15 mL, 20 mg/5 mL, 100 mg/30 mL (*otc*)	Various, *Colace* (Roberts), *Diocto* (Various), *Docu* (Hi-Tech Pharmacal), *Silace* (Silax)
GLYCERIN	
Suppositories: Glycerin (*otc*)	Various, *Sani-Supp* (G & W), *Colace* (Roberts)
Liquid: 4 mL/applicator (*otc*)	*Fleet Babylax* (Fleet)
LACTULOSE	
Syrup: 10 g lactulose/15 mL (< 1.6 g galactose, < 1.2 g lactose, and ≤ 1.2 g other sugars) (*Rx*)	Various, *Cephulac*, *Chronulac* (Aventis), *Cholac* (Alra), *Constilac* (Alra), *Constulose*, *Enulose* (Alpharma), *Duphalac* (Solvay Pharm.)
MINERAL OIL	
Liquid: mineral oil (*otc*)	Various
Emulsion: Mineral oil with an emulsifier (*otc*)	*Kondremul Plain* (Heritage Consumer)
POLYCARBOPHIL	
Tablets: 500 and 625 mg (*otc*)	*FiberNorm* (G & W), *Konsyl Fiber* (Konsyl)
Tablets, chewable: 625 mg (as calcium) (*otc*)	*Equalactin* (Numark), *Mitrolan* (Whitehall-Robins)
Tablets: 625 mg (as calcium) (*otc*)	*Bulk Forming Fiber Laxative* (Goldline Consumer), *Fiber-Lax* (Rugby), *FiberCon* (Lederle)

PSYLLIUM	
Powder: Psyllium (*otc*)	Various, *Fiberall Tropical Fruit Flavor, Fiberall Orange Flavor* (Heritage Consumer), *Genfiber, Genfiber, Orange Flavor* (Goldline Consumer), *Hydrocil Instant* (Numark), *Konsyl, Konsyl-D, Konsyl-Orange, Konsyl Easy Mix Formula* (Konsyl Pharm.), *Metamucil, Metamucil Sugar Free, Metamucil Orange Flavor* (Procter & Gamble), *Modane Bulk* (Savage), *Natural Fiber Laxative* (Apothecary), *Reguloid, Reguloid, Orange, Reguloid, Sugar Free Orange* (Rugby), *Syllact* (Wallace)
Wafers: Psyllium (*otc*)	*Metamucil* (Procter & Gamble)
Granules: Psyllium (*otc*)	*Serutan* (Menley & James)
SALINE LAXATIVES	
Granules: Magnesium sulfate (*otc*)	*Epsom Salt (Various)*
Suspension: Magnesium hydroxide (*otc*)	*Milk of Magnesia, Milk of Magnesia, Concentrated (Various), Phillips' Milk of Magnesia, Phillips' Milk of Magnesia, Concentrated* (Bayer)
Solution: Magnesium citrate (*otc*)	*Magnesium Citrate Solution* (Humco)
Solution: Sodium phosphates (*otc*)	Various, *Fleet Phospho-soda* (Fleet)
SENNOSIDES	
Tablets: 6, 8.6, 15, 17, and 25 mg (*otc*)	*ex•lax, ex•lax, chocolated, Maximum Relief ex•lax* (Novartis Consumer), *Black-Draught* (Monticello), *Senokot* (Purdue Frederick), *Senna-Gen* (Zenith-Goldline), *SenokotXTRA* (Purdue Fredrick)
Granules: 15 mg/5 mL and 20 mg/5 mL	*Black-Draught* (Monticello), *Senokot* (Purdue Frederick)
Liquid: 25 mg sennosides A and B/15 mL and 33.3 mg/mL senna concentrate (*otc*)	*Agoral* (Numark), *Fletcher's Castoria* (Mentholatum)
Syrup: 8.8 mg/5 mL sennosides (*otc*)	*Senokot* (Purdue Frederick)
ENEMAS	
Disposable enemas	*Fleet, Fleet Bisacodyl, Fleet Mineral Oil* (Fleet), *Therevac-SB, Therevac-Plus* (Jones Medical)
LAXATIVE COMBINATIONS	
Capsules and tablets: 50 mg docusate sodium, 8.6 mg senna concentrate (*otc*)	*Senokot-S Tablets* (Purdue Frederick)
100 mg docusate sodium, 30 mg casanthranol (*otc*)	Various, *Doxidan Capsules* (Pharmacia), *DSS 100 Plus* (Magno-Humphries), *Genasoft Plus Softgels, Peri-Dos Softgels* (Goldline), *Peri-Colace* (Roberts), *Nature's Remedy* (Block Drug)
150 mg cascara sagrada (*otc*)	*Nature's Remedy Tablets* (Block Drug)
Liquids, syrups, emulsions, suspensions: 60 mg docusate sodium and 30 mg casanthranol/15 mL (*otc*)	*Diocto C* (Various), *Peri-Colace* (Roberts), *DOK-Plus* (Major)
Mineral oil in emulsifying base (*otc*)	*Liqui-Doss* (Ferndale)
≈ 900 mg magnesium hydroxide and 3.75 mL mineral oil/ 15 mL (*otc*)	*Haley's M-O* (Bayer)
90 mg/15 mL casantrhanol with senna extract, rhubarb, methyl salicylate, and menthol (*otc*)	*Black-Draught* (Monticello)
30 mg casanthranol, 60 mg docusate sodium/15 mL (*otc*)	*Silace-C* (Silarx)
15 mL equiv. to 30 mL milk of magnesia and 5 mL aromatic cascara fluid extract (*otc*)	*Concentrated Milk of Magnesia-Cascara* (Roxane)
Granules: 3.25 g psyllium, 0.74 g senna, 1.8 mg sodium, 35.5 mg potassium/rounded teaspoonful (*otc*)	*Perdiem Overnight Relief* (Novartis Consumer)
MISCELLANEOUS BOWEL EVACUANTS	
Miscellaneous Bowel Evacuants (*otc*)	*Evac-Q-Kwik* (Savage), *Fleet Prep Kit 1, 2, and 3* (Fleet), *X-Prep Liquid, X-Prep Bowel Evacuant Kit-1, X-Prep Bowel Kit-2* (Gray), *Tridate Bowel Cleansing System* (Lafayette)
MISCELLANEOUS BULK-PRODUCING LAXATIVES	
Powder: 2 mg methylcellulose per heaping tbsp (*otc*)	*Citrucel, Citrucel Sugar Free* (GlaxoSmithKline)
Powder: Powdered cellulose (*otc*)	*Unifiber* (Niche)
Tablets, coated: 750 mg malt soup extract (*otc*)	*Maltsupex* (Wallace)
Powder: 8 g malt soup extract/scoop (*otc*)	*Maltsupex* (Wallace)

Liquid: 16 g malt soup extract/tbsp (*otc*)	*Maltsupex* (Wallace)

Indications

Constipation: Treatment of constipation.

Rectal/Bowel examinations: Certain stimulant, lubricant, and saline laxatives are used to evacuate the colon for rectal and bowel examinations.

Prophylaxis: Laxatives, generally **fecal softeners** or **mineral oil**, are useful prophylactically in patients who should not strain during defecation (ie, following anorectal surgery, MI).

Lactulose (certain brands): Prevention and treatment of portal-systemic encephalopathy, including the stages of hepatic precoma and coma.

Psyllium: Useful in patients with irritable bowel syndrome and diverticular disease.

Polycarbophil: For constipation or diarrhea associated with conditions such as irritable bowel syndrome and diverticulosis; acute nonspecific diarrhea.

Mineral oil (enema): Relief of fecal impaction.

Docusate sodium: Prevention of dry, hard stools.

Unlabeled uses: **Psyllium** appears to be useful in the reduction of cholesterol levels as an adjunct to a dietary program.

Administration and Dosage

BISACODYL: Swallow whole; do not chew. Do not take within 1 hour of antacids or milk.

Tablets –

Adults and children ≥ 12 years of age: 10 to 15 mg (usually 10 mg) in a single dose once daily.

Children (6 to < 12 years of age): 5 mg once daily.

Suppositories –

Adults: 10 mg once daily.

Children (6 to < 12 years of age): 5 mg once daily.

CASCARA SAGRADA:

Tablets – 1 tablet at bedtime.

Liquid – 5 mL.

CASTOR OIL:

Liquid –

Adults: Daily dose range, 15 to 60 mL.

Children (2 to 12 years of age): 5 to 15 mL.

Infants: 2.5 to 7.5 mL.

Emulsion –

Adults: 67%, 15 to 60 mL; 95%, 45 mL (should be mixed with ½ to 1 glass liquid).

Children (2 to 12 years of age): 67%, 15 mL; 95%, 5 to 10 mL (should be mixed with ½ to 1 glass liquid).

DOCUSATE CALCIUM *(Dioctyl Calcium Sulfosuccinate):*

Adults and children ≥ 12 years of age – 240 mg daily until bowel movements are normal.

DOCUSATE SODIUM *(Dioctyl Sodium Sulfosuccinate; DSS):* Give in milk, fruit juice, or infant formula to mask taste. In enemas, add 50 to 100 mg (5 to 10 mL liquid) to a retention or flushing enema.

Adults and older children – 50 to 500 mg.

Children (6 to 12 years of age) – 40 to 120 mg.

Children (3 to 6 years of age) – 20 to 60 mg.

Children (< 3 years of age) – 10 to 40 mg.

GLYCERIN:

Suppositories – Insert 1 suppository high in the rectum and retain 15 to 30 minutes; it need not melt to produce laxative action.

Rectal liquid – With gentle, steady pressure, insert stem with tip pointing towards navel. Squeeze unit until nearly all the liquid is expelled, then remove. A small amount of liquid will remain in unit.

LACTULOSE:

Chronulac, Constilac, Duphalac, Constulose –

Treatment of constipation: 15 to 30 mL (10 to 20 g lactulose) daily, increased to 60 mL/day, if necessary.

Cephulac, Cholac, Enulose – Prevent and treat portal-systemic encephalopathy

Oral:

Adults – 30 to 45 mL 3 or 4 times daily. Adjust dosage every day or two to produce 2 or 3 soft stools daily. Hourly doses of 30 to 45 mL may be used to induce rapid laxation in the initial phase of therapy. When the laxative effect has been achieved, reduce dosage to recommended daily dose. Improvement may occur within 24 hours, but may not begin before 48 hours or later. Continuous long-term therapy is indicated to lessen severity and prevent recurrence of portal-systemic encephalopathy.

Children – Recommended initial daily oral dose in infants is 2.5 to 10 mL in divided doses. For older children and adolescents, the total daily dose is 40 to 90 mL. If the initial dose causes diarrhea, reduce immediately. If diarrhea persists, discontinue use.

May be more palatable when mixed with fruit juice, water, or milk.

Rectal: Administer to adults during impending coma or coma stage of portal-systemic encephalopathy when the danger of aspiration exists or when endoscopic or intubation procedures interfere with oral administration. The goal of treatment is reversal of the coma stage so the patient can take oral medication. Reversal of coma may occur within 2 hours of the first enema. Start recommended oral doses before enema is stopped entirely.

Lactulose may be given as a retention enema via a rectal balloon catheter. Do not use cleansing enemas containing soap suds or other alkaline agents.

Mix 300 mL lactulose with 700 mL water or physiologic saline and retain for 30 to 60 minutes. The enema may be repeated every 4 to 6 hours. If the enema is inadvertently evacuated too promptly, it may be repeated immediately.

MINERAL OIL:

Dose –

Adults and children ≥ 12 years of age: 15 to 45 mL, take at bedtime; *Kondremul*, 30 to 75 mL.

Children 6 to < 12 years of age: 5 to 15 mL; *Kondremul*, 10 to 25 mL.

POLYCARBOPHIL:

Adults and children ≥ 12 years of age – 1 g 1 to 4 times daily or as needed. Do not exceed 4 g in 24 hours.

Children 6 to < 12 years of age – 500 mg ≤ 4 times daily or as needed. Do not exceed 2 g/day.

Children < 6 years of age – Products vary. Consult product labeling for specific guidelines.

For severe diarrhea, repeat dose every 30 min; do not exceed maximum daily dose.

When using as a laxative, drink 8 oz water or other liquid with each dose.

PSYLLIUM: Refer to respective package inserts for particular dosing.

SALINE LAXATIVES:

Magnesium sulfate –

Adults: 10 to 15 g in glass of water.

Children: 5 to 10 g in glass of water.

Magnesium hydroxide –

Adults: Recommended dosage varies from product to product, ranging from 10 to 60 mL/day. See individual package labeling for specific dosing information.

Children (≥ 2 years of age): 5 to 30 mL, depending on age (must be at least 2 years of age).

Magnesium citrate –

Adults: 1 glassful (≈ 240 mL) as needed.

Children: ½ the adult dose as needed; repeat if necessary.

Sodium phosphates –

Adults: 20 to 30 mL mixed with ½ glass cool water.

Children: 5 to 15 mL.

SENNOSIDES: The following dosages are for senna concentrate *only*. For other forms of senna, consult labeling. Dosages are different.

Tablets (6 and 8.6 mg) –

Adults: 2 tablets, up to 8/day.

Children: 1 tablet, up to 4/day.

Tablets (15 mg) –

Adults: 1 tablet at bedtime, up to 4/day.

Granules –

Adults: 1 tsp, up to 4 tsp/day.

Children: ½ tsp, up 2 tsp/day.

Suppositories –

Adults: 1 at bedtime; repeat in 2 hours if necessary.

Children: ½ suppository at bedtime.

Liquid –

Adults: 15 to 30 mL with or after meals or at bedtime.

Children (6 to 15 years of age): 10 to 15 mL at bedtime.

Children (2 to 5 years of age): 5 to 10 mL at bedtime.

Syrup –

Adults: 10 to 15 mL at bedtime (up to 30 mL/day).

Children (5 to 15 years of age): 5 to 10 mL at bedtime (up to 20 mL/day).

Children (1 to 5 years of age): 2.5 to 5 mL at bedtime (up to 10 mL/day).

Children (1 month to 1 year of age): 1.25 to 2.5 mL at bedtime (up to 5 mL/day).

MISCELLANEOUS BULK-PRODUCING LAXATIVES:

Citrucel –

Adults and children ≥ 12 years: 1 heaping tbsp (19 g) in 8 oz cold water 1 to 3 times daily.

Children (6 to < 12 years of age): ½ the adult dose in 8 oz cold water once daily.

Unifiber – Dose is 1 tbsp in 3 or 4 oz of fruit juice, milk, or water, or mix with soft foods such as applesauce, mashed potatoes, or pudding. Can be taken up to 3 times daily if needed or as recommended by a doctor.

Maltsupex –

Tablets: Adults, 12 to 36 g/day. Initially, 4 tablets 4 times daily (meals and bedtime).

Powder: 16 g = 1 heaping tablespoon.

Adults, up to 32 g twice daily for 3 or 4 days, then 16 to 32 g at bedtime. Children 6 to 12 years, up to 16 g twice daily for 3 or 4 days; 2 to 6 years, 8 g twice daily for 3 or 4 days. For infants < 2 years, consult a doctor.

Liquid: Adults, 2 tbsp twice daily for 3 or 4 days, then 1 to 2 tbsp at bedtime. Children 6 to 12 years, 1 tbsp twice daily for 3 or 4 days; 2 to 6 years, ½ tbsp twice daily for 3 or 4 days. For infants < 2 years, consult a doctor.

Actions

Pharmacology:

Pharmacologic Actions of Laxatives

	Laxatives	Onset of action (hrs)	Site of action	Mechanism of action	Comments
Saline	Dibasic sodium phosphate[1,2] Magnesium citrate Magnesium hydroxide Magnesium sulfate Monobasic sodium phosphate[1,2] Sodium biphosphate[1]	0.5-3	Small & large intestine	Attract/Retain water in intestinal lumen increasing intraluminal pressure; cholecystokinin release	May alter fluid and electrolyte balance. Sulfate salts are considered the most potent.

Pharmacologic Actions of Laxatives

	Laxatives	Onset of action (hrs)	Site of action	Mechanism of action	Comments
Stimulant/Irritant	Cascara	6-8	Colon	Direct action on intestinal mucosa or nerve plexus, alters water and electrolyte secretion	May prefer castor oil when more complete evacuation is required.
	Bisacodyl tablets Casanthranol Senna	6-10			
	Bisacodyl suppository	0.25-1			
Bulk-Producing	Methylcellulose Polycarbophil Psyllium	12-72	Small & large intestine	Holds water in stool to increase bulk-stimulating peristalsis; forms emollient gel	Safe; minimal side effects. Take with plenty of water (240 mL/dose).
Emollient	Mineral oil	6-8	Colon	Retards colonic absorption of fecal water; softens stool	May decrease absorption of fat-soluble vitamins.
Fecal Softeners/ Surfactants	Docusate[3]	12-72	Small & large intestine	Facilitates admixture of fat and water to soften stool	Beneficial in anorectal conditions where passage of a firm stool is painful.
Hyperosmotic	Glycerin suppository	0.25-1	Colon	Local irritation; hyperosmotic action	Sodium stearate in preparation causes the local irritation.
	Lactulose	24-48	Colon	Osmotic effect retains fluid in the colon, lowering the pH and increasing colonic peristalsis	Also indicated in portal-systemic encephalopathy.
Miscellaneous	Castor oil	2-6	Small intestine	Direct action on intestinal mucosa or nerve plexus, alters water and electrolyte secretion	Castor oil is converted to ricinoleic acid (active component) in the gut.

[1] Onset of action for rectal preparations is 2 to 15 min.
[2] Colon is site of action for rectal preparations.
[3] Site of action for potassium salt is in the colon.

Contraindications

Hypersensitivity to any ingredient; nausea, vomiting, or other symptoms of appendicitis; fecal impaction; intestinal obstruction; undiagnosed abdominal pain; patients who require a low galactose diet (**lactulose**).

Do not give **docusate sodium** if **mineral oil** is being given.

Warnings

Fluid and electrolyte balance: Excessive laxative use may lead to significant fluid and electrolyte imbalance. Monitor patients periodically.

Preparations containing sodium should be used cautiously by individuals on a sodium-restricted diet, and in the presence of edema, CHF, renal failure, or borderline hypertension.

Megacolon, bowel obstruction, imperforate anus, or CHF: Do not use sodium phosphate and sodium biphosphate in these patients; hypernatremic dehydration may occur.

Abuse/Dependency: Chronic use of laxatives, particularly stimulants, may lead to laxative dependency, which in turn may result in fluid and electrolyte imbalances, steatorrhea, osteomalacia, vitamin and mineral deficiencies, and a poorly functioning colon. Also known as laxative abuse syndrome (LAS), it is difficult to diagnose.

Cathartic colon: Cathartic colon, a poorly functioning colon, results from the chronic abuse of stimulant cathartics.

Melanosis coli: Melanosis coli is a darkened pigmentation of the colonic mucosa resulting from chronic use of anthraquinone derivatives (**casanthrol, cascara sagrada, senna**).

Lipid pneumonitis: Lipid pneumonitis may result from oral ingestion and aspiration of mineral oil, especially when the patient reclines. The young, elderly, debilitated, and dysphagic are at greatest risk.

Electrocautery procedures: A theoretical hazard may exist for patients being treated with **lactulose** who may undergo electrocautery procedures during proctoscopy or colonoscopy. Accumulation of H_2 gas in significant concentration in the presence of an electrical spark may result in an explosion. Although this complication has not been reported with lactulose, patients should have a thorough bowel cleansing with a nonfermentable solution.

Renal function impairment: Up to 20% of the magnesium in magnesium salts may be absorbed. Do not use products containing phosphate, sodium, magnesium, or potassium salts in the presence of renal dysfunction.

Pregnancy: Category B. (**Lactulose, magnesium sulfate**). *Category* C. (**Casanthranol, cascara sagrada, danthron, docusate sodium, docusate calcium, docusate potassium, mineral oil, senna**). Do not use **castor oil** during pregnancy; its irritant effect may induce premature labor. Mineral oil may decrease absorption of fat-soluble vitamins. Improper use of saline cathartics can lead to dangerous electrolyte imbalance. If needed, limit use to bulk-forming or surfactant laxatives.

Lactation: Anthraquinone derivatives (eg, **casanthranol, cascara sagrada, danthron**) are excreted in breast milk resulting in a potential increased incidence of diarrhea in the nursing infant. Sennosides A and B (eg, **senna**) are not excreted in breast milk. It is not known whether **docusate calcium, docusate potassium, docusate sodium, lactulose**, and **mineral oil** are excreted in breast milk.

Children: Physical manipulation of a glycerin suppository in infants often initiates defecation; hence, adverse effects are minimal. Do not administer enemas to children < 2 years of age.

Precautions

Monitoring: In the overall management of portal-systemic encephalopathy, there is serious underlying liver disease with complications such as electrolyte disturbance (eg, hypokalemia, hypernatremia), which may require other specific therapy. Elderly, debilitated patients who receive **lactulose** for > 6 months should have serum electrolytes (potassium, chloride) and carbon dioxide measured periodically.

Diabetic patients: **Lactulose** syrup contains galactose (< 1.6 g/15 mL) and lactose (< 1.2 g/15 mL). Use with caution in diabetic patients.

Concomitant laxative use: Do not use other laxatives, especially during the initial phase of therapy for portal-systemic encephalopathy; the resulting loose stools may falsely suggest adequate **lactulose** dosage.

Rectal bleeding or response failure: Rectal bleeding or failure to respond to therapy may indicate a serious condition that may require further medical attention.

Discoloration: Discoloration of acid urine to yellow-brown or black may occur with cascara sagrada or senna. Pink-red, red-violet, or red-brown discoloration of alkaline urine may occur with phenolphthalein, cascara sagrada, or senna.

Impaction or obstruction: Impaction or obstruction may be caused by bulk-forming agents if temporarily arrested in their passage through the alimentary canal (eg, patients with esophageal strictures). Administer bulk-forming agents with at least 240 mL fluid.

Drug Interactions

Drugs that may interact with laxatives include mineral oil, milk or antacids, H_2 antagonists, proton pump inhibitors, lipid soluble vitamins (A, D, E, and K), and tetracycline.

Adverse Reactions

Excessive bowel activity (griping, diarrhea, nausea, vomiting); perianal irritation; weakness; dizziness; fainting; palpitations; sweating; bloating; flatulence; abdominal cramps.

Esophageal, gastric, small intestinal, and rectal obstruction caused by the accumulation of mucilaginous components of bulk laxatives have occurred.

Large doses of mineral oil may cause anal seepage, resulting in itching (pruritus ani), irritation, hemorrhoids, and perianal discomfort.

Lactulose – Gaseous distention with flatulence, belching, abdominal discomfort such as cramping (≈ 20%); nausea; vomiting. Excessive dosage can lead to diarrhea.

POLYETHYLENE GLYCOL-ELECTROLYTE SOLUTION (PEG-ES)

Oral solution: 146 mg NaCl, 168 mg sodium bicarb, 1.29 g sodium sulfate decahydrate, 75 mg KCl, 6 g PEG 3350, 30 mg polysorbate-80/100 mL (*Rx*)	*OCL* (Abbott)
Powder for oral solution: 1 gal: 227.1 g PEG 3350, 21.5 g sodium sulfate, 6.36 g sodium bicarb, 5.53 g NaCl, 2.82 g KCl (*Rx*)	*CoLyte* (Schwarz Pharma)
4 L: 240 g PEG 3350, 22.72 g sodium sulfate, 6.72 g sodium bicarb, 5.84 g NaCl, 2.98 g KCl. (*Rx*)	
Powder for oral solution: 236 g PEG 3350, 22.74 g sodium sulfate, 6.74 g sodium bicarb, 5.86 g NaCl, 2.97 g KCl; 227.1 g PEG 3350, 21.5 g sodium sulfate, 6.36 g sodium bicarb, 5.53 g NaCl, 2.82 g KCl (*Rx*)	*GoLYTELY* (Braintree Labs)
Powder for reconstitution: 420 g PEG 3350, 5.72 g sodium bicarb, 11.2 g NaCl, 1.48 g KCl (*Rx*)	*NuLytely* (Braintree)

Indications

For bowel cleansing prior to GI examination.

Unlabeled uses: PEG electrolyte solutions are useful in the management of acute iron overdose in children.

Administration and Dosage

The patient should fast ≈ 3 to 4 hours prior to ingestion of the solution; solid foods should never be given < 2 hours before solution is administered.

One method is to schedule patients for midmorning exam, allowing 3 hours for drinking and 1 hour to complete bowel evacuation. Another method is to give the solution the evening before the exam, particularly if the patient is to have a barium enema. No foods except clear liquids are permitted after solution administration.

Adult dosage: Adult dosage is 4 L orally of solution prior to GI exam. May be given via a nasogastric tube to patients unwilling or unable to drink the preparation. Drink 240 mL every 10 minutes until 4 L are consumed or until the rectal effluent is clear. Rapid drinking of each portion is preferred to drinking small amounts continuously. Nasogastric tube administration is at the rate of 20 to 30 mL/min (1.2 to 1.8 L/hour). The first bowel movement should occur in ≈ 1 hour.

Actions

Pharmacology: Oral solution induces diarrhea (onset, 30 to 60 minutes) that rapidly cleanses the bowel, usually within 4 hours. Polyethylene glycol 3350 (PEG 3350), a nonabsorbable solution, acts as an osmotic agent.

Contraindications

GI obstruction; gastric retention; bowel perforation; toxic colitis, megacolon, or ileus.

Warnings

Pregnancy: Category C.

Children: Safety and efficacy for use in children have not been established.

Several studies in infants and children ranging in age from 3 to 14 years of age showed that the use of PEG-electrolyte solutions are safe and effective in bowel evacuation.

Precautions

Regurgitation/Aspiration: Observe unconscious or semiconscious patients with impaired gag reflex and those who are otherwise prone to regurgitation or aspiration during use, especially if given via a nasogastric tube. If GI obstruction or perforation is suspected, rule out these contraindications before administration.

Severe bloating: If a patient experiences severe bloating, distention, or abdominal pain, slow or temporarily discontinue administration until symptoms abate.

Severe ulcerative colitis: Use with caution.

Drug Interactions

Oral medication given within 1 hour of start of therapy may be flushed from the GI tract and not absorbed.

Adverse Reactions

Nausea, abdominal fullness, bloating (≤ 50%); abdominal cramps, vomiting, anal irritation (less frequent).

POLYETHYLENE GLYCOL (PEG) SOLUTION

Powder for Oral Solution: 255 g PEG 3350, 527 g PEG 3350 (*Rx*)	*MiraLax* (Braintree Labs.)

For complete prescribing information, refer to the Laxatives group monograph.

Indications

For the treatment of occasional constipation. Do not use for > 2 weeks.

Administration and Dosage

The usual dose is 17 g of powder/day in 8 ounces of water. Each bottle is supplied with a measuring cap marked to contain 17 g of laxative powder when filled to the indicated line.

Two to 4 days (48 to 96 hours) may be required to produce a bowel movement.

LOOP DIURETICS

BUMETANIDE	
Tablets: 0.5, 1, and 2 mg (*Rx*) **Injection:** 0.25 mg/mL (*Rx*)	Various, *Bumex* (Roche)
ETHACRYNIC ACID	
Tablets: 25 and 50 mg (*Rx*)	*Edecrin* (Merck)
Powder for Injection: 50 mg (as ethacrynate sodium) per vial (*Rx*)	*Edecrin Sodium* (Merck)
FUROSEMIDE	
Tablets: 20, 40, and 80 mg (*Rx*) **Oral Solution:** 10 mg/mL (*Rx*) **Injection:** 10 mg/mL (*Rx*)	Various, *Lasix* (Hoechst-Roussel)
TORSEMIDE	
Tablets: 5, 10, 20, and 100 mg (*Rx*) **Injection:** 10 mg/mL (*Rx*)	*Demadex* (Boehringer Mannheim)

Warning:
These agents are potent diuretics; excess amounts can lead to a profound diuresis with water and electrolyte depletion.

Indications

Edema: Edema associated with CHF, hepatic cirrhosis, and renal disease, including the nephrotic syndrome. Particularly useful when greater diuretic potential is desired.

Parenteral administration is indicated when a rapid onset of diuresis is desired (eg, acute pulmonary edema), when GI absorption is impaired or when oral use is not practical for any reason. As soon as it is practical, replace with oral therapy.

Hypertension (furosemide, oral; torsemide, oral): Alone or in combination with other antihypertensive drugs.

Ethacrynic acid:

Ascites – Short-term management of ascites due to malignancy, idiopathic edema, and lymphedema.

Congenital heart disease, nephrotic syndrome – Short-term management of hospitalized pediatric patients, other than infants.

Pulmonary edema, acute – Adjunctive therapy.

Administration and Dosage

BUMETANIDE:

Oral – 0.5 to 2 mg/day, given as a single dose. If diuretic response is not adequate, give a second or third dose at 4- to 5-hour intervals, up to a maximum daily dose of 10 mg. An intermittent dose schedule, given on alternate days or for 3 to 4 days with rest periods of 1 to 2 days in between, is the safest and most effective method for the continued control of edema. In patients with hepatic failure, keep the dose to a minimum, and if necessary, increase the dose carefully.

Parenteral – Initially, 0.5 to 1 mg IV or IM. Administer IV over a period of 1 to 2 minutes. If the initial response is insufficient, give a second or third dose at intervals of 2 to 3 hours; do not exceed a daily dosage of 10 mg. End parenteral treatment and start oral treatment as soon as possible.

Renal function impairment – In patients with severe chronic renal insufficiency, a continuous infusion of bumetanide (12 mg over 12 hours) may be more effective and less toxic than intermittent bolus therapy.

ETHACRYNIC ACID:

Oral –

Initial therapy: Give minimally effective dose (usually, 50 to 200 mg/day) on a continuous or intermittent dosage schedule to produce gradual weight loss of 2.2 to 4.4 kg/day (1 to 2 lb/day). Adjust dose in 25 to 50 mg increments. Higher doses, up to 200 mg twice daily, achieved gradually, are most often required in patients with severe, refractory edema.

Children: Initial dose is 25 mg. Make careful increments of 25 mg to achieve maintenance. Dosage for infants has not been established.

Maintenance therapy: Administer intermittently after an effective diuresis is obtained using an alternate daily schedule or more prolonged periods of diuretic therapy interspersed with rest periods.

Parenteral – Do not give SC or IM because of local pain and irritation. The usual IV dose for the average adult is 50 mg, or 0.5 to 1 mg/kg. Give slowly through the tubing of a running infusion or by direct IV injection over several minutes. Usually, only 1 dose is necessary; occasionally, a second dose may be required; use a new injection site to avoid thrombophlebitis. A single IV dose, not exceeding 100 mg, has been used. Insufficient pediatric experience precludes recommendation for this age group.

FUROSEMIDE:

Oral –

Edema: 20 to 80 mg/day as a single dose. Depending on response, administer a second dose 6 to 8 hours later. If response is not satisfactory, increase by increments of 20 or 40 mg, no sooner than 6 to 8 hours after previous dose, until desired diuresis occurs. This dose should then be given once or twice daily (eg, at 8 am and 2 pm). Dosage may be titrated up to 600 mg/day in patients with severe edema.

Mobilization of edema may be most efficiently and safely accomplished with an intermittent dosage schedule; the drug is given 2 to 4 consecutive days each week. With doses > 80 mg/day, clinical and laboratory observations are advisable.

Hypertension: 40 mg twice a day; adjust according to response. If the patient does not respond, add other antihypertensive agents. Reduce dosage of other agents by at least 50% as soon as furosemide is added to prevent excessive drop in blood pressure.

Infants and children: 2 mg/kg. If diuresis is unsatisfactory, increase by 1 or 2 mg/kg, no sooner than 6 to 8 hours after previous dose. Doses > 6 mg/kg are not recommended. For maintenance therapy, adjust dose to the minimum effective level. A dose range of 0.5 to 2 mg/kg twice daily has also been recommended.

CHF and chronic renal failure: It has been suggested that doses as high as 2 to 2.5 g/day or more are well tolerated and effective in these patients.

Parenteral –

Edema: Initial dose: 20 to 40 mg IM or IV. Give the IV injection slowly (1 to 2 minutes). If needed, another dose may be given in the same manner 2 hours later. The dose may be raised by 20 mg and given no sooner than 2 hours after previous dose, until desired diuretic effect is obtained. This dose should then be given once or twice daily. Administer high-dose parenteral therapy as a controlled infusion at a rate ≤ 4 mg/min.

Acute pulmonary edema: The usual initial dose is 40 mg IV (over 1 to 2 minutes). If response is not satisfactory within 1 hour, increase to 80 mg IV (over 1 to 2 minutes).

Infants and children: 1 mg/kg IV or IM given slowly under close supervision. If diuretic response after the initial dose is not satisfactory, increase the dosage by 1 mg/kg, no sooner than 2 hours after previous dose, until desired effect is obtained. Doses > 6 mg/kg are not recommended.

CHF and chronic renal failure: It has been suggested that doses as high as 2 to 2.5 g/day or more are well tolerated and effective in these patients. For IV bolus injections, the maximum should not exceed 1 g/day given over 30 minutes.

TORSEMIDE: Torsemide may be given at any time in relation to a meal.

Because of high bioavailability, oral and IV doses are therapeutically equivalent, so patients may be switched to and from the IV form with no change in dose. Administer the IV injection slowly over a period of 2 minutes.

Congestive heart failure/chronic renal failure – The usual initial dose is 10 or 20 mg once daily oral or IV. If the diuretic response is inadequate, titrate the dose upward by approximately doubling until the desired diuretic response is obtained. Single doses > 200 mg have not been adequately studied.

Hepatic cirrhosis – The usual initial dose is 5 or 10 mg once daily oral or IV, administered together with an aldosterone antagonist or a potassium-sparing diuretic. If the diuretic response is inadequate, titrate the dose upward by approximately doubling until the desired diuretic response is obtained. Single doses > 40 mg have not been adequately studied.

Hypertension – The usual initial dose is 5 mg once daily. If the 5 mg dose does not provide adequate reduction in blood pressure within 4 to 6 weeks, the dose may be increased to 10 mg once daily.

Actions

Pharmacology: Furosemide and ethacrynic acid inhibit primarily reabsorption of sodium and chloride, not only in proximal and distal tubules, but also the loop of Henle. In contrast, bumetanide is more chloruretic than natriuretic and may have an additional action in the proximal tubule; it does not appear to act on the distal tubule. Torsemide acts from within the lumen of the thick ascending portion of the loop of Henle, where it inhibits the $Na^+/K^+/2Cl^-$-carrier system.

Pharmacokinetics: These agents are metabolized and excreted primarily through the urine. Protein binding of these agents exceeds 90%. Furosemide is metabolized ≈ 30% to 40%, and its urinary excretion is 60% to 70%. Oral administration of bumetanide revealed that 81% was excreted in urine, 45% of it as unchanged drug. Torsemide is cleared from the circulation by both hepatic metabolism (≈ 80% of total clearance) and excretion into the urine (≈ 20% of total clearance).

Pharmacokinetic Parameters of the Loop Diuretics

Diuretic	Bioavailability (%)	Half-life (min)	Onset of action (min)	Peak (min)	Duration (hr)	Dosage (mg)	Relative potency	Doses/ day
Bumetanide								
Oral	72-96	60-90[5]	30-60	60-120	4-6	0.5-2	≈ 40	1
IV			within minutes	15-30	0.5-1	0.5-1	≈ 40	1-3
Ethacrynic acid								
Oral	≈100	60	≤ 30	120	6-8	50-100	0.6-0.8	1-2
IV			≤ 5	15-30	2	50	0.6-0.8	1-2
Furosemide								
Oral	60-64[1]	≈ 120[2]	≤ 60	60-120[3]	6-8	20-80	1	1-2
IV or IM			≤ 5[4]	30	2	20-40	1	
Torsemide								
Oral	≈ 80	210	≤ 60	60-120	6-8	5-20	2-4	1
IV			≤ 10	≤ 60	6-8	5-20	2-4	1

[1] Decreased in uremia and nephrosis.
[2] Prolonged in renal failure, uremia and in neonates.
[3] Decreased in CHF.
[4] Somewhat delayed after IM administration.
[5] Prolonged in renal disease.

Contraindications

Anuria; hypersensitivity to these compounds or to sulfonylureas; infants (ethacrynic acid); patients with hepatic coma or in states of severe electrolyte depletion until the condition is improved or corrected (bumetanide).

Warnings

Dehydration: Excessive diuresis may result in dehydration and reduction in blood volume with circulatory collapse and the possibility of vascular thrombosis and embolism, particularly in elderly patients.

Hepatic cirrhosis and ascites: In these patients, sudden alterations of electrolyte balance may precipitate hepatic encephalopathy and coma. Do not institute therapy until the basic condition is improved.

Ototoxicity: Tinnitus, reversible and irreversible hearing impairment, deafness, and vertigo with a sense of fullness in the ears have been reported. Deafness is usually reversible and of short duration (1 to 24 hours); however, irreversible hearing impairment has occurred. Usually, ototoxicity is associated with rapid injection, with severe renal impairment, with doses several times the usual dose, and with concurrent use with other ototoxic drugs.

Systemic lupus erythematosus: Systemic lupus erythematosus may be exacerbated or activated.

Thrombocytopenia: Because there have been rare spontaneous reports of thrombocytopenia with **bumetanide,** observe regularly for possible occurrence.

Hypersensitivity reactions: Patients with known sulfonamide sensitivity may show allergic reactions to **furosemide**, **torsemide**, or **bumetanide**. Bumetanide use following instances of allergic reactions to furosemide suggests a lack of cross-sensitivity. Refer to Management of Acute Hypersensitivity Reactions.

Renal function impairment: If increasing azotemia, oliguria, or reversible increases in BUN or creatinine occur during treatment of severe progressive renal disease, discontinue therapy.

Pregnancy: Category B (ethacrynic acid, torsemide); *Category C* (furosemide, bumetanide). Since furosemide may increase the incidence of patent ductus arteriosus in preterm infants with respiratory-distress syndrome, use caution when administering before delivery.

Lactation: **Furosemide** appears in breast milk.

Children: Safety and efficacy for use of **torsemide** in children, **bumetanide** in children < 18 years of age, and **ethacrynic acid** in infants (oral) and children (IV) have not been established.

Furosemide – Furosemide stimulates renal synthesis of prostaglandin E_2 and may increase the incidence of patent ductus arteriosus when given in the first few weeks of life, to premature infants with respiratory-distress syndrome.

Precautions

Monitoring: Observe for blood dyscrasias, liver or kidney damage, or idiosyncratic reactions. Perform frequent serum electrolyte, calcium, glucose, uric acid, CO_2, creatinine, and BUN determinations during the first few months of therapy and periodically thereafter.

Cardiovascular effects: Too vigorous a diuresis, as evidenced by rapid and excessive weight loss, may induce an acute hypotensive episode. In elderly cardiac patients, avoid rapid contraction of plasma volume and the resultant hemoconcentration to prevent thromboembolic episodes, such as cerebral vascular thromboses and pulmonary emboli.

Electrolyte imbalance: Electrolyte imbalance may occur, especially in patients receiving high doses with restricted salt intake. Perform periodic determinations of serum electrolytes.

Hypokalemia – Hypokalemia prevention requires particular attention to the following: Patients receiving digitalis and diuretics for CHF, hepatic cirrhosis, and ascites; in aldosterone excess with normal renal function; potassium-losing nephropathy; certain diarrheal states; or where hypokalemia is an added risk to the patient (eg, history of ventricular arrhythmias).

Hypomagnesemia – Loop diuretics increase the urinary excretion of magnesium.

Hypocalcemia – Serum calcium levels may be lowered (rare cases of tetany have occurred).

Hyperuricemia: Asymptomatic hyperuricemia can occur, and rarely, gout may be precipitated.

Glucose: Increases in blood glucose and alterations in glucose tolerance tests (fasting and 2 hour postprandial sugar) have been observed.

Lipids: Increases in LDL and total cholesterol and triglycerides with minor decreases in HDL cholesterol may occur.

Photosensitivity: Photosensitization (photoallergy or phototoxicity) may occur.

Drug Interactions

Loop diuretics may affect the following drugs: Aminoglycosides; anticoagulants; chloral hydrate; digitalis glycosides; lithium; nondepolarizing neuromuscular blockers; propranolol; sulfonylureas; theophyllines. Loop diuretics may be affected by the following drugs: Charcoal; cisplatin; clofibrate; hydantoins; NSAIDs; probenecid; salicylates; thiazide diuretics.

Drug/Food interactions: The bioavailability of **furosemide** is decreased and its degree of diuresis reduced when administered with food. Simultaneous food intake with **torsemide** delays the time to C_{max} by about 30 minutes, but overall bioavailability and diuretic activity are unchanged.

Adverse Reactions

Adverse reactions associated with loop diuretics include nausea; vomiting; diarrhea; gastric irritation; headache; fatigue; dizziness; thrombocytopenia; rash; orthostatic hypotension; hyperuricemia; hyperglycemia; electrolyte imbalance (decreased chloride, potassium and sodium); dehydration.

Bumetanide: Adverse reactions may include impaired hearing, ear discomfort, dry mouth, pain, renal failure, weakness, arthritic pain, muscle cramps, ECG changes, chest pain, hives, pruritus, itching, sweating, hyperventilation.

Ethacrynic acid: Adverse reactions may include anorexia, pain, GI bleeding, severe neutropenia, agranulocytosis, fever, chills, confusion, fatigue, malaise, sense of fullness in the ears, blurred vision, tinnitus, hearing loss (irreversible), rash.

Furosemide: Adverse reactions may include anorexia, cramping, constipation, blurred vision, hearing loss, restlessness, fever, anemia, purpura, thrombocytopenia, agranulocytosis, photosensitivity, urticaria, pruritus, thrombophlebitis, muscle spasm, weakness.

Torsemide: Adverse reactions may include excessive urination.

MACROLIDES

AZITHROMYCIN	
Tablets: 250 mg (as dihydrate) and 600 mg (*Rx*)	*Zithromax* (Pfizer)
Powder for oral suspension: 100 mg and 200 mg/5 mL, 1 g/packet (*Rx*)	
Powder for injection: 500 mg (*Rx*)	
CLARITHROMYCIN	
Tablets: 250 and 500 mg (*Rx*)	*Biaxin* (Abbott)
Tablets, extended release: 500 mg (*Rx*)	*Biaxin XL* (Abbott)
Granules for oral suspension: 125 and 250 mg/5 mL (*Rx*)	*Biaxin* (Abbott)
DIRITHROMYCIN	
Tablets, enteric coated: 250 mg (*Rx*)	*Dynabac* (Sanofi)
ERYTHROMYCIN BASE	
Tablets, enteric coated: 250, 333, and 500 mg (*Rx*)	*E-Mycin* (Knoll), *Ery-Tab* (Abbott), *E-Base* (Barr)
Tablets with polymer-coated particles: 333 and 500 mg (*Rx*)	*PCE Dispertab* (Abbott)
Tablets, film coated: 250 and 500 mg (*Rx*)	*Erythromycin Filmtabs* (Abbott)
Capsules, delayed release: 250 mg (*Rx*)	Various, *Eryc* (Warner Chilcott)
ERYTHROMYCIN ESTOLATE	
Tablets: 500 mg (as estolate)	*Ilosone* (Lilly)
Capsules: 250 mg (as estolate)	Various, *Ilosone Pulvules* (Lilly)
Suspension: 235 and 250 mg (as estolate)/5 mL	Various, *Ilosone* (Lilly)
ERYTHROMYCIN LACTOBIONATE	
Powder for injection: 500 mg and 1 g (as lactobionate) (*Rx*)	Various, *Erythrocin* (Abbott)
ERYTHROMYCIN GLUCEPTATE	
Injection: 1 g (as gluceptate) (*Rx*)	*Ilotycin Gluceptate* (Lilly)
ERYTHROMYCIN ETHYLSUCCINATE	
Tablets, chewable: 200 mg (as ethylsuccinate) (*Rx*)	*EryPed* (Abbott)
Tablets: 400 mg (as ethylsuccinate) (*Rx*)	Various, *E.E.S. 400* (Abbott)
Suspension: 200 and 400 mg (as ethylsuccinate)/5 mL (*Rx*)	Various, *E.E.S. 200* (Abbott), *E.E.S. 400* (Abbott), *EryPed 200* (Abbott), *EryPed 400* (Abbott)
Drops, suspension: 100 mg (as ethylsuccinate)/2.5 mL (*Rx*)	*EryPed Drops* (Abbott)
Powder for oral suspension: 200 mg (as ethylsuccinate)/ 5 mL when reconstituted (*Rx*)	*E.E.S. Granules* (Abbott)
ERYTHROMYCIN STEARATE	
Tablets, film coated: 250 and 500 mg (*Rx*)	Various, *Erythrocin Stearate* (Abbott)
TROLEANDOMYCIN	
Capsules: 250 mg (*Rx*)	*Tao* (Pfizer)

Indications

For specific approved indications, refer to the Administration and Dosage sections.

Administration and Dosage

AZITHROMYCIN: Administer at least 1 hour before or 2 hours after a meal. Do not give with food. Azithromycin *tablets* can be taken with or without food.

Adults –

Mild-to-moderate acute bacterial exacerbations of chronic obstructive pulmonary disease, community-acquired pneumonia of mild severity, pharyngitis/tonsillitis (as second-line therapy), and uncomplicated skin and skin structure infections: 500 mg as a single dose on the first day followed by 250 mg once daily on days 2 through 5.

Genital ulcer disease caused by Haemophilus ducreyi (chancroid): Single 1 g dose.

Nongonococcal urethritis and cervicitis due to Chlamydia trachomatis: Single 1 g dose.

Gonococcal urethritis/cervitis caused by C. *trachomatis:* Single 2 g dose.

Uncomplicated gonococcal infections of the cervix, urethra, and rectum caused by Neisseria gonorrhoeae: Single 1 g dose (plus a single dose of 400 mg oral cefixime, 125 mg IM ceftriaxone, 500 mg oral ciprofloxacin, or 400 mg oral ofloxacin).

Gonococcal pharyngitis: Single 1 g dose (plus a single dose of 125 mg IM ceftriaxone, 500 mg ciprofloxacin, or 400 mg ofloxacin).

Chlamydial infections caused by C. *trachomatis:* Single 1 g dose.

Children –

Acute otitis media/community-acquired pneumonia: The recommended dose for oral suspension is 10 mg/kg as a single dose on the first day (not to exceed 500 mg/day, followed by 5 mg/kg on days 2 through 5 (not to exceed 250 mg/day). See the following table.

Pediatric Dosage Guidelines for Otitis Media (≥ 6 months of age)						
Dosing calculated on 10 mg/kg on day 1 dose, followed by 5 mg/kg on days 2 to 5						
Weight		Amount of 100 mg/5 mL suspension		Amount of 200 mg/5 mL suspension		Total mL per treatment course
kg	lbs	Day 1	Days 2 to 5	Day 1	Days 2 to 5	
10	22	5 mL	2.5 mL			15 mL
20	44			5 mL	2.5 mL	15 mL
30	66			7.5 mL	3.75 mL	22.5 mL
40	88			10 mL	5 mL	30 mL

Chlamydial infections caused by C. *trachomatis (≥ 45 kg and < 8 years of age or ≥ 8 years of age):* 1 g orally in single dose.

Pharyngitis/tonsillitis: The recommended dose for children with pharyngitis/tonsillitis is 12 mg/kg qd for 5 days (not to exceed 500 mg/day). See the following.

Pediatric Dosage Guidelines for Pharyngitis/Tonsillitis (≥ 2 years of age)			
Dosing calculated on 12 mg/kg once daily on days 1 through 5			
Weight		Amount of 200 mg/5 mL suspension	
kg	lbs	Days 1 to 5	Total mL per treatment course
8	18	2.5 mL	12.5 mL
17	37	5 mL	25 mL
25	55	7.5 mL	37.5 mL
33	73	10 mL	50 mL
40	88	12.5	62.5 mL

Parenteral – Infuse injections over a period of > 60 minutes. Do not administer azithromycin for injection as a bolus or IM injection.

Community-acquired pneumonia: 500 mg as a single daily dose IV for ≥ 2 days. Follow IV therapy by the oral route at a single daily dose of 500 mg to complete a 7- to 10-day course of therapy.

Pelvic inflammatory disease (PID): 500 mg as a single daily dose for 1 or 2 days. Follow IV therapy by the oral route at a single daily dose of 250 mg to complete a 7-day course of therapy. If anaerobic microorganisms are suspected of contributing to the infection, administer an antimicrobial agent with anaerobic activity in combination with azithromycin.

The infusate concentration and rate of infusion for azithromycin for injection should be either 1 mg/mL over 3 hours or 2 mg/mL over 1 hour.

CLARITHROMYCIN: Clarithromycin may be given with or without meals.

Helicobacter pylori –

Clarithromycin and Omeprazole Dosage Regimens for Active Duodenal Ulcer Associated with *H. pylori* Infection (28-Day Therapy)	
Days 1 to 14	Days 15 to 28
500 mg clarithromycin tablet 3 times daily plus omeprazole 2 × 20 mg every morning	Omeprazole 20 mg every morning

Clarithromycin and Ranitidine Bismuth Citrate Dosage Regimens for Active Duodenal Ulcer Associated with *H. pylori* Infection (28-Day Therapy)	
Days 1 to 14	Days 15 to 28
500 mg clarithromycin tablet 3 times daily plus ranitidine bismuth citrate 400 mg tablet twice daily	Ranitidine bismuth citrate 400 mg tablet twice daily

H. pylori eradication to reduce the risk of duodenal ulcer recurrence triple therapy:

Clarithromycin/Lansoprazole/Amoxicillin – 500 mg clarithromycin, 30 mg lansoprazole, and 1 g amoxicillin every 12 hours for 14 days.

Clarithromycin/Omeprazole/Amoxicillin – 500 mg clarithromycin, 20 mg omeprazole, and 1 g amoxicillin every 12 hours for 10 days. In patients with an ulcer present at the time of initiation of therapy, an additional 18 days of omeprazole 20 mg once daily is recommended for ulcer healing and symptom relief.

Adults –

Clarithromycin Dosage Guidelines				
	Tablets		Extended-release tablets	
Infection	Dosage (q 12 hr)	Duration (days)	Dosage (q 24 hr)	Duration (days)
Pharyngitis/Tonsillitis	250 mg	10	-	-
Acute maxillary sinusitis	500 mg	14	2 × 500 mg	14
Acute exacerbation of chronic bronchitis caused by:				
Haemophilus parainfluenzae	500 mg	7	2 × 500 mg	7
Streptococcus pneumoniae	250 mg	7 to 14	2 × 500 mg	7
Moraxella catarrhalis	250 mg	7 to 14	2 × 500 mg	7
Haemophilus influenzae	500 mg	7 to 14	2 × 500 mg	7
Community-acquired pneumonia caused by:				
S. pneumoniae	250 mg	7 to 14	2 × 500 mg	7
Mycoplasma pneumoniae	250 mg	7 to 14	2 × 500 mg	7
H. influenzae	250 mg	7	2 × 500 mg	7
H. parainfluenzae	-	-	2 × 500 mg	7
M. catarrhalis	-	-	2 × 500 mg	7
Chlamydia pneumoniae	250 mg	7 to 14	2 × 500 mg	7
Uncomplicated skin and skin structure infection	250 mg	7 to 14	-	-

Mycobacterial infections – Recommended as the primary agent for the treatment of disseminated *Mycobacterium avium* complex (MAC). Use in combination with other antimycobacterial drugs that have shown an in vitro activity against MAC. Continue therapy for life if clinical and mycobacterial improvements are observed.

Dosage for mycobacterial infection:

Adults – 500 mg twice daily.

Children – 7.5 mg/kg twice daily up to 500 mg twice daily. Refer to the Pediatric Dosing table.

Children – Usual recommended daily dosage is 15 mg/kg/day divided every 12 hours for 10 days.

Pediatric Dosage Guidelines (based on body weight)				
Dosing calculated on 7.5 mg/kg q 12 h				
Weight		Dose (q 12 h)	125 mg/5 mL (q 12 h)	250 mg/5 mL (q 12 h)
kg	lb			
9	20	62.5 mg	2.5 mL	1.25 mL
17	37	125 mg	5 mL	2.5 mL
25	55	187.5 mg	7.5 mL	3.75 mL
33	73	250 mg	10 mL	5 mL

Renal/Hepatic function impairment – In the presence of severe renal impairment (Ccr < 30 mL/min) with or without co-existing hepatic impairment, halved doses or prolongation of dosing intervals may be needed.

DIRITHROMYCIN: Administer with food or within 1 hour of eating. Do not cut, crush, or chew the tablets.

Recommended Dosage Schedule for Dirithromycin (≥ 12 years of age)			
Infection (mild-to-moderate severity)	Dose	Frequency	Duration (days)
Acute bacterial exacerbations of chronic bronchitis caused by *H. influenzae*, *M. catarrhalis*, or *S. pneumoniae*.	500 mg	once a day	5 to 7
Secondary bacterial infection of acute bronchitis caused by *M. catarrhalis* or *S. pneumoniae*.	500 mg	once a day	7
Community-acquired pnemonia caused by *Legionella pneumophila*, *M. pneumoniae*, or *S. pneumoniae*.	500 mg	once a day	14
Pharyngitis/Tonsillitis caused by *Streptococcus pyogenes*.	500 mg	once a day	10
Uncomplicated skin and skin structure infections caused by *Staphylococcus aureus* (methicillin-susceptible) or *S. pyogenes*.	500 mg	once a day	5 to 7

ERYTHROMYCIN, IV:

Erythromycin IV – Erythromycin IV is indicated when oral use is impossible, or when severity of the infection requires immediate high serum levels. Replace IV therapy with oral as soon as possible.

Continuous infusion: Continuous infusion is preferable, but intermittent infusion in 20- to 60-minute periods at intervals of ≤ 6 hours is also effective. Because of irritative properties of erythromycin, IV push is unacceptable.

Severe infections – 15 to 20 mg/kg/day. Up to 4 g/day in very severe infections.

ERYTHROMYCIN, ORAL: Dosages and product strengths are expressed as erythromycin base equivalents. Because of differences in absorption and biotransformation, varying quantities of each salt form are required to produce the same free erythromycin serum levels.

Optimal serum levels of erythromycin are reached when erythromycin base or stearate is taken in the fasting state or immediately before meals. Erythromycin ethylsuccinate, estolate, and enteric-coated erythromycin may be administered without regard to meals.

Usual dosage –

Adults: 250 mg (or 400 mg ethylsuccinate) every 6 hours, or 500 mg every 12 hours, or 333 mg every 8 hours. May increase up to ≥ 4 g/day, according to severity of infection. If twice-daily dosage is desired, the recommended dose is 500 mg every 12 hours. Twice-daily dosing is not recommended when doses > 1 g daily are administered.

Children: 30 to 50 mg/kg/day in divided doses.

Erythromycin Uses and Dosages	
Indication (Organism)	Dosage (Stated as erythromycin base)
Labeled uses:	
Upper respiratory tract infections of mild-to-moderate severity	
S. pyogenes (group A beta-hemolytic streptococcus)	250 to 500 mg 4 times/day or 20 to 50 mg/kg/day for children (not to exceed the adult dose) in divided doses for 10 days.
S. pneumoniae	250 to 500 mg every 6 hours.
H. influenzae (used concomitantly with a sulfonamide)	Erythromycin ethylsuccinate: 50 mg/kg/day for children (not to exceed 6 g/day). Sulfisoxazole: 150 mg/kg/day. Combination given for 10 days.
Lower respiratory tract infections of mild to moderate severity	
S. pyogenes (group A beta-hemolytic streptococcus)	250 to 500 mg 4 times/day or 20 to 50 mg/kg/day for children (not to exceed the adult dose) in divided doses for 10 days.
S. pneumoniae	250 to 500 mg every 6 hours.

Erythromycin Uses and Dosages	
Indication (Organism)	Dosage (Stated as erythromycin base)
Respiratory tract infections M. *pneumoniae* (Eaton agent, PPLO)	500 mg every 6 hours for 5 to 10 days. Treat severe infections for up to 3 weeks.
Skin and skin structure infections of mild to moderate severity S. *pyogenes*	250 to 500 mg 4 times/day or 20 to 50 mg/kg/day for children (not to exceed the adult dose) in divided doses for 10 days.
S. *aureus* (resistant organisms may emerge)	250 mg every 6 hours or 500 mg every 12 hours, maximum 4 g/day.
Pertussis (whooping cough) *Bordetella pertussis*: Effective in eliminating the organism from the nasopharynx of infected patients. May be helpful in prophylaxis of pertussis in exposed individuals.	40 to 50 mg/kg/day for children (not to exceed the adult dose) in divided doses for 5 to 14 days, or 500 mg 4 times/day for 10 days.
Diphtheria *Corynebacterium diphtheriae*: Adjunct to antitoxin to prevent establishment of carriers and to eradicate organism in carriers.	500 mg every 6 hours for 10 days.
Erythrasma *Corynebacterium minutissiumum*	250 mg 3 times daily for 21 days.
Intestinal amebiasis *Entamoeba histolyticia*: Oral erythromycin only.	*Adults:* 250 mg 4 times daily for 10 to 14 days. *Children:* 30 to 50 mg/kg/day in divided doses for 10 to 14 days.
Pelvic inflammatory disease (PID), acute N. *gonorrhoeae*: Erythromycin lactobionate IV followed by oral erythromycin.[1]	500 mg IV every 6 hours for 3 days, then 250 mg orally every 6 hours for 7 days.
Conjunctivitis of the newborn, pneumonia of infancy, urogenital infections during pregnancy	50 mg/kg/day for children (not to exceed the adult dose) in 4 divided doses for 10 to ≥ 14 days (conjunctivitis) or ≥ 21 days (pneumonia)
C. *trachomatis*	500 mg 4 times daily for 7 days or 250 mg 4 times daily on an empty stomach for ≥ 14 days (urogenital infections).
Urethral, endocervical, or rectal infections, uncomplicated C. *trachomatis*[1]	500 mg ≥ 4 times daily for 7 days or 250 mg 4 times daily for 14 days if patient cannot tolerate high-dose erythromycin.[2]
Nongonococcal urethritis *Ureaplasma urealyticum*[1]	500 mg 4 times daily for at least 7 days or 250 mg orally 4 times daily for 14 days if patient cannot tolerate high-dose erythromycin.[2]
Primary syphilis *Treponema pallidum*: Oral erythromycin only[1]	20 to 40 g in divided doses over 10 to 15 days.
Legionnaire's disease *Legionella pneumophila*: No controlled clinical efficacy studies have been conducted, but data suggest effectiveness	1 to 4 g daily in divided doses for 10 to 14 days.
Rheumatic fever S. *pyogenes* (group A beta-hemolytic streptococci): Prevention of initial or recurrent attacks.[1]	250 mg 2 times daily.
Bacterial endocarditis (in penicillin-allergic patients with valvular heart disease who are to undergo dental procedures or surgical procedures of the upper respiratory tract).	

Erythromycin Uses and Dosages	
Indication (Organism)	Dosage (Stated as erythromycin base)
Alpha-hemolytic streptococcus (viridans)[1]	Adults: 1 g 1 to 2 hours prior to procedure, then 500 mg 6 hours after initial dose.[3] Children: 20 mg/kg 2 hours prior to procedure, then 10 mg/kg 6 hours after initial dose.[3]
Listeria monocytogenes	*Adults:* 250 mg every 6 hours or 500 mg every 12 hours, maximum 4 g/day.
Unlabeled uses:	
Campylobacter jejuni: Has been successful in severe or prolonged diarrhea associated with *Campylobacter enteritis* or enterocolitis.[2]	500 mg 4 times a day for 7 days.
Lymphogranuloma venereum: Genital, inguinal, or anorectal.[2]	500 mg 4 times a day for 21 days.
Haemophilus ducreyi (*chancroid*): Treat until ulcers or lymph nodes are healed.[2]	500 mg 4 times a day for 7 days.
T. pallidum:	
Early syphilis (primary or secondary)	500 mg 4 times a day for 14 days.
Prior to elective colorectal surgery, to reduce wound complications	Combination of erythromycin base and neomycin is a popular preoperative preparation.
Clostridium tetani:	
Tetanus[1]	500 mg every 6 hours for 10 days.
Granuloma inguinale	
Calymmatobacterium granulomatis[2,4]	500 mg orally 4 times daily for ≥ 21 days.

[1] Use as alternative drug in penicillin or tetracycline hypersensitivity or when penicillin or tetracycline are contraindicated or not tolerated.
[2] CDC 1998 Guidelines for Sexually Transmitted Diseases Treatment. *MMWR*. 1998;47:1-117.
[3] American Heart Association statement. *JAMA*. 1990;264:2919-2922.
[4] Use as alternate therapy to trimethoprim-sulfamethoxazole or doxycycline.

ERYTHROMYCIN ETHYLSUCCINATE: Expressed in base equivalents, 400 mg erythromycin ethylsuccinate produces the same free erythromycin serum levels as 250 mg of erythromycin base, stearate, or estolate.

TROLEANDOMYCIN: Continue therapy for 10 days when used for streptococcal infection.

Adults – 250 to 500 mg 4 times a day.

Children – 125 to 250 mg (6.6 to 11 mg/kg) every 6 hours.

Actions

Pharmacology: Macrolide antibiotics reversibly bind to the P site of the 50S ribosomal subunit of susceptible organisms and inhibit RNA-dependent protein synthesis by stimulating the dissociation of peptidyl t-RNA from ribosomes. They may be bacteriostatic or bactericidal, depending on such factors as drug concentration.

Macrolides are weak bases; their activity increases in alkaline pH. Macrolides enter pleural fluid, ascitic fluid, middle-ear exudates, and sputum. When meninges are inflamed, macrolides may enter the CSF. They are used for respiratory, genital, GI tract, and skin and soft tissue infections, especially when beta-lactam antibiotics or tetracyclines are contraindicated.

Despite differing structures, macrolides have similar antibacterial spectrum, mechanisms of action and resistance, but relatively different pharmacokinetics (see table).

Pharmacokinetics:

Various Pharmacokinetic Parameters of Macrolides									
Macrolide	Route of administration	Protein binding (%)	Bioavailability (%)	Effect of food	C_{max}* (mcg/mL)	T_{max}* (hr)	Half-life (hr)	Metabolism	Elimination
Azithromycin	Oral IV	51 (0.02 mcg/L) 7 (2 mcg/L)	≈ 40	Food increases absorption, C_{max} by 23% and suspension by 56%; take on empty stomach.	0.5 1.14[3] 3.63[4]	2.2	68[1]	Some hepatic but mainly excreted unchanged	6% excreted unchanged in urine; primarily excreted unchanged in bile
Clarithromycin	Oral	40-70	≈ 50	Food delays onset of absorption and formation of metabolite; does not affect extent of bioavailability. Take without regard to meals.	1-3	2-3	3-7	Metabolized to active metabolite (14-OH clarithromycin)	Primarily renal; rate approximates normal GFR
Dirithromycin	Oral	15-30[2]	≈ 10	Take with food or within an hour of eating.	0.3 - 0.4[2]	3.9 - 4.1[2]	2-36	Nonenzymatic conversion to erythromycylamine	81%-97% fecal/hepatic[2]
Erythromycin	Oral IV	70-80 (96 estolate)	> 35	Base or stearate: Take on an empty stomach. Estolate, ethylsuccinate, delayed release base: Take without regard to meals.	0.3-2	1.6	1.6	Hepatic; demethylation	< 5% (oral) and 12% to 15% (IV) excreted unchanged in urine; significant quantity excreted in bile
Troleandomycin	Oral				2	2			20% excreted in urine; significant quantity excreted in bile

* C_{max} = Maximum concentration; T_{max} = Time to reach maximum concentration.
[1] Average terminal half-life.
[2] Value listed for erythromycylamine, the active moiety.
[3] At a concentration of 1 mg/mL.
[4] At a concentration of 2 mg/mL.

Microbiology:

Organisms Generally Susceptible to Macrolides In Vitro						
	Organisms (✓ = generally susceptible)	Azithromycin	Clarithromycin	Dirithromycin	Erythromycin	Troleandomycin[1]
Gram-positive aerobes	*Staphylococcus aureus*	✓	✓	✓	✓	
	Streptococcus pyogenes	✓	✓	✓	✓	✓
	Streptococcus pneumoniae	✓	✓	✓	✓	✓
	Streptococcus agalactiae	✓	✓	✓	✓	
	Streptococcus sp.	✓	✓	✓		
	Streptococcus viridans	✓	✓	✓	✓	
	Listeria monocytogenes			✓	✓	
	Corynebacterium diphtheriae				✓	
	Corynebacterium minutissimum				✓	

Organisms Generally Susceptible to Macrolides In Vitro						
	Organisms (✓ = generally susceptible)	Azithromycin	Clarithromycin	Dirithromycin	Erythromycin	Troleandomycin[1]
Gram-negative aerobes	*Haemophilus influenzae*	✓	✓	✓	†[2]	
	Haemophilus ducreyi	✓				
	Moraxella catarrhalis	✓	✓	✓	✓	
	Bordetella pertussis	✓	✓	✓	✓	
	Legionella pneumophila	✓	✓	✓	✓	
	Neisseria gonorrhoeae	✓	✓		✓	
	Pasteurella multocida		✓			
Anaerobes	*Prevotella* (formerly *Bacteroides*) *bivius*	✓				
	Prevotella (formerly *Bacteroides*) *melaninogenicus*		✓			
	Clostridium perfringens		✓			
	Propionibacterium acnes		✓	✓		
	Peptococcus niger		✓			
	Peptostreptococcus sp.	✓				
Other	*Borrelia burgdorferi*	✓				
	Chlamydia trachomatis	✓	✓		✓	
	Mycobacterium kansasii		✓			
	Mycoplasma pneumoniae	✓	✓	✓	✓	
	Treponema pallidum	✓			✓	
	Ureaplasma urealyticum	✓			✓	
	Entamoeba histolytica				✓	
	Chlamydia pneumoniae (TWAR strain)	✓	✓			
	Mycoplasma hominis	✓				
	Mycobacterium avium		✓			
	Mycobacterium intracellulare		✓			
	Helicobacter pylori		✓			
	Clostridium tetani				✓	

[1] Data is limited for troleandomycin.
[2] Many strains resistant to erythromycin alone; may be susceptible to erythromycin plus a sulfonamide.

The in vitro spectrum of erythromycin covers primarily gram-positive microorganisms and gram-negative cocci.

Azithromycin is less active than **erythromycin** against most *Staphylococcus* and *Streptococcus* sp, but it is more potent against other organisms, including many gram-negative bacteria considered resistant to erythromycin. Azithromycin may expand the therapeutic range traditionally assigned to macrolides.

Clarithromycin exhibits the same spectrum of in vitro activity as erythromycin, but appears to have significantly increased potency against those organisms.

Troleandomycin, an acetylated ester of oleandomycin, is less active than erythromycin and offers no advantage. It also can cause hepatotoxicity.

Contraindications

Hypersensitivity to any of the macrolide antibiotics; patients receiving astemizole, cisapride, or pimozide; known, suspected, or potential bacteremias (**dirithromycin**); pre-existing liver disease (**erythromycin estolate**).

Warnings

Pseudomembranous colitis: Pseudomembranous colitis has occurred with nearly all antibacterial agents and may range in severity from mild to life-threatening. Consider this diagnosis in patients who present with diarrhea subsequent to the administration of antibacterial agents.

Cardiac effects: Ventricular arrhythmias in individuals with prolonged QT intervals have occurred with macrolide products.

Acute porphyria: Do not use **clarithromycin** in combination with ranitidine bismuth citrate in patients with a history of acute porphyria.

Azithromycin:

Pneumonia – Do not use oral **azithromycin** in patients with pneumonia who are judged to be inappropriate for oral therapy because of moderate-to-severe illness or risk factors such as any of the following: Nosocomially acquired infections; known or suspected bacteremia; conditions requiring hospitalization; cystic fibrosis; significant underlying health problems that may compromise patients' ability to respond to their illness (including immunodeficiency or functional asplenia); elderly or debilitated patients.

Hypersensitivity – Rare serious allergic reactions, including angioedema, anaphylaxis, and dermatologic reactions including Stevens-Johnson syndrome and toxic epidermal necrolysis have occurred in patients on **azithromycin** therapy.

Dirithromycin:

Bacteremias – Dirithromycin should not be used in patients with known, suspected or potential bacteremias as serum levels are inadequate to provide antibacterial coverage of the blood stream.

Erythromycin:

Hepatotoxicity – Erythromycin administration has been associated with the infrequent occurrence of cholestatic hepatitis. This effect is most common with erythromycin estolate; however, it has also occurred with other erythromycin salts.

Although initial symptoms have developed after a few days of treatment, they generally have followed 1 or 2 weeks of continuous therapy. Symptoms reappear promptly, usually within 48 hours after the drug is readministered to sensitive patients. The syndrome seems to result from a form of sensitization, occurs chiefly in adults, and is reversible when medication is discontinued.

Myasthenia gravis – **Erythromycin** may aggravate the weakness of patients with myasthenia gravis.

Troleandomycin:

Hepatic effects – Troleandomycin has been associated with allergic cholestatic hepatitis. Some patients receiving troleandomycin for > 2 weeks or in repeated courses have developed jaundice accompanied by right upper quadrant pain, fever, nausea, vomiting, eosinophilia, and leukocytosis. These have reversed on drug discontinuance. Readministration reproduces hepatotoxicity, often within 24 to 48 hours.

Renal/Hepatic function impairment:

Clarithromycin – In the presence of severe renal impairment (creatinine < 30 mL/min) with or without coexisting hepatic impairment, decreased dosage or prolonged dosing intervals may be appropriate.

Azithromycin and troleandomycin – Exercise caution when administering to patients with impaired renal or hepatic function.

Erythromycin – Erythromycin is principally excreted by the liver. Exercise caution in administering to patients with impaired hepatic function.

Dirithromycin – No dosage adjustment should be necessary in patients with impaired renal function, including dialysis patients. In patients with mild hepatic impairment, mean peak serum concentration, AUC and volume of distribution increased somewhat with multiple-dose administration; however, based on the magnitude of these changes, no dosage adjustment should be necessary in patients with mildly impaired hepatic function.

Elderly:

Clarithromycin – Studies show age-related decreases in renal function. Consider dosage adjustment in elderly patients with severe renal impairment.

Azithromycin – Dosage adjustment does not appear to be necessary for older patients with normal renal and hepatic function.

Dirithromycin – No dosage adjustment should be necessary in elderly patients.

Pregnancy: *Category* B (azithromycin, erythromycin); *Category* C (clarithromycin, dirithromycin, troleandomycin).

Lactation:

Clarithromycin, dirithromycin, and azithromycin – It is not known whether these agents are excreted in breast milk.

Erythromycin – Erythromycin is excreted in breast milk, and may concentrate (observed milk:plasma ratio of 0.5 to 3). Erythromycin is considered compatible with breastfeeding by the American Academy of Pediatrics.

Children:

Dirithromycin – Safety and efficacy in children < 12 years of age have not been established.

Clarithromycin – Safety and efficacy in children < 6 months of age have not been established.

Azithromycin – Safety and efficacy in children < 6 months of age (acute otitis media, community-acquired pneumonia) or < 2 years of age (pharyngitis/tonsillitis) have not been established.

IV use: Safety and efficacy of azithromycin for IV injection in children or adolescents < 16 years of age have not been established.

Precautions

Azithromycin:

Local IV site reactions – Local IV site reactions have been reported with the IV administration of azithromycin. The incidence and severity of these reactions were the same when 500 mg was given over 1 hour (2 mg/mL as 250 mL infusion) or over 3 hours (1 mg/mL as 500 mL infusion). All volunteers who received infusate concentrations > 2 mg/mL experienced local IV site reactions; therefore, avoid higher concentrations.

Drug Interactions

Clarithromycin: Drugs that may be affected by clarithromycin include anticoagulants, astemizole, benzodiazepines, buspirone, carbamazepine, cisapride, cyclosporine, digoxin, disopyramide, ergot alkaloids, HMG-CoA reductase inhibitors, omeprazole, ranitidine bismuth citrate, tacrolimus, theophylline, and zidovudine. Also consider all drug interactions with erythromycin. Drugs that may affect clarithromycin include fluconazole, ranitidine bismuth citrate, pimozide, rifamycins, and omeprazole.

Azithromycin: Drugs that may interact with azithromycin include antacids, cyclosporine, HMG-CoA reductase inhibitors, pimozide, tacrolimus, theophyllines, and warfarin. Also consider all drug interactions with erythromycin.

Dirithromycin: Drugs that may be affected by dirithromycin include antacids. Drugs that may affect dirithromycin include antacids, pimozide, and H_2 antagonists. Also consider all drug interactions with erythromycin.

Erythromycin: Drugs that may be affected by erythromycin include alfentanil, anticoagulants, astemizole, benzodiazepines, buspirone, carbamazepine, cisapride, cyclosporine, digoxin, disopyramide, ergot alkaloids, felodipine, fluoroquinolones, HMG-CoA reductase inhibitors, lincosamides, methylprednisolone, penicillins, and theophyllines. Drugs that may affect erythromycin include antacids, pimozide, rifamycins, and theophyllines.

Troleandomycin: Drugs that may be affected by troleandomycin include astemizole, benzodiazepines, buspirone, carbamazepine, cisapride, oral contraceptives, cyclosporine, ergot alkaloids, methylprednisolone, tacrolimus, and theophyllines. Drugs that may affect troleandomycin include rifamycins.

Drug/Food interactions:

Clarithromycin – Following tablet administration, food delays both the onset of clarithromycin absorption and the formulation of 14 OH clarithromycin, but does not affect bioavailability. Following the suspension, food decreases mean peak clarithromycin levels and extent of absorption.

Azithromycin – When azithromycin suspension was administered with food, the rate of absorption (C_{max}) was increased by 56% while the extent of absorption (AUC) was unchanged. Take 1 hour before or 2 hours after a meal. Do not take with food.

Dirithromycin – Dirithromycin should be administered with food or within an hour of eating. After administration of two 250 mg tablets 1 or 4 hours before food and immediately after a standard breakfast indicated an increase in absorption of erythromycylamine when dirithromycin was administered after food, while a significant decrease in C_{max} (33%) and AUC (31%) occurred when administered 1 hour before food.

Erythromycin – Antimicrobial effectiveness of erythromycin stearate and certain formulations of erythromycin base may be reduced. Take at least 2 hours before or after a meal. Erythromycin estolate and ethylsuccinate and the base in a delayed release form may be administered without regard to meals.

Adverse Reactions

Clarithromycin – Adverse reactions occurring in ≥ 3% of patients include diarrhea, nausea, abdominal pain, rash, increased BUN, and abnormal taste.

Azithromycin – Adverse reactions occurring in ≥ 3% of patients include diarrhea/loose stools, vomiting, nausea, abdominal pain, increased ALT and AST, increased serum creatinine, and increased bilirubin.

Dirithromycin – Adverse reactions occurring in ≥ 3% of patients include abdominal pain/discomfort, diarrhea/loose stools, nausea, vomiting, increased platelet count, and headache.

Erythromycin – Adverse reactions occurring in ≥ 3% of patients include abdominal pain/discomfort, diarrhea/loose stools, nausea, increased platelet count, and headache.

Hepatic – Hepatotoxicity is most commonly associated with erythromycin estolate.

Local – Venous irritation and phlebitis have occurred with parenteral administration, but the risk of such reactions may be reduced if the infusion is given slowly, in dilute solution, by continuous IV infusion or intermittent infusion over 20 to 60 minutes.

MESALAMINE (5-aminosalicylic acid, 5-ASA)

Tablets, delayed release: 400 mg (*Rx*)	*Asacol* (Procter & Gamble)
Capsules, controlled release: 250 mg (*Rx*)	*Pentasa* (Aventis)
Suppositories: 500 mg (*Rx*)	*Rowasa* (Solvay)
Rectal suspension: 4 g/60 mL (*Rx*)	*Rowasa* (Solvay)

Indications

Chronic inflammatory bowel disease:

Oral – Remission and treatment of mildly to moderately active ulcerative colitis.

Rectal – Treatment of active mild to moderate distal ulcerative colitis, proctosigmoiditis, or proctitis.

Administration and Dosage

Oral:

Tablets – 800 mg 3 times daily for a total dose of 2.4 g/day for 6 weeks.

Capsules – 1 g 4 times daily for a total dose of 4 g for up to 8 weeks.

Suppository: One suppository (500 mg) 2 times daily. Retain the suppository in the rectum for 1 to 3 hours or more if possible to achieve maximum benefit. While the effect may be seen within 3 to 21 days, the usual course of therapy is 3 to 6 weeks depending on symptoms and sigmoidoscopic findings.

Suspension: The usual dosage of mesalamine suspension enema in 60 mL units is 1 rectal instillation (4 g) once a day, preferably at bedtime, and retained for ≈ 8 hours. While the effect may be seen within 3 to 21 days, the usual course of therapy is 3 to 6 weeks depending on symptoms and sigmoidoscopic findings.

Actions

Pharmacology: Sulfasalazine is split by bacterial action in the colon into sulfapyridine and mesalamine (5-ASA).

The mechanism of action of mesalamine (and sulfasalazine) is unknown, but appears to be topical rather than systemic, and it is possible that mesalamine diminishes inflammation by blocking cyclooxygenase and inhibiting prostaglandin production in the colon.

Pharmacokinetics:

Absorption/Distribution –

Rectal: Mesalamine administered rectally as a suspension enema is poorly absorbed from the colon and is excreted principally in the feces during subsequent bowel movements. At steady state, ≈ 10% to 30% of the daily 4 g dose can be recovered in cumulative 24 hour urine collections.

Oral:

Tablets – Mesalamine tablets are coated with an acrylic-based resin that delays release of mesalamine until it reaches the terminal ileum and beyond. Approximately 28% is absorbed after oral ingestion, leaving the remainder available for topical action and excretion in the feces. Mesalamine from oral mesalamine tablets appears to be more extensively absorbed than that released from sulfasalazine.

Capsules – Mesalamine capsules are designed to release therapeutic quantities of the drug throughout the GI tract; 20% to 30% of mesalamine is absorbed. Plasma mesalamine concentration peaked at ≈ 1 mcg/mL 3 hours after administration of a 1 g dose and declined in a biphasic manner. Mean terminal half-life was 42 minutes after IV administration.

Metabolism/Excretion –

Rectal: Whatever the metabolic site, most absorbed mesalamine is excreted in urine as the N-acetyl-5-ASA metabolite. While the elimination half-life of mesalamine is short (0.5 to 1.5 hours), the acetylated metabolite exhibits a half-life of 5 to 10 hours.

Oral:

Tablets – Following oral administration, the absorbed mesalamine is rapidly acetylated in the gut mucosal wall and by the liver. It is excreted mainly by the kidneys as N-acetyl-5-ASA. The half-lives of elimination for mesalamine and the metabolite are usually ≈ 12 hours, but are variable ranging from 2 to 15 hours.

Capsules – Elimination of free mesalamine and salicylates in feces increased proportionately with the dose. N-acetyl-5-ASA was the primary compound excreted in the urine (19% to 30%).

Contraindications

Hypersensitivity to mesalamine, salicylates, or any component of the formulation.

Warnings

Intolerance/Colitis exacerbation: Mesalamine has been implicated in the production of an acute intolerance syndrome or exacerbation of colitis characterized by cramping, acute abdominal pain and bloody diarrhea, and occasionally fever, headache, malaise, pruritus, conjunctivitis, and rash. Symptoms usually abate when mesalamine is discontinued.

Pancolitis: While using mesalamine, some patients have developed pancolitis.

Hypersensitivity reactions: Most patients who were hypersensitive to sulfasalazine were able to take mesalamine enemas without evidence of any allergic reaction. Nevertheless, exercise caution when mesalamine is initially used in patients known to be allergic to sulfasalazine.

Renal function impairment: Renal impairment, including minimal change nephropathy, and acute and chronic interstitial nephritis, has occurred.

Pregnancy: *Category B.* Mesalamine is known to cross the placental barrier.

Lactation: Low concentrations of mesalamine and higher concentrations of N-acetyl-5-ASA have been detected in breast milk.

Children: Safety and efficacy for use in children have not been established.

Precautions

Pericarditis: Pericarditis has occurred rarely with mesalamine-containing products including sulfasalazine.

Adverse Reactions

Adverse reactions may include abdominal pain/cramps/discomfort; colitis exacerbation; constipation; diarrhea; dyspepesia; eructation; flatulence/gas; nausea; vomiting; asthenia; chills; dizziness; fever; headache; malaise/fatigue/weakness; sweating; pharyngitis; rhinitis; pruritus; rash/spots; arthralgia; back pain; hypertonia; myalgia; chest pain; dysmenorrhea; edema; flu syndrome; pain.

METHOTREXATE

Tablets: 2.5 mg (as sodium)	Various, *Rheumatrex Dose Pack* (STADA Pharm)
Tablets: 5, 7.5, 10, and 15 mg	*Trexall* (Barr)

Warning:

Severe reactions: Because of the possibility of severe toxic reactions, fully inform patient of the risks involved and assure constant supervision.

Deaths: Deaths have occurred with the use of methotrexate.

In rheumatoid arthritis treatment: Restrict use to patients with severe, recalcitrant, disabling disease, which is not adequately responsive to other forms of therapy, and only after established diagnosis and appropriate consultation.

Pregnancy: Fetal death or congenital anomalies have occurred; do not use in women of childbearing potential unless benefits outweigh possible risks. Pregnant rheumatoid arthritis patients should not receive methotrexate.

Periodic monitoring: Periodic monitoring for toxicity, including CBC with differential and platelet counts, and liver and renal function tests is mandatory. Periodic liver biopsies may be indicated in some situations. Monitor patients at increased risk for impaired methotrexate elimination (eg, renal dysfunction, pleural effusions, ascites) more frequently.

Liver: Methotrexate (MTX) causes hepatotoxicity, fibrosis, and cirrhosis but generally only after prolonged use. Acutely, liver enzyme elevations are frequent, usually transient and asymptomatic, and also do not appear predictive of subsequent hepatic disease. Liver biopsy after sustained use often shows histologic changes, and fibrosis and cirrhosis have been reported; these latter lesions often are not preceded by symptoms or abnormal liver function tests.

MTX-induced lung disease: MTX-induced lung disease, a potentially dangerous lesion, may occur acutely at any time during therapy and has been reported at doses as low as 7.5 mg/week. It is not always fully reversible. Pulmonary symptoms (especially a dry, nonproductive cough) may require treatment interruption and careful investigation.

Marked bone marrow depression: Marked bone marrow depression may occur, with resultant anemia, leukopenia, or thrombocytopenia.

Unexpectedly severe (sometimes fatal) marrow suppression and GI toxicity have been reported with coadministration of methotrexate (usually in high dosage) and some NSAIDs.

GI: Diarrhea and ulcerative stomatitis require interruption of therapy; hemorrhagic enteritis and death from intestinal perforation may occur.

Renal use: Use MTX in patients with impaired renal function with extreme caution and at reduced dosages, because renal dysfunction will prolong elimination.

Indications

Severe, active, classical, or definite rheumatoid arthritis: (ARA criteria) in selected adults who have had an insufficient therapeutic response to, or are intolerant of, an adequate trial of first line therapy including full dose NSAIDs and usually a trial of at least 1 or more disease-modifying antirheumatic drugs.

Administration and Dosage

Initial therapy may be instituted with the MTX 2.5 mg tablet dose pack, designated to initiate therapy with a 7.5 mg weekly dose. The dose pack is not recommended for titration to higher weekly doses, if they are necessary. Individualize dose. An initial test dose may be given prior to the regular dosing schedule to detect any extreme sensitivity to adverse effects. Maximal myelosuppression usually occurs in 7 to 10 days.

Recommended starting dosage schedules: Single oral doses of 7.5 mg/week or divided oral dosages of 2.5 mg at 12-hour intervals for 3 doses given as a course once weekly.

Dosages in each schedule may be adjusted gradually to achieve an optimal response but not ordinarily to exceed a total weekly dose of 20 mg. Limited experience shows a significant increase in the incidence and severity of serious toxic reactions, especially bone marrow suppression, at doses greater than 20 mg/week. Once response has been achieved, reduce each schedule, if possible, to the lowest possible effective dose.

Therapeutic response usually begins within 3 to 6 weeks and the patient may continue to improve for another 12 weeks or more.

Optimal duration of therapy is unknown. Limited data indicate that initial clinical improvement is maintained at least 2 years with continued therapy. When MTX is discontinued, the arthritis usually worsens within 3 to 6 weeks.

Actions

Pharmacology: The mechanism of action in rheumatoid arthritis is unknown; it may affect immune function. Two reports describe in vitro MTX inhibition of DNA precursor uptake by stimulated mononuclear cells and another (in animals) describes partial correction by MTX of spleen cell hyporesponsiveness and suppressed interleukin-2 production.

Contraindications

Pregnant and lactating patients (see Warnings); alcoholism, alcoholic liver disease or other chronic liver disease; overt or laboratory evidence of immunodeficiency syndromes; preexisting blood dyscrasias, such as bone marrow hypoplasia, leukopenia, thrombocytopenia, or significant anemia; hypersensitivity to MTX.

Warnings

Pregnancy: Category X. MTX can cause fetal death or teratogenic effects when administered to a pregnant woman and is contraindicated in pregnant patients with rheumatoid arthritis. Do not start women of childbearing potential on MTX until pregnancy is excluded and fully counsel them on the serious risk to the fetus should they become pregnant while undergoing treatment. Avoid pregnancy if either partner is receiving MTX: During and for a minimum of 3 months after therapy for male patients, and during and for at least 1 ovulatory cycle after therapy for female patients.

Lactation: Because of the potential for serious adverse reactions from MTX in breastfed infants, it is contraindicated in nursing mothers.

Children: Safety and efficacy in children have not been established other than in cancer chemotherapy.

Precautions

Monitoring: Monitor hematology at least monthly, and liver and renal function every 1 to 3 months during therapy. During initial or changing doses, or periods of increased risk of elevated MTX blood levels (eg, dehydration), more frequent monitoring may be indicated. Stop MTX immediately if there is a significant drop in blood counts.

Aspirin, NSAIDs, or low dose steroids may be continued, although the possibility of increased toxicity with concomitant use of NSAIDs including salicylates has not been fully explored. Studies of MTX in patients with rheumatoid arthritis have usually included concomitant NSAIDs without apparent problems. Note, however, that doses used in rheumatoid arthritis (7.5 to 15 mg/week) are somewhat lower than those used in psoriasis; larger doses could lead to unexpected toxicity.

Physicians and pharmacists should emphasize that the dose is taken weekly. Mistaken daily use has led to fatal toxicity. Encourage patients to read the Patient Instructions in the Dose Pack. Do not write or refill prescriptions on a PRN basis.

Adverse Reactions

Elevated liver function tests (15%); nausea/vomiting (10%); thrombocytopenia (platelet count < $100,000/mm^3$); stomatitis (3% to 10%).

METOCLOPRAMIDE

Tablets: 5 and 10 mg (*Rx*)	Various, *Reglan* (Robins), *Maxolon* (GlaxoSmith-Kline)
Syrup: 5 mg/5 mL (*Rx*)	Various, *Reglan* (Robins)
Concentrated solution: 10 mg/mL (*Rx*)	*Metoclopramide Intensol* (Roxane)
Injection: 5 mg/mL (*Rx*)	Various, *Octamide PFS* (Adria), *Reglan* (Robins)

Indications

Diabetic gastroparesis: Relief of symptoms associated with acute and recurrent diabetic gastroparesis (diabetic gastric stasis). Usual manifestations of delayed gastric emptying (ie, nausea, vomiting, heartburn, persistent fullness after meals, anorexia) respond within different time intervals. Significant relief of nausea occurs early and improves over 3 weeks. Relief of vomiting and anorexia may precede the relief of abdominal fullness by ≥ 1 week.

Oral:

Symptomatic gastroesophageal reflux – Short-term (4 to 12 weeks) therapy for adults with symptomatic documented gastroesophageal reflux who fail to respond to conventional therapy.

Parenteral: For prevention of nausea and vomiting associated with emetogenic cancer chemotherapy.

Prophylaxis of postoperative nausea and vomiting when nasogastric suction is undesirable.

Single doses may facilitate small bowel intubation when the tube does not pass the pylorus with conventional maneuvers.

Stimulates gastric emptying and intestinal transit of barium in cases where delayed emptying interferes with radiological examination of the stomach or small intestine.

Unlabeled uses: Used to improve lactation. Doses of 30 to 45 mg/day have increased milk secretion, possibly by elevating serum prolactin levels (see Warnings). Also for treatment of postoperative gastric bezoars (10 mg 3 or 4 times daily).

Administration and Dosage

Diabetic gastroparesis: 10 mg 30 minutes before each meal and at bedtime for 2 to 8 weeks.

Determine initial route of administration by the severity of symptoms. With only the earliest manifestations of diabetic gastric stasis, initiate oral administration. If symptoms are severe, begin with parenteral therapy. Administer 10 mg IV over 1 to 2 minutes. Parenteral administration up to 10 days may be required before symptoms subside, then oral administration may be instituted. Reinstitute therapy at the earliest manifestation.

Symptomatic gastroesophageal reflux: 10 to 15 mg orally up to 4 times daily 30 minutes before each meal and at bedtime. If symptoms occur only intermittently or at specific times of the day, single doses up to 20 mg prior to the provoking situation may be preferred rather than continuous treatment. Occasionally, patients who are more sensitive to the therapeutic or adverse effects of metoclopramide (eg, elderly) will require only 5 mg/dose. Guide therapy directed at esophageal lesions by endoscopy. Therapy > 12 weeks has not been evaluated and cannot be recommended.

Prevention of postoperative nausea and vomiting: Inject IM near the end of surgery. The usual adult dose is 10 mg; however, doses of 20 mg may be used.

Prevention of chemotherapy-induced emesis: Infuse slowly IV over not less than 15 minutes, 30 minutes before beginning cancer chemotherapy; repeat every 2 hours for 2 doses, then every 3 hours for 3 doses.

The initial 2 doses should be 2 mg/kg if highly emetogenic drugs such as cisplatin or dacarbazine are used alone or in combination. For less emetogenic regimens, 1 mg/kg/dose may be adequate.

If extrapyramidal symptoms occur, administer 50 mg diphenhydramine IM.

IV admixture: When diluted in a parenteral solution, administer IV slowly over a period of not less than 15 minutes.

Direct IV injection: Inject undiluted metoclopramide slowly IV allowing 1 to 2 minutes for 10 mg, because a transient but intense feeling of anxiety and restlessness followed by drowsiness may occur with rapid administration.

Facilitation of small bowel intubation – If the tube has not passed the pylorus with conventional maneuvers in 10 minutes, administer a single undiluted dose slowly IV over 1 to 2 minutes.

Recommended single dose –

Adults: 10 mg (2 mL).

Children (6 to 14 years of age): 2.5 to 5 mg (0.5 to 1 mL).

Children (< 6 years of age): 0.1 mg/kg.

Radiological examinations – In patients where delayed gastric emptying interferes with radiological examination of the stomach or small intestine, a single dose may be administered slowly IV over 1 to 2 minutes.

Rectal administration: For outpatient treatment when oral dosing is not possible, suppositories containing 25 mg metoclopramide have been extemporaneously compounded (5 pulverized oral tablets in polyethylene glycol). Administer 1 suppository 30 to 60 minutes before each meal and at bedtime.

Renal/Hepatic function impairment: Because metoclopramide is excreted principally through the kidneys, in those patients whose Ccr is < 40 mL/min, initiate therapy at ≈ ½ the recommended dosage. Depending on clinical efficacy and safety considerations, the dosage may be increased or decreased as appropriate.

Metoclopramide undergoes minimal hepatic metabolism, except for simple conjugation. Its safe use has been described in patients with advanced liver disease whose renal function was normal.

Admixture compatibilities/incompatibilities:

Physically and chemically compatible up to 48 hours – Cimetidine; mannitol; potassium acetate; potassium chloride; potassium phosphate.

Physically compatible up to 48 hours – Ascorbic acid; benztropine; cytarabine; dexamethasone sodium phosphate; diphenhydramine; doxorubicin; heparin sodium; hydrocortisone sodium phosphate; lidocaine; magnesium sulfate; multivitamin infusion (must be refrigerated) vitamin B complex with ascorbic acid.

Incompatible – Cephalothin; chloramphenicol; sodium bicarbonate.

Actions

Pharmacology: Metoclopramide stimulates motility of the upper GI tract without stimulating gastric, biliary, or pancreatic secretions. Its mode of action is unclear.

Pharmacokinetics:

Absorption/Distribution – Metoclopramide is rapidly and well absorbed. Onset of action is 1 to 3 minutes following an IV dose, 10 to 15 minutes following IM administration, and 30 to 60 minutes following an oral dose. Effects persist for 1 to 2 hours.

Relative to an IV dose of 20 mg, the absolute oral bioavailability of metoclopramide is ≈ 80%. Peak plasma concentrations occur at ≈ 1 to 2 hours after a single oral dose. Similar time to peak is observed after individual doses at steady-state. The area under the drug concentration-time curve increases linearly with doses from 20 to 100 mg; peak concentrations also increase linearly with dose. The whole body volume of distribution is high (≈ 3.5 L/kg), which suggests extensive distribution of drug to the tissues.

Metabolism/Excretion – Approximately 85% of an orally administered dose appears in the urine within 72 hours. Of the 85% eliminated in the urine, about one-half is present as free or conjugated metoclopramide. The average elimination half-life in individuals with normal renal function is 5 to 6 hours. The drug is not extensively bound to plasma proteins (about 30%).

Contraindications

When stimulation of GI motility might be dangerous (eg, in the presence of GI hemorrhage, mechanical obstruction, or perforation); pheochromocytoma (the drug may cause a hypertensive crisis, probably because of release of catecholamines from the tumor; control such crises with phentolamine); sensitivity or intolerance to metoclopramide; epileptics or patients receiving drugs likely to cause extrapyramidal reactions (the frequency and severity of seizures or extrapyramidal reactions may be increased).

Warnings

Depression: Depression has occurred in patients with and without a history of depression. Give metoclopramide to patients with a prior history of depression only if the expected benefits outweigh the potential risks.

Extrapyramidal symptoms: Extrapyramidal symptoms, manifested primarily as acute dystonic reactions, occur in ≈ 0.2% to 1% of patients treated with the usual adult dosages of 30 to 40 mg/day. These usually are seen during the first 24 to 48 hours of treatment, occur more frequently in children and young adults, and are even more frequent at the higher doses used in prophylaxis of vomiting caused by cancer chemotherapy. If symptoms occur, they usually subside following 50 mg diphenhydramine IM. Benztropine 1 to 2 mg IM may also be used to reverse these reactions.

Parkinson-like symptoms: Parkinson-like symptoms have occurred, more commonly within the first 6 months after beginning treatment with metoclopramide but occasionally after longer periods. These symptoms generally subside within 2 to 3 months following discontinuance of metoclopramide. Give metoclopramide cautiously, if at all, to patients with preexisting Parkinson's disease, because such patients may experience exacerbation of parkinsonian symptoms when taking metoclopramide.

Tardive dyskinesia: Tardive dyskinesia, a syndrome consisting of potentially irreversible, involuntary, dyskinetic movements, may develop in patients treated with metoclopramide. Metoclopramide itself, however, may suppress (or partially suppress) the signs of tardive dyskinesia, thereby masking the underlying disease process. Therefore, the use of metoclopramide for the symptomatic control of tardive dyskinesia is not recommended.

Hypertension: In one study of hypertensive patients, IV metoclopramide released catecholamines. Use caution in hypertensive patients.

Anastomosis or closure of the gut: Giving a promotility drug such as metoclopramide could theoretically put increased pressure on suture lines following a gut anastomosis or closure.

Carcinogenesis: Elevated prolactin levels persist during chronic administration. Approximately one-third of human breast cancers are prolactin-dependent in vitro; use caution if metoclopramide is contemplated in a patient with previously detected breast cancer. Although galactorrhea, amenorrhea, gynecomastia, and impotence have occurred with prolactin-elevating drugs, the clinical significance of elevated serum prolactin levels is unknown.

Pregnancy: *Category B.*

Lactation: Metoclopramide is excreted into breast milk and may concentrate at about twice the plasma level at 2 hours postdose. There appears to be no risk to the nursing infant with maternal doses ≤ 45 mg/day.

Children: Infants and children (21 days to 3.3 years of age) with symptomatic gastroesophageal reflux have been treated with metoclopramide at a dosage of 0.5 mg/kg/day; symptoms improved, the duration of the disease was shortened, and surgery was avoided.

Methemoglobinemia has occurred in premature and full-term neonates given metoclopramide orally, IV or IM, 1 to 4 mg/kg/day for 1 to ≥ 3 days; this did not occur at 0.5 mg/kg/day. Reverse methemoglobinemia by IV administration of methylene blue.

Precautions

Hypoglycemia: Gastroparesis (gastric stasis) may be responsible for poor diabetic control. Exogenously administered insulins may act before food has left the stomach, leading to hypoglycemia.

Hazardous tasks: May cause drowsiness; observe caution while driving or performing other tasks requiring alertness, coordination or physical dexterity.

Drug Interactions

Drugs that may affect metoclopramide include levodopa, anticholinergics, and narcotic analgesics. Drugs that may be affected by metoclopramide include alcohol, cimetidine, cyclosporine, digoxin, levodopa, MAO inhibitors, and succinylcholine.

Adverse Reactions

Adverse reactions occurring in ≥ 3% of patients include restlessness; drowsiness; fatigue; lassitude; akathisia; dizziness; anxiety; dystonia; insomnia; headache; myoclonus; confusion; convulsive seizures; hallucinations; nausea; bowel disturbances, primarily diarrhea.

METRONIDAZOLE

Tablets: 250 mg and 500 mg (*Rx*)	Various, *Flagyl* (Searle)
Capsules: 375 mg (*Rx*)	*Flagyl 375* (Searle)
Powder for injection, lyophilized: 500 mg (as HCl) (*Rx*)	*Flagyl I.V.* (Schiapparelli Searle)
Injection, ready-to-use: 500 mg/100 mL (*Rx*)	Various, *Metronidazole* (Abbott), *Flagyl I.V. RTU* (Schiapparelli Searle)

Metronidazole also is available for topical and intravaginal use and also is used orally as an amebicide.

Warning:
Metronidazole is carcinogenic in rodents. Avoid unnecessary use.

Indications

Anaerobic infections: Treatment of serious infections caused by susceptible anaerobic bacteria. Effective in *Bacteroides fragilis* infections resistant to clindamycin, chloramphenicol, and penicillin.

Intra-abdominal infections – Intra-abdominal infections (peritonitis, intra-abdominal abscess, and liver abscess) caused by *Bacteroides* sp. (*B. fragilis, B. distasonis, B. ovatus, B. thetaiotaomicron, B. vulgatus*), *Clostridium* sp., *Eubacterium* sp., *Peptostreptococcus* sp., and *Peptococcus* sp.

Skin and skin structure infections – Skin and skin structure infections, caused by *Bacteroides* sp. including the *B. fragilis* group, *Clostridium* sp., *Peptococcus* sp., *Peptostreptococcus* sp., and *Fusobacterium* sp.

Gynecologic infections – Gynecologic infections (endometritis, endomyometritis, tubo-ovarian abscess, and postsurgical vaginal cuff infection), caused by *Bacteroides* sp. including the *B. fragilis* group, *Clostridium* sp., *Peptococcus* sp., and *Peptostreptococcus* sp.

Bacterial septicemia – Bacterial septicemia caused by *Bacteroides* sp. including the *B. fragilis* group and *Clostridium* sp.

Bone and joint infections – Bone and joint infections caused by *Bacteroides* sp. including the *B. fragilis* group, as adjunctive therapy.

CNS infections – CNS infections (meningitis and brain abscess), caused by *Bacteroides* sp. including the *B. fragilis* group.

Lower respiratory tract infections – Lower respiratory tract infections (pneumonia, empyema, and lung abscess) caused by *Bacteroides* sp. including the *B. fragilis* group.

Endocarditis – Endocarditis caused by *Bacteroides* sp. including the *B. fragilis* group.

Prophylaxis: Preoperative, intraoperative, and postoperative IV metronidazole may reduce the incidence of postoperative infection in patients undergoing elective colorectal surgery which is classified as contaminated or potentially contaminated.

Metronidazole also is indicated for amebiasis and trichomoniasis, intravaginally for bacterial vaginosis, and topically for acne rosacea.

Unlabeled uses: The CDC has recommended the use of oral metronidazole for bacterial vaginosis (500 mg twice daily for 7 days). Single-dose therapy for bacterial vaginosis (2 g) also appears to be as effective as multiple-dose therapy.

Administration and Dosage

May cause GI upset; take with food. Avoid alcoholic beverages.

Anaerobic bacterial infections: In the treatment of most serious anaerobic infections, metronidazole is usually administered IV initially.

Loading dose – 15 mg/kg infused over 1 hour ($\approx$ 1 g for a 70 kg adult).

Maintenance dose – 7.5 mg/kg infused over 1 hour every 6 hours ($\approx$ 500 mg for a 70 kg adult). Administer the first maintenance dose 6 hours following the initiation of loading dose. Do not exceed a maximum of 4 g in 24 hours.

The usual duration of therapy is 7 to 10 days; however, infections of the bone and joints, lower respiratory tract, and endocardium may require longer treatment.

Administer by slow IV, continuous or intermittent drip infusion only. Do not give by direct IV bolus injection because of the low pH (0.5 to 2) of the reconstituted product. The drug must be further diluted and neutralized for infusion.

Oral – Following IV therapy, use oral metronidazole when conditions warrant. The usual adult oral dosage is 7.5 mg/kg every 6 hours. Do not exceed a maximum of 4 g in 24 hours.

Prophylaxis: To prevent postoperative infection in contaminated or potentially contaminated colorectal surgery, the recommended adult dosage is 15 mg/kg infused over 30 to 60 minutes and completed ≈ 1 hour before surgery, followed by 7.5 mg/kg infused over 30 to 60 minutes at 6 and 12 hours after the initial dose.

It also has been suggested that a dose of 1500 mg infused at the beginning of surgery achieves significantly higher concentrations against *B. fragilis* than the 500 mg infusion and may be beneficial in ensuring adequate metronidazole levels.

Hepatic disease: Hepatic disease patients metabolize metronidazole slowly; accumulation of metronidazole and its metabolites occurs. Therefore, reduce doses below those usually recommended.

Renal disease: Do not specifically reduce the dose in anuric patients because accumulated metabolites may be rapidly removed by dialysis.

Actions

Pharmacology: Metronidazole, a nitroimidazole, is active against various anaerobic bacteria and protozoa.

Pharmacokinetics:

Absorption – Metronidazole is well absorbed after oral administration. Peak serum levels occur at about 1 to 2 hours. Food delays peak serum levels up to 2 hours.

Distribution – Metronidazole has a large apparent volume of distribution. It diffuses well into all tissues.

Excretion – The major route of elimination of metronidazole and its metabolites is via the urine (60% to 80% of the dose); fecal excretion accounts for 6% to 15% of the dose. Renal clearance is ≈ 10 mL/min/1.73 m^2. Metronidazole has an average elimination half-life in healthy subjects of 8 hours. Patients with Ccr < 10 mL/min (not receiving dialysis) will accumulate both metabolites. Metronidazole and its 2 major metabolites are removed by hemodialysis. Metronidazole is also removed by peritoneal dialysis.

Contraindications

Hypersensitivity to metronidazole or other nitroimidazole derivatives; pregnancy (first trimester in patients with trichomoniasis).

Warnings

Neurologic effects: Seizures (associated with high cumulative doses) and peripheral neuropathy (characterized by numbness or paresthesia of an extremity) have occurred. In some cases, neuropathy is not reversible.

Hepatic function impairment: Patients with severe hepatic disease metabolize metronidazole slowly. Accumulation of the drug and its metabolites may occur.

Elderly: Because the pharmacokinetics of metronidazole may be altered in the elderly, monitoring of serum levels may be necessary to adjust the dosage accordingly.

Pregnancy: *Category* B. Restrict metronidazole for trichomoniasis in the second and third trimesters to those in whom local palliative treatment has been inadequate to control symptoms.

Lactation: Safety for use in nursing mothers has not been established. A nursing mother should express and discard any breast milk produced while on the drug and resume nursing 24 to 48 hours after the drug is discontinued.

Children: Safety and efficacy in children have not been established, except for the treatment of amebiasis. Newborns demonstrate a diminished capacity to eliminate metronidazole; half-life may be as high as 22 hours.

Precautions

Crohn's disease: Crohn's disease patients are known to have an increased incidence of GI and certain extraintestinal cancers.

Candidiasis: Candidiasis may present more prominent symptoms during therapy and requires treatment with a candicidal agent.

Hematologic effects: Metronidazole is a nitroimidazole; use with care in patients with evidence or history of blood dyscrasia. Perform total and differential leukocyte counts before and after therapy.

Amebic liver abscess: Metronidazole does not obviate the need for aspiration of pus.

Drug Interactions

Drugs that may affect metronidazole include barbiturates and cimetidine. Drugs that may be affected by metronidazole include anticoagulants, disulfiram, ethanol, hydantoins, and lithium.

Drug/Lab test interactions: The drug may interfere with chemical analyses for AST, ALT, LDH, triglycerides, and hexokinase glucose.

Adverse Reactions

Adverse reactions may include dysuria; cystitis; polyuria; incontinence; proliferation of *Candida* in the vagina; dyspareunia; darkened urine; seizures and peripheral neuropathy; dizziness; vertigo; incoordination; ataxia; confusion; irritability; depression; weakness; insomnia; headache; syncope; nausea; diarrhea; epigastric distress; constipation; proctitis; glossitis; stomatitis; unpleasant metallic taste; urticaria; erythematous rash; flushing; nasal congestion.

OCTREOTIDE ACETATE

Injection: 0.05, 0.1, 0.2, 0.5, 1 mg/mL (*Rx*)	*Sandostatin* (Novartis)
10 mg/5 mL, 20 mg/5 mL, 30 mg/5 mL (*Rx*)	*Sandostatin LAR Depot* (Novartis)

Indications

Sandostatin and Sandostatin LAR Depot: Acromegaly; carcinoid tumors.

Vasoactive intestinal peptide tumors (VIPomas) – Treatment of the profuse watery diarrhea associated with VIP-secreting tumors.

Unlabeled uses:

GI fistula – To reduce output from GI fistulas. Dosage ranges from 50 to 200 mcg every 8 hours.

Variceal bleeding – Dosage ranges from 25 to 50 mcg/hr via continuous IV infusion. Duration is from 18 hours to 5 days.

Diarrheal states – Because octreotide prolongs intestinal transit time, it is beneficial in relieving diarrhea associated with a variety of conditions including the following: AIDS-related diarrhea (100 to 500 mcg SC 3 times daily); idiopathic secretory diarrhea; short bowel (ileostomy) syndrome (IV infusion of 25 mcg/hr or SC 50 mcg twice daily); diabetes; pancreatic cholera syndrome; diarrhea caused by chemotherapy/radiation therapy in cancer patients (50 to 100 mcg SC 3 times daily for 1 to 3 days).

Pancreatic fistula – To reduce output from pancreatic fistulas. Dosages range from 50 to 200 mcg every 8 hours.

Irritable bowel syndrome – 100 mcg single dose to 125 mcg SC twice daily.

Dumping syndrome – 50 to 150 mcg/day.

Administration and Dosage

Sandostatin administration: Octreotide may be administered SC or IV. SC injection is the usual route of administration for control of symptoms. Pain with SC use may be reduced by using the smallest volume that will deliver the desired dose. Avoid multiple injections at the same site within short periods of time. Rotate sites in a systematic manner. The initial dosage usually is 50 mcg administered 2 or 3 times daily. Upward dose titration usually is required.

Although not an approved method of administration, continuous subcutaneous infusion (CSI) has been used to administer octreotide. Advantages to CSI include patient convenience, increased compliance, decreased injection site pain, minimization of GI side effects and continuous octreotide serum levels.

Sandostatin LAR Depot administration: Do not administer IV or SC. Administer immediately after mixing. Administer intragluteally at 4-week intervals. Avoid deltoid injections because of significant discomfort at the injection site.

Acromegaly:

Sandostatin – Dosage may be initiated at 50 mcg 3 times daily. IGF-I levels every 2 weeks can be used to guide titration. The goal is to achieve growth hormone levels < 5 ng/mL or IGF-I levels < 1.9 U/mL in males and < 2.2 U/mL in females. The dose most commonly found to be effective is 100 mcg 3 times daily, but some require up to 500 mcg 3 times daily for maximum efficacy. Doses > 300 mcg/day seldom result in additional benefit. If an increase in dose fails to provide additional benefit, reduce the dose. Reevaluate IGF-I or growth hormone levels at 6-month intervals.

Sandostatin LAR Depot – Patients currently receiving *Sandostatin* injection can be switched directly to *Sandostatin LAR Depot* in a dose of 20 mg given IM intragluterally at 4-week intervals for 3 months. Avoid detoid injections because of significant discomfort at injection site. Alternate gluteal injection sites to avoid irritation.

Administration of *Sandostatin LAR Depot* at intervals > 4 weeks is not recommended.

Carcinoid tumors: The suggested daily dosage of octreotide during the first 2 weeks of therapy ranges from 100 to 600 mcg/day in 2 to 4 divided doses (mean daily dosage is 300 mcg). Experience with doses > 750 mcg/day is limited.

VIPomas: Daily dosages of 200 to 300 mcg in 2 to 4 divided doses are recommended during the initial 2 weeks of therapy (range, 150 to 750 mcg) to control symptoms of the disease. On an individual basis, dosage may be adjusted to achieve a therapeutic response, but usually doses > 450 mcg/day are not required.

Sandostatin LAR Depot: Patients not currently receiving octreotide acetate should begin therapy with *Sandostatin* injection given SC. The suggested daily dosage for carcinoid tumors during the first 2 weeks of therapy ranges from 100 to 600 mcg/day in 2 to 4 divided doses. Some patients may require ≤ 1500 mcg/day. The suggested daily dosage for VIPomas is 200 to 300 mcg in 2 to 4 divided doses; dosage may be adjusted on an individual basis to control symptoms but usually doses > 450 mcg/day are not required.

Continue *Sandostatin* injection for ≥ 2 weeks. Thereafter, patients who are considered "responders" to octreotide acetate and who tolerate the drug may be switched to *Sandostatin LAR Depot* in the dosage regimen described below.

Patients currently receiving *Sandostatin* can be switched to *Sandostatin LAR Depot* in a dosage of 20 mg given IM intragluteally at 4-week intervals for 2 months. Avoid deltoid injections because of significant discomfort at the injection site. Because of the need for serum octreotide to reach therapeutically effective levels following initial injection of *Sandostatin LAR Depot*, carcinoid tumor and VIPoma patients should continue to receive *Sandostatin* SC for at least 2 weeks in the same dosage used before the switch. Failure to continue SC injections for this period may result in exacerbation of symptoms.

After 2 months of a 20 mg dosage of *Sandostatin LAR Depot*, dosage may be increased to 30 mg every 4 weeks if symptoms are not adequately controlled. Patients who achieve good control on a 20 mg dose may have the dose lowered to 10 mg for a trial period. If symptoms recur, increase dosage to 20 mg every 4 weeks. However, many patients can be satisfactorily maintained at a 10 mg dosage every 4 weeks. A dose of 10 mg is not recommended as a starting dose.

Doses > 30 mg are not recommended because there is no information on their usefulness.

Despite good overall control of symptoms, patients with carcinoid tumors and VIPomas often experience periodic exacerbation of symptoms. During these periods they may be given *Sandostatin* SC for a few days at the dosage they were receiving prior to switching to *Sandostatin LAR Depot*. When symptoms are again controlled, the *Sandostatin* SC can be discontinued.

Administration of *Sandostatin LAR Depot* at intervals > 4 weeks are not recommended because there is no adequate information on whether such patients could be adequately controlled.

Actions

Pharmacology: Octreotide acetate is a more potent inhibitor of growth hormone, glucagon, and insulin than somatostatin. Like somatostatin, it also suppresses LH response to GnRH, decreases splanchnic blood flow, and inhibits release of serotonin, gastrin, vasoactive intestinal peptide, secretin, motilin, and pancreatic polypeptide. Octreotide substantially reduces growth hormone or IGF-I (somatomedin C) levels in patients with acromegaly. Single doses inhibit gallbladder contractility and decrease bile secretion in healthy volunteers. In clinical trials, the incidence of gallstone or biliary sludge formation was markedly increased. Octreotide also suppresses secretion of thyroid stimulating hormone.

Pharmacokinetics:

Absorption/Distribution – After SC injection, octreotide is absorbed rapidly and completely from the injection site. Peak concentrations of 5.5 ng/mL (100 mcg dose) were reached 0.4 hours after dosing. IV and SC doses are bioequivalent.

The distribution of octreotide from plasma was rapid (alpha half-life = 0.2 hours), the volume of distribution (Vd) was estimated to be 13.6 L and total body clearance was 10 L/hr. In blood, the distribution into the erythrocytes was found to be negligible and about 65% was bound in the plasma in a concentration-independent manner. Binding was mainly to lipoprotein and, to a lesser extent, to albumin.

Metabolism/Excretion – The elimination half-life was 1.7 hours compared with 1 to 3 minutes with the natural hormone. The duration of action is variable but extends up to 12 hours depending upon the type of tumor. About 32% of the dose is excreted unchanged in the urine. In elderly patients, dose adjustments may be necessary due to a significant increase in the half-life (46%) and a significant decrease in the clearance (26%) of octreotide.

In patients with severe renal failure requiring dialysis, clearance was reduced to about half that found in healthy subjects (from approximately 10 to 4.5 L/hr). The effect of hepatic diseases on the disposition of octreotide is unknown.

Contraindications

Sensitivity to this drug or any of its components.

Warnings

Biliary tract effects: Single doses have inhibited gallbladder contractility and decreased bile secretion in healthy volunteers. In clinical trials (primarily patients with acromegaly or psoriasis), the incidence of biliary tract abnormalities was 52% (27% gallstones, 22% sludge without stones, 3% biliary duct dilatation). Incidence of stones or sludge in patients who received the drug for ≥ 12 months was 48%. Among patients treated for ≤ 1 month, < 2% developed gallstones. The incidence of gallstones did not appear related to age, sex, or dose.

Renal function impairment: In patients with severe renal failure requiring dialysis, octreotide half-life may be increased, necessitating adjustment of maintenance dose.

Elderly: Dose adjustments may be necessary because of a significant increase in the half-life (46%) and a significant decrease in the clearance (26%) of octreotide.

Pregnancy: Category B. Use during pregnancy only if clearly needed.

Lactation: Exercise caution when octreotide is administered to a nursing woman.

Children: The youngest patient to receive the drug was 1 month of age. Doses of 1 to 10 mcg/kg were well tolerated in young patients. A single case of an infant (nesidioblastosis) was complicated by a seizure thought to be independent of octreotide.

Precautions

Monitoring: Laboratory tests that may be helpful as biochemical markers in determining and following patient response depend on the specific tumor. Based on diagnosis, measurement of the following substances may be useful in monitoring the progress of therapy:

Acromegaly – Growth hormone, IGF-I. Responsiveness to octreotide may be evaluated by determining growth hormone levels at 1- to 4-hour intervals for 8 to 12 hours post dose; alternatively, a single measurement of IGF-I level may be made 2 weeks after drug initiation or dosage change.

Carcinoid – 5-HIAA (urinary 5-hydroxyindole acetic acid), plasma serotonin, plasma Substance P.

VIPoma – VIP (plasma vasoactive intestinal peptide).

Perform baseline and periodic total or free T_4 measurements during chronic use.

Hypo- or hyperglycemia: Hypo- or hyperglycemia that may occur during therapy usually is mild, but may result in overt diabetes mellitus or necessitate dose changes in insulin or other hypoglycemic agents.

Hypothyroidism: In acromegalic patients, 12% developed biochemical hypothyroidism, only 6% developed goiter, and 4% required initiation of thyroid replacement therapy while receiving octreotide. Baseline and periodic assessment of thyroid function (TSH, total or free T_4) is recommended during chronic therapy.

Cardiac effects: In acromegalics, bradycardia (< 50 bpm) developed in 21%; conduction abnormalities and arrhythmias each occurred in 9% of patients during therapy.

Other ECG changes observed included QT prolongation, axis shifts, early repolarization, low voltage, R/S transition, and early wave progression.

Pancreatitis: Several cases of pancreatitis occurred in patients receiving octreotide.

Dietary fat: Dietary fat absorption may be altered in some patients. Perform periodic quantitative 72-hour fecal fat and serum carotene determinations to aid in the assessment of possible drug-induced aggravation of fat malabsorption.

Drug Interactions

Cyclosporine: A single case of a transplant rejection episode (renal/whole pancreas) in a patient immunosuppressed with cyclosporine was reported.

Drug/Food interactions: Octreotide may alter the absorption of dietary fats in some patients. In addition, depressed vitamin B_{12} levels and abnormal Schilling's tests have been observed in some patients receiving octreotide; monitoring of vitamin B_{12} levels is recommended during chronic therapy.

Adverse Reactions

Adverse reactions include the following: Sinus bradycardia (> 20%); conduction abnormalities, arrhythmias (in acromegliacs), headache, injection site pain, hyperglycemia, hypoglycemia (in acromegliacs), biochemical hypothyroidism (in acromegliacs), loose stools, nausea, abdominal discomfort, vomiting, flatulence, abnormal stools, abdominal distention, constipation (≥ 3%).

OPIUM

Liquid: 10 mg anhydrous morphine equiv./mL (c-II)	*Opium Tincture, Deodorized* (Ranbaxy)
2 mg anhydrous morphine equiv./5 mL (c-III)	*Paregoric* (Various)

Indications

Diarrhea: For treatment of diarrhea.

Unlabeled uses:

Neonatal abstinence syndrome – Treatment of opioid-related drug withdrawal (neonates). Diluted opium tincture is the preferred treatment for neonatal withdrawal in newborns. Paregoric contains benzoic acid (an oxidative product of benzyl alcohol), usually camphor, and other ingredients that may have potentially toxic effects.

Management of short bowel syndrome – Used to slow gastric emptying and delay bowel transit time in short bowel syndrome.

Administration and Dosage

Caution: Opium tincture contains 25 times more morphine than paregoric. Do not confuse opium tincture with paregoric; this may lead to a potentially fatal overdose of morphine.

Opium tincture:

Adults – 0.6 mL (single dose < 1 mL) 4 times daily, maximum of 6 mL/day.

Paregoric:

Adults – 5 to 10 mL 1 to 4 times daily.

Children – 0.25 to 0.5 mL/kg 1 to 4 times daily.

Actions

Pharmacology:

Narcotic Agonist Comparative Pharmacology[1]

Drug	Analgesic	Antitussive	Constipation	Respiratory depression	Sedation	Emesis	Physical dependence
Phenanthrenes							
Codeine	+	+++	+	+	+	+	+
Hydrocodone	+	+++	nd[2]	+	nd[2]	nd[2]	+
Hydromorphone	++	+++	+	++	+	+	++
Levorphanol	++	++	++	++	++	+	++
Morphine	++	+++	++	++	++	++	++
Oxycodone	++	+++	++	++	++	++	++
Oxymorphone	++	+	++	+++	nd[2]	+++	+++
Phenylpiperidines							
Alfentanil	++	nd[2]	nd[2]	nd[2]	nd[2]	nd[2]	nd[2]
Fentanyl	++	nd[2]	nd[2]	+	nd[2]	+	nd[2]
Meperidine	++	+	+	++	+	nd[2]	++
Sufentanil	+++	nd[2]	nd[2]	nd[2]	nd[2]	nd[2]	nd[2]
Diphenylheptanes							
Levomethadyl	++	nd[2]	++	nd[2]	nd[2]	+	+
Methadone	++	++	++	++	+	+	+
Propoxyphene	+	nd[2]	nd[2]	+	+	+	+
Anilidopiperidines							
Remifentanil	+++	nd[2]	+	++	nd[2]	++	+

[1] Table adapted from Catalano RB. The medical approach to management of pain caused by cancer. *Semin Oncol.* 1975;2:379-392 and Reuler JB, et al. The chronic pain syndrome: misconceptions and management. *Ann Intern Med.* 1980;93:588-596.

[2] nd – No data available.

Pharmacokinetics:

Pharmacokinetics of Narcotic Agonist Analgesics[1]						
					Approximate equi-analgesic doses[3] (mg)	
Drug	Onset (minutes)	Peak (hours)	Duration[2] (hours)	t½ (hours)	Parenteral	Other
Alfentanil	immediate	nd[4]	nd[4]	1 to 2[5]	IM 0.4 to 0.8	nd[4]
Codeine	10 to 30	0.5 to 1	4 to 6	3	IM 120 to 130 SC 120	Oral 180 to 200[6]
Fentanyl	7 to 8	nd[4]	1 to 2	1.5 to 6	IM 0.1 to 0.2	Transdermal 25 mcg/h
Hydrocodone	nd[4]	nd[4]	4 to 6	3.3 to 4.5	nd[4]	Oral 30
Hydromorphone	15 to 30	0.5 to 1	4 to 5	2 to 3	IM 1.3 to 1.5 SC 1 to 1.5	Oral 7.5
Levomethadyl	2 to 4 h	1.5 to 2	48 to 72	2 to 6 days	nd[4]	nd[4]
Levorphanol	30 to 90	0.5 to 1	6 to 8	11 to 16	IM 2 SC 2	Oral 4
Meperidine	10 to 45	0.5 to 1	2 to 4	3 to 4	IM 75 SC 75 to 100	Oral 300[6]
Methadone	30 to 60	0.5 to 1	4 to 6[7]	15 to 30	IM 10 SC 8 to 10	Oral 10 to 20
Morphine	15 to 60[8]	0.5 to 1	3 to 7	1.5 to 2	IM 10 SC 10	Oral 30 to 60
Oxycodone	15 to 30	1	4 to 6	nd[4]	IM 10 to 15 SC 10 to 15	Oral 30[6]
Oxymorphone	5 to 10	0.5 to 1	3 to 6	nd[4]	IM 1 SC 1 to 1.5	Rectal 5, 10
Propoxyphene (PO)	30 to 60	2 to 2.5	4 to 6	6 to 12	nd[4]	Oral 130[9]
Remifentanil	1	1 min	short[10]	≈ 3 to 10 min	nd[4]	nd[4]
Sufentanil	1.3 to 3[5]	nd[4]	nd[4]	2.5	IM 0.01 to 0.04	nd[4]

[1] Caution: Recommended doses do not apply for adult patients with body weight < 50 kg. Recommended doses do not apply to patients with renal or hepatic insufficiency or other conditions affecting drug metabolism and kinetics.
[2] After IV administration, peak effects may be more pronounced but duration is shorter. Duration of action may be longer with the oral route.
[3] Based on morphine 10 mg IM or SC. The initial dose of the new drug is given at ½ to ⅔ of the calculated dose because opioid-specific tolerance may occur, and the new drug may have more relative effectiveness (and more side effects) than the drug being discontinued.
[4] nd – No data available.
[5] Data based on IV administration.
[6] Starting doses lower (codeine, 30 mg; oxycodone, 5 mg; meperidine, 50 mg).
[7] Duration and half-life increase with repeated use because of cumulative effects.
[8] Data based on intrathecal or epidural administration.
[9] Starting doses lower (propoxyphene, 65 to 130 mg). In equimolar doses (100 mg of napsylate equals 65 mg of HCl).
[10] The duration of action does not increase with prolonged administration.

Contraindications

Opium: Opium tincture in children; diarrhea caused by poisoning until the toxic material has been eliminated.

Warnings

Caution: Opium tincture contains 25 times more morphine than paregoric. Do not confuse opium tincture with paregoric; this may lead to a potentially fatal overdose of morphine. It is best to dispense to the nursery diluted opium tincture that contains a concentration of morphine equivalent to the concentration in paregoric.

PANCREATIC ENZYMES

PANCRELIPASE	
Tablets: 8000 units lipase, 30,000 units protease, 30,000 units amylase (*Rx*)	*Pancrelipase* (Various), *Viokase* (Axcan Scandipharm)
Capsules: 1200 units lipase, 15,000 units protease, 15,000 units amylase (*Rx*)	*Ku-Zyme* (Schwarz Pharma)
2400 units lipase, 30,000 units protease, 30,000 units amylase(*Rx*)	*Kutrase* (Schwarz Pharma)
4000 units lipase, 12,000 units protease, 12,000 units amylase (*Rx*)	*Pancrease MT 4* (McNeil)
4500 units lipase, 25,000 units protease, 20,000 units amylase (*Rx*)	*Pancrease* (McNeil), *Lipram* (Global), *Ultrase* (Axcan Scandipharm)
8000 units lipase, 30,000 units protease, 30,000 units amylase (*Rx*)	*Ku-Zyme HP* (Schwarz Pharma)
10,000 units lipase, 30,000 units protease, 30,000 units amylase (*Rx*)	*Lipram-PN10* (Global), *Pancrease MT 10* (McNeil)
10,000 units lipase, 37,500 units protease, 33,200 units amylase (*Rx*)	*Creon 10* (Solvay)
12,000 units lipase, 24,000 units protease, 24,000 units amylase (*Rx*)	*Zymase* (Organon)
12,000 units lipase, 39,000 units protease, 39,000 units amylase (*Rx*)	*Lipram-UL12* (Global), *Ultrase MT 12* (Axcan Scandipharm)
16,000 units lipase, 48,000 units protease, 48,000 units amylase (*Rx*)	*Lipram-PN16* (Global), *Pancrease MT 16* (McNeil)
18,000 units lipase, 58,500 units protease, 58,500 units amylase (*Rx*)	*Lipram-UL18* (Global), *Ultrase MT 18* (Axcan Scandipharm)
20,000 units lipase, 44,000 units protease, 56,000 units amylase (*Rx*)	*Pancrease MT 20* (McNeil)
20,000 units lipase, 65,000 units protease, 65,000 units amylase (*Rx*)	*Lipram-UL20* (Global), *Ultrase MT 20* (Axcan Scandipharm)
20,000 units lipase, 75,000 units protease, 66,400 units amylase (*Rx*)	*Creon 20* (Solvay), *Lipram-CR20* (Global)
Powder: 16,800 units lipase, 70,000 units protease, 70,000 units amylase per 0.7 g (*Rx*)	*Viokase* (Axcan Scandipharm)
PANCREATIN	
Tablets: 2400 mg pancreatin, 4800 units lipase, 60,000 units protease, 60,000 units amylase (*Rx*)	*Hi-Vegi-Lip* (Freeda)
2400 mg pancreatin, 12,000 units lipase, 60,000 units protease, 60,000 units amylase (*Rx*)	*4X Pancreatin 600 mg* (Vitaline)
7200 mg pancreatin, 22,500 units lipase, 180,000 units protease, 180,000 units amylase (*Rx*)	*8X Pancreatin 900 mg* (Vitaline)

Indications

Enzyme replacement therapy in patients with deficient exocrine pancreatic secretions, cystic fibrosis, chronic pancreatitis, postpancreatectomy, ductal obstructions caused by cancer of the pancreas or common bile duct, pancreatic insufficiency and for steatorrhea of malabsorption syndrome and postgastrectomy (Billroth II and Total), or post-GI surgery (eg, Billroth II gastroenterostomy).

Presumptive test for pancreatic function, especially in pancreatic insufficiency caused by chronic pancreatitis.

Administration and Dosage

Microspheres/Microtablets: To protect enteric coating, do not crush or chew the microspheres or microtablets. When swallowing capsules is difficult, they may be opened and shaken onto a small quantity of soft, non-hot food (eg, applesauce, gelatin) that does not require chewing. Swallow immediately without chewing as the proteolytic action may cause irritation of the mucosa. Follow with a glass of juice or water to ensure complete swallowing of the microspheres/microtablets. Contact of the microspheres/microtablets with foods with a pH > 5.5 can dissolve the protective enteric shell. Use any mixture of food or liquid with the microspheres/microtablets immediately; do not store.

Brand interchange: These products are not bioequivalent. Therefore, do not substitute one brand for another without first consulting the physician.

PANCRELIPASE: Adjust dosage according to the severity of the exocrine pancreatic enzyme deficiency. Estimate dosage by assessing which dose minimizes steatorrhea and maintains good nutritional status. The assessment of the endpoints in children is aided by charting growth curves.

Capsules and tablets –

Children:

< 6 months of age – Dosage not established.

6 months to 1 year of age – 2000 units lipase per meal.

1 to 6 years of age – 4000 to 8000 units lipase with each meal and 4000 units with snacks.

7 to 12 years of age – 4000 to 12,000 units lipase (or more if necessary) with each meal and with snacks.

Adults: 4000 to 48,000 units lipase with each meal and with snacks.

In patients with pancreatectomy or obstruction of pancreatic ducts, administer 8000 to 16,000 units lipase at 2 hour intervals or as directed by physician (*Viokase*). In severe deficiencies, the dose may be increased to 64,000 to 88,000 units lipase with meals or the frequency of administration may be increased to hourly intervals if nausea, cramps, or diarrhea do not occur.

Powder (in cystic fibrosis) – 0.7 g with meals.

PANCREATIN: Take 1 to 2 tablets with meals or snacks. Adjust according to individual requirements for control of steatorrhea.

Actions

Pharmacology: Pancreatin and pancrelipase hydrolyze fats to glycerol and fatty acids, change protein into proteoses and derived substances, and convert starch into dextrins and sugars. Administration reduces the fat and nitrogen content in the stool. These agents exert their primary effects in the duodenum and upper jejunum. Pancreatic enzymes normally are secreted in great excess. There is a 10-fold reserve for exocrine pancreatic enzyme secretion. Generally, steatorrhea and malabsorption occur only after a ≥ 90% reduction in secretion of lipase and proteolytic enzymes. It has been estimated that ≈ 8000 units/hr of lipase should be delivered into the duodenum postprandially. Even if all of the enzymes taken orally reached the proximal intestine in active form, ingestion of 24,000 units of lipase (8000 units/hr) for 3 postprandial hours would be required. If one could deliver sufficient pancreatic enzymes to the small intestine, malabsorption could be corrected. It rarely is possible to achieve complete relief of steatorrhea, although major improvement in fat absorption can be achieved in most patients.

There are many factors that may influence the ability to deliver pancreatic enzymes to the duodenum, including asynchrony of gastric emptying of food and enzyme, sensitivity of pancreatic enzymes to permanent inactivation by gastric acid and pepsin secreted in response to the meal, and acidic precipitation of bile acids.

Pancreatic lipase is irreversibly inactivated at pH ≤ 4. An enteric coating may prevent destruction or inactivation by gastric pepsin and acid pH, but may inhibit enzyme delivery to the duodenum. Cimetidine or antacids may increase the amount of pancreatin in the duodenum by decreasing its destruction by the gastric acid.

Pancreatic Extract Activity

		Minimal USP standards (USP units/mg)		
Enzyme concentrate	Source	Lipase	Protease	Amylase
Pancrelipase	Porcine	24	100	100
Pancreatin	Bovine, porcine, or vegetable	2	25	25

Warnings

Replacement therapy: Pancreatic exocrine replacement therapy should not delay or supplant treatment of the primary disorder.

Pregnancy: Category C. Give to a pregnant woman only if clearly needed.

Lactation: It is not known whether pancreatin is excreted in breast milk. Exercise caution when administering to a nursing mother.

Precautions

Excessive doses: Excessive doses may cause nausea, abdominal cramps, or diarrhea. Extremely high doses have been associated with hyperuricosuria and hyperuricemia.

Pork sensitivity: Use pork products with caution in patients sensitive to pork. Discontinue use if symptoms of sensitivity appear and initiate symptomatic and supportive treatment if necessary. Individuals previously sensitized to trypsin, pancreatin, or pancrelipase may have allergic reactions.

Irritation of skin/mucous membranes: Do not spill powder on hands because it may irritate skin. The dust of finely powdered concentrates irritates the nasal mucosa and the respiratory tract. Inhalation of airborne powder can precipitate an asthma attack. Asthma also can occur in patients sensitized to pancreatic enzyme concentrates.

Drug Interactions

Pancreatic enzymes may interact with antacids and iron.

Adverse Reactions

The most frequently reported adverse reactions are GI in nature. Less frequently, allergic-type reactions also have been observed. Perianal irritation and, rarely, inflammation (with large doses) may occur with pancreatin.

PEGINTERFERON ALFA-2B

Powder for injection, lyophilized: 100, 160, 240, and 300 mcg/mL (*Rx*)	*PEG-Intron* (Schering)

Warning:

Alpha interferons, including peginterferon alfa-2b, cause or aggravate fatal or life-threatening neuropsychiatric, autoimmune, ischemic, and infectious disorders. Closely monitor patients with periodic clinical and laboratory evaluations. Withdraw from therapy patients with persistently severe or worsening signs or symptoms of these conditions. In many but not all cases, these disorders resolve after stopping peginterferon alfa-2b therapy.

Indications

Chronic hepatitis C: As monotherapy for the treatment of chronic hepatitis C in patients not previously treated with interferon alpha who have compensated liver disease and are ≥ 18 years of age. The safety and effectiveness of peginterferon alfa-2b in combination with ribavirin for the treatment of chronic hepatitis C have not been established.

Unlabeled uses: Renal carcinoma.

Administration and Dosage

Patients should self-inject only if the physician determines that it is appropriate and patients agree to medical follow-up as necessary and receive training in proper injection technique.

Peginterferon alfa-2b is administered SC once weekly for 1 year. Administer the dose on the same day of each week. Base initial dosing on weight, as described in the following table.

Recommended Dosing of Peginterferon Alfa-2b

Vial strength[1] to use (mcg/mL)	Weight (kg)	Amount of peginterferon alfa-2b to administer (mcg)	Volume of peginterferon alfa-2b to administer (mL)
100	37 to 45	40	0.4
	46 to 56	50	0.5
160	57 to 72	64	0.4
	73 to 88	80	0.5
240	89 to 106	96	0.4
	107 to 136	120	0.5
300	137 to 160	150	0.5

[1] When reconstituted as directed.

Assess serum hepatitis C virus (HCV) RNA levels after 24 weeks of treatment. Consider discontinuation of treatment in any patient who has not achieved an HCV RNA below the limit of detection of the assay after 24 weeks of therapy with peginterferon alfa-2b.

There are no safety and efficacy data for treatment ≥ 48 weeks or for retreatment of patients who relapse following peginterferon alfa-2b therapy.

Dose reduction: If a serious adverse reaction develops during the course of treatment discontinue or modify the dosage of peginterferon alfa-2b to 50% of the starting dosage until the adverse reaction abates or decreases in severity. If persistent or recurrent intolerance develops despite adequate dosage adjustment, discontinue treatment with peginterferon alfa-2b. For dose modification in the event of neutropenia and thrombocytopenia, refer to the following table.

Guidelines for Dose Modifications of Peginterferon Alfa-2b for Neutropenia and Thrombocytopenia		
	Dose reduction	Permanent discontinuation
Neutrophil count	$< 0.75 \times 10^9$/L	$< 0.50 \times 10^9$/L
Platelet count	$< 80 \times 10^9$/L	$< 50 \times 10^9$/L

Actions

Pharmacology: The biological activity of peginterferon alfa-2b is derived from its interferon alfa-2b moiety. Interferons exert their cellular activities by binding to specific membrane receptors on the cell surface and initiate a complex sequence of intracellular events.

Pharmacokinetics:

Absorption/Distribution – Maximal serum concentrations (C_{max}) occur between 15 and 44 hours postdose and are sustained for ≤ 48 to 72 hours.

Metabolism/Excretion – The mean peginterferon alfa-2b elimination half-life is ≈ 40 hours (range, 22 to 60 hours) in patients with HCV infection. The apparent clearance of peginterferon alfa-2b is estimated to be ≈ 22 mL/hr•kg. Renal elimination accounts for 30% of the clearance.

Pegylation of interferon alfa-2b produces a product (peginterferon alfa-2b) whose clearance is lower than that of nonpegylated interferon alfa-2b. When compared to interferon alfa-2b, peginterferon alfa-2b (1 mcg/kg) has an ≈ 7-fold lower mean apparent clearance and a 5-fold greater mean half life permitting a reduced dosing frequency.

Contraindications

Hypersensitivity to peginterferon alfa-2b or any component of the product; autoimmune hepatitis; decompensated liver disease.

Warnings

Hypersensitivity reactions: Serious, acute hypersensitivity reactions (eg, urticaria, angioedema, bronchoconstriction, anaphylaxis) have been rarely observed during alpha interferon therapy.

Renal function impairment: Closely monitor patients with impairment of renal function for signs and symptoms of interferon toxicity and adjust doses of peginterferon alfa-2b accordingly. Use peginterferon alfa-2b with caution in patients with Ccr < 50 mL/min.

Elderly: Treatment with alpha interferons, including peginterferon alfa-2b, is associated with CNS, cardiac, and systemic (flu-like) adverse effects. Because these adverse reactions may be more severe in the elderly, exercise caution in the use of interferon alfa-2b in this population.

Pregnancy: Category C. Peginterferon alfa-2b should be assumed to have abortifacient potential. Use during pregnancy only if the potential benefit justifies the potential risk to the fetus. Therefore, peginterferon alfa-2b is recommended for use in fertile women only when they are using effective contraception during the treatment period.

Lactation: It is not known whether the components of interferon alfa-2b are excreted in human milk.

Children: Safety and efficacy in pediatric patients < 18 years of age have not been established.

Precautions

Neuropsychiatric events: Life-threatening or fatal neuropsychiatric events, including suicide, suicidal and homicidal ideation, depression, relapse of drug addiction/overdose, and aggressive behavior have occurred in patients with and without a previous psychiatric disorder during peginterferon alfa-2b treatment and follow-up. Psychoses and hallucinations have been observed in patients treated with alpha interferons.

Bone marrow toxicity: Peginterferon alfa-2b suppresses bone marrow function, sometimes resulting in severe cytopenias. Discontinue peginterferon alfa-2b in patients who develop severe decreases in neutrophil or platelet counts. Very rarely, alpha interferons may be associated with aplastic anemia.

Colitis: Fatal and nonfatal ulcerative and hemorrhagic colitis have been observed within 12 weeks of the start of alpha-interferon treatment. Abdominal pain, bloody diarrhea, and fever are the typical manifestations. Immediately discontinue peginterferon alfa-2b in patients who develop these symptoms and signs. The colitis usually resolves within 1 to 3 weeks of discontinuation of alpha interferons.

Pancreatitis: Fatal and nonfatal pancreatitis have been observed in patients treated with alpha interferon. Suspend peginterferon alfa-2b therapy in patients with signs and symptoms suggestive of pancreatitis and discontinue in patients diagnosed with pancreatitis.

Pulmonary disorders: Dyspnea, pulmonary infiltrates, pneumonitis, and pneumonia, some resulting in patient deaths, have been associated with peginterferon alfa-2b or alpha-interferon therapy. Closely monitor patients with pulmonary infiltrates or pulmonary function impairment.

Immunogenicity: One percent of patients receiving peginterferon alfa-2b developed low-titer (≤ 64) neutralizing antibodies to interferon alfa-2b. The clinical and pathological significance of the appearance of serum neutralizing antibodies is unknown.

Special risk:

Endocrine disorders – Peginterferon alfa-2b causes or aggravates hypothyroidism and hyperthyroidism. Hyperglycemia has been observed in patients treated with interferon alfa-2b. Diabetes mellitus has been observed in patients treated with alpha interferons.

Cardiovascular events – Cardiovascular events, including hypotension, arrhythmia, tachycardia, cardiomyopathy, and MI, have been observed in patients treated with peginterferon alfa-2b.

Autoimmune disorders – Development or exacerbation of autoimmune disorders (eg, thyroiditis, thrombocytopenia, rheumatoid arthritis, interstitial nephritis, systemic lupus erythematosus, psoriasis) have been observed in patients receiving peginterferon alfa-2b.

Ophthalmologic disorders – Retinal hemorrhages, cotton wool spots, and retinal artery or vein obstruction have been observed after treatment with peginterferon alfa-2b or alpha interferons.

Lab test abnormalities: Peginterferon alfa-2b may cause severe decreases in neutrophil and platelet counts and abnormality of TSH. In 10% of patients treated with peginterferon alfa-2b, ALT levels rose 2- to 5-fold above baseline. The elevations were transient and were not associated with deterioration of other liver functions.

Patients on peginterferon alfa-2b therapy should have hematology and blood chemistry testing before the start of treatment and then periodically thereafter.

Drug Interactions

It is not known if peginterferon alfa-2b therapy causes clinically significant drug interactions with drugs metabolized by the liver in patients with hepatitis C.

Adverse Reactions

Adverse reactions occurring in ≥ 3% of patients include the following: Headache; depression; anxiety/emotional lability/irritability; insomnia; dizziness; alopecia; pruritus; dry skin; sweating increased; rash; flushing; nausea; anorexia; diarrhea; abdominal pain; vomiting; dyspepsia; thrombocytopenia; neutropenia; pharyngitis; sinusitis; coughing; musculoskeletal pain; fatigue; injection site inflammation/reaction; influenza-like symptoms; rigors; fever; weight decrease; viral infection; right upper quadrant pain; malaise; hepatomegaly; hypertonia; hypothyroidism.

POTASSIUM-SPARING DIURETICS

Actions

Pharmacology: In the kidney, potassium is filtered at the glomerulus and then absorbed parallel to sodium throughout the proximal tubule and thick ascending limb of the loop of Henle, so that only minor amounts reach the distal convoluted tubule. As a result, potassium appearing in urine is secreted at the distal tubule and collecting duct. The potassium-sparing diuretics interfere with sodium reabsorption at the distal tubule, thus decreasing potassium secretion. They exert a weak diuretic and antihypertensive effect when used alone. Their major use is to enhance the action and counteract the kaliuretic effect of thiazide and loop diuretics.

Spironolactone – Spironolactone, a competitive inhibitor of aldosterone, binds to aldosterone receptors of the distal tubule and prevents the formation of a protein important in sodium transport. It is effective in primary and secondary hyperaldosteronism. Spironolactone is effective in lowering systolic and diastolic blood pressure in primary hyperaldosteronism and essential hypertension, although aldosterone secretion may be normal in benign essential hypertension.

Amiloride and triamterene – **Amiloride** and **triamterene** not only inhibit sodium reabsorption induced by aldosterone, but they also inhibit basal sodium reabsorption. They are not aldosterone antagonists, but act directly on the renal distal tubule, cortical collecting tubule and collecting duct. They induce a reversal of polarity of the transtubular electrical-potential difference and inhibit active transport of sodium and potassium. Amiloride may inhibit sodium, potassium-ATPase.

Potassium-Sparing Diuretics: Pharmacological and Pharmacokinetic Properties

Parameters	Amiloride	Spironolactone	Triamterene
Pharmacology			
Tubular site of action	Proximal = distal	Distal	Distal
Mechanism of action	Na^+, K^+–ATPase inhibition; Na^+/H^+ exchange mechanism inhibition (proximal tubule)	Aldosterone antagonism	Membrane effect
Action:			
Onset (hours)	2	24 to 48	2 to 4
Peak (hours)	6 to 10	48 to 72	6 to 8
Duration (hours)	24	48 to 72	12 to 16
Pharmacokinetics			
Bioavailability	15% to 25%	> 90%	30% to 70%
Protein binding	23%	≥ 98%[1]	50% to 67%
Half-life (hours)	6 to 9	20[2]	3
Active metabolites	none	canrenone	hydroxytriamterene sulfate
Peak plasma levels (hours)	3 to 4	canrenone: 2 to 4	3
Excreted unchanged in urine	≈ 50%[3]	†[4]	≈ 21%
Dosage			
Daily dose (mg)	5 to 20	25 to 400	200 to 300

[1] Canrenone > 98%.
[2] 10 to 35 hours for canrenone.
[3] 40% excreted in stool within 72 hours.
[4] Metabolites primarily excreted in urine, but also in bile.

AMILORIDE HCl

Tablets: 5 mg (*Rx*)	*Midamor* (Merck)

Indications

Adjunctive treatment with thiazide or loop diuretics in CHF or hypertension to: Help restore normal serum potassium in patients who develop hypokalemia on the kaliuretic diuretic; prevent hypokalemia in patients who would be at particular risk if hypokalemia were to develop (eg, digitalized patients or patients with significant cardiac arrhythmias).

Unlabeled uses: Amiloride (10 to 20 mg/day) may be useful in reducing lithium-induced polyuria without increasing lithium levels as is seen with thiazide diuretics.

Administration and Dosage

Administer with food.

Concomitant therapy: Add amiloride 5 mg/day to the usual antihypertensive or diuretic dosage of a kaliuretic diuretic. Increase dosage to 10 mg/day, if necessary; doses > 10 mg are usually not needed. If persistent hypokalemia is documented with 10 mg, increase the dose to 15 mg, then 20 mg, with careful titration of the dose and careful monitoring of electrolytes.

In patients with CHF, potassium loss may decrease after an initial diuresis; reevaluate the need or dosage for amiloride. Maintenance therapy may be intermittent.

Single drug therapy: The starting dose is 5 mg/day. Increase to 10 mg/day, if necessary; doses > 10 mg are usually not needed. If persistent hypokalemia is documented with 10 mg, increase the dose to 15 mg, then 20 mg, with careful monitoring of electrolytes.

Contraindications

Hypersensitivity to amiloride; serum potassium > 5.5 mEq/L; antikaliuretic therapy or potassium supplementation; renal function impairment patients receiving spironolactone or triamaterene.

Warnings

Hyperkalemia: Amiloride may cause hyperkalemia (serum potassium > 5.5 mEq/L) that, if uncorrected, is potentially fatal. Monitor serum potassium carefully. Symptoms of hyperkalemia include paresthesias, muscular weakness, fatigue, flaccid paralysis of the extremities, bradycardia, shock, and ECG abnormalities.

Diabetes mellitus: Avoid use of amiloride in diabetic patients. If it is used, monitor serum electrolytes and renal function frequently. Discontinue use ≥ 3 days before glucose tolerance testing.

Metabolic or respiratory acidosis: Cautiously institute amiloride in severely ill patients in whom respiratory or metabolic acidosis may occur, such as patients with cardiopulmonary disease or poorly controlled diabetes. Monitor acid-base balance frequently. Shifts in acid-base balance alter the ratio of extracellular/intracellular potassium; the development of acidosis may be associated with rapid increases in serum potassium.

Renal function impairment: Anuria, acute or chronic renal insufficiency and evidence of diabetic nephropathy are contraindications because potassium retention is accentuated and may result in the rapid development of hyperkalemia. Do not give to patients with evidence of renal impairment (BUN > 30 mg/dL or serum creatinine > 1.5 mg/dL) or diabetes mellitus without continuous monitoring of serum electrolytes, creatinine, and BUN levels.

Hepatic function impairment: In patients with preexisting severe liver disease, hepatic encephalopathy (manifested by tremors, confusion, and coma, and increased jaundice) may occur. Because amiloride is not metabolized by the liver, drug accumulation is not anticipated in patients with hepatic dysfunction, but accumulation can occur if hepatorenal syndrome develops.

Pregnancy: Category B.

Lactation: It is not known whether amiloride is excreted in breast milk.

Children: Safety and efficacy for use in children have not been established.

Precautions

Electrolyte imbalance and BUN increases: Hyponatremia and hypochloremia may occur when amiloride is used with other diuretics. Increases in BUN levels usually accompany vigorous fluid elimination, especially when diuretic therapy is used in seriously ill patients, such as those who have hepatic cirrhosis with ascites and metabolic alkalosis, or those with resistant edema.

Drug Interactions

Drugs that may interact include digoxin, potassium preparations, ACE inhibitors, and NSAIDs.

Adverse Reactions

Possible adverse reactions include headache, nausea, anorexia, diarrhea, vomiting.

SPIRONOLACTONE

Tablets: 25, 50, and 100 mg (*Rx*)	Various, *Aldactone* (Searle)

Indications

Primary hyperaldosteronism: Diagnosis of primary hyperaldosteronism.

Short-term preoperative treatment of patients with primary hyperaldosteronism.

Long-term maintenance therapy for patients with discrete aldosterone-producing adrenal adenomas who are poor operative risks, or who decline surgery.

Long-term maintenance therapy for patients with bilateral micronodular or macronodular adrenal hyperplasia (idiopathic hyperaldosteronism).

Edematous conditions when other therapies are inappropriate or inadequate:

CHF – Management of edema and sodium retention; also indicated with digitalis.

Cirrhosis of the liver accompanied by edema or ascites – For maintenance therapy in conjunction with bed rest and the restriction of fluid and sodium.

Nephrotic syndrome.

Essential hypertension: Usually in combination with other drugs.

Hypokalemia: Hypokalemia and the prophylaxis of hypokalemia in patients taking digitalis.

Unlabeled uses: Spironolactone has been used in the treatment of hirsutism (50 to 200 mg/day) due to its antiandrogenic properties. One study suggested that a lower dosage (50 mg twice/day on days 4 through 21 of the menstrual cycle) may help minimize the risk of metrorrhagia that occurs with higher doses.

Symptoms of premenstrual syndrome (PMS) have been relieved at a dosage of 25 mg 4 times daily beginning on day 14 of the menstrual cycle.

The combination of spironolactone (2 mg/kg/day) and testolactone (20 to 40 mg/kg/day) for ≥ 6 months may be effective for short-term treatment of familial male precocious puberty.

Spironolactone 100 mg/day appears effective in short-term treatment of acne vulgaris.

Administration and Dosage

Spironolactone may be administered in single or divided doses.

Diagnosis of primary hyperaldosteronism: As initial diagnostic measure to provide presumptive evidence of primary hyperaldosteronism in patients on normal diets, as follows:

Long test – 400 mg/day for 3 to 4 weeks. Correction of hypokalemia and hypertension provides presumptive evidence for diagnosis of primary hyperaldosteronism.

Short test – 400 mg/day for 4 days. If serum potassium increases but decreases when spironolactone is discontinued, consider a presumptive diagnosis of primary hyperaldosteronism.

Maintenance therapy for hyperaldosteronism: 100 to 400 mg/day in preparation for surgery. For patients unsuitable for surgery, employ the drug for long-term maintenance therapy at lowest possible dose.

Edema:

Adults (CHF, hepatic cirrhosis, nephrotic syndrome) – Initially, 100 mg/day (range, 25 to 200 mg/day). When given as the sole diuretic agent, continue for ≥ 5 days at the initial dosage level, then adjust to the optimal level. If after 5 days an adequate diuretic response has not occurred, add a second diuretic, which acts more proximally in the renal tubule. Because of the additive effect of spironolactone with such diuretics, an enhanced diuresis usually begins on the first day of combined treatment; combined therapy is indicated when more rapid diuresis is desired. Spironolactone dosage should remain unchanged when other diuretic therapy is added.

Children – 3.3 mg/kg/day (1.5 mg/lb/day) administered in single or divided doses.

Essential hypertension:

Adults – Initially, 50 to 100 mg/day in single or divided doses. May also be combined with diuretics, which act more proximally, and with other antihypertensive agents. Continue treatment for ≥ 2 weeks because the maximal response may not occur sooner. Individualize dosage.

Children – A dose of 1 to 2 mg/kg twice/day has been recommended.

Hypokalemia: 25 to 100 mg/day. Useful in treating diuretic-induced hypokalemia when oral potassium supplements or other potassium-sparing regimens are considered inappropriate.

Contraindications

Anuria; acute renal insufficiency; significant impairment of renal function; hyperkalemia; patients receiving amiloride or triamterene.

Warnings

Hyperkalemia: Carefully evaluate patients for possible fluid and electrolyte balance disturbances. Hyperkalemia may occur with impaired renal function or excessive potassium intake and can cause cardiac irregularities that may be fatal. Ordinarily, do not give potassium supplements with spironolactone.

Renal function impairment: Use of spironolactone may cause a transient elevation of BUN, especially in patients with preexisting renal impairment. The drug may cause mild acidosis.

Carcinogenesis: Spironolactone was a tumorigen in chronic toxicity studies in rats.

Pregnancy: Spironolactone or its metabolites may cross the placental barrier.

Lactation: Canrenone, a metabolite of spironolactone, appears in breast milk. The labeling suggests that an alternative method of infant feeding be instituted when using spironolactone; however, the American Academy of Pediatrics considers the drug to be compatible with breastfeeding.

Precautions

Hyponatremia: Hyponatremia may be caused or aggravated by spironolactone, especially in combination with other diuretics. Symptoms include dry mouth, thirst, lethargy, drowsiness.

Gynecomastia: Gynecomastia may develop and appears to be related to dosage and duration of therapy. It is normally reversible when therapy is discontinued.

Reversible hyperchloremic metabolic acidosis: Reversible hyperchloremic metabolic acidosis, usually in association with hyperkalemia, occurs in some patients with decompensated hepatic cirrhosis, even in the presence of normal renal function.

Drug Interactions

Drugs that may affect spironolactone include ACE inhibitors, salicylates, and food. Drugs that may be affected by spironolactone include anticoagulants, digitalis glycosides, mitotane, digoxin, and potassium preparations.

Adverse Reactions

Adverse reactions are usually reversible upon discontinuation of the drug.

Possible adverse reactions include cramping; diarrhea; gastric bleeding; ulceration; gastritis; vomiting; drowsiness; lethargy; headache; mental confusion; ataxia; irregular menses; carcinoma of the breast.

TRIAMTERENE

Capsules: 50 and 100 mg *(Rx)* — *Dyrenium* (Wellspring Pharmaceuticals)

Indications

Edema: Edema associated with CHF, hepatic cirrhosis, and the nephrotic syndrome; steroid-induced edema, idiopathic edema, and edema due to secondary hyperaldosteronism.

May be used alone or with other diuretics, either for additive diuretic effect or antikaliuretic (potassium-sparing) effect. It promotes increased diuresis in patients resistant or only partially responsive to other diuretics because of secondary hyperaldosteronism.

Administration and Dosage

Individualize dosage.

When used alone, the usual starting dose is 100 mg twice/daily after meals. When combined with other diuretics or antihypertensives, decrease the total daily dosage of each agent initially, and then adjust to the patient's needs. Do not exceed 300 mg/day.

Contraindications

Patients receiving spironolactone or amiloride; anuria; severe hepatic disease; hyperkalemia; hypersensitivity to triamterene; severe or progressive kidney disease or dysfunction, with the possible exception of nephrosis; preexisting elevated serum potassium (impaired renal function, azotemia) or patients who develop hyperkalemia while on triamterene.

Warnings

Hyperkalemia: Abnormal elevation of serum potassium levels (≥ 5.5 mEq/L) can occur. Hyperkalemia is more likely to occur in patients with renal impairment and diabetes (even without evidence of renal impairment), and in the elderly or severely ill. Because uncorrected hyperkalemia may be fatal, serum potassium levels must be monitored at frequent intervals, especially when dosages are changed or with any illness that may influence renal function.

When triamterene is added to other diuretic therapy, or when patients are switched to triamterene from other diuretics, discontinue potassium supplementation.

Hypersensitivity reactions: Monitor patients regularly for blood dyscrasias, liver damage, or other idiosyncratic reactions.

Renal function impairment: Perform periodic BUN and serum potassium determinations to check kidney function, especially in patients with suspected or confirmed renal insufficiency and in elderly or diabetic patients; diabetic patients with nephropathy are especially prone to develop hyperkalemia.

Hepatic function impairment: Triamterene is extensively metabolized in the liver. The overall diuretic response may not be affected.

Pregnancy: Category B.

Lactation: If the drug is essential, the patient should stop nursing.

Children: Safety and efficacy have not been established.

Precautions

Electrolyte imbalance: In CHF, renal disease, or cirrhosis, electrolyte imbalance may be aggravated or caused by diuretics. The use of full doses of a diuretic when salt intake is restricted can result in a low salt syndrome.

Renal stones: Triamterene has been found in renal stones with other usual calculus components. Use cautiously in patients with histories of stone formation.

Hematologic effects: Triamterene is a weak folic acid antagonist. Because cirrhotics with splenomegaly may have marked variations in hematological status, it may contribute to the appearance of megaloblastosis in cases where folic acid stores have been depleted. Perform periodic blood studies in these patients.

Metabolic acidosis: Triamterene may cause decreasing alkali reserve with a possibility of metabolic acidosis.

Diabetes mellitus: Triamterene may raise blood glucose levels for adult-onset diabetes; dosage adjustments of hypoglycemic agents may be necessary. Concurrent use with chlorpropamide may increase the risk of severe hyponatremia.

Photosensitivity: Photosensitization is likely to occur; avoid prolonged exposure to sunlight.

Drug Interactions

Drugs that may affect triamterene include ACE inhibitors, cimetidine, and indomethacin. Drugs that may be affected by triamterene include amantadine and potassium preparations. Triamterene will interfere with the fluorescent measurement of quinidine serum levels.

Adverse Reactions

Diarrhea; nausea; vomiting; jaundice; liver enzyme abnormalities. Azotemia; elevated BUN/creatinine; increased serum uric acid levels (in patients predisposed to gouty arthritis); thrombocytopenia; megaloblastic anemia; weakness; dizziness; hypokalemia; headache; dry mouth; anaphylaxis.

PROTON PUMP INHIBITORS

OMEPRAZOLE	
Capsules, delayed release: 10 mg, 20 mg (Rx)	*Prilosec* (AstraZeneca)
LANSOPRAZOLE	
Capsules, delayed release: 15 mg, 30 mg (Rx)	*Prevacid* (TAP Pharm.)
RABEPRAZOLE	
Tablets, delayed release: 20 mg (Rx)	*Aciphex* (Eisai/Janssen)
PANTOPRAZOLE	
Tablets, delayed release: 20 and 40 mg (Rx)	*Protonix* (Wyeth-Ayerst)
Powder for injection, freeze-dried: 40 mg/vial (Rx)	*Protonix I.V.* (Wyeth-Ayerst)
ESOMEPRAZOLE	
Capsules, delayed release: 20 mg, 40 mg (Rx)	*Nexium* (AstraZeneca)

Indications

Gastric ulcers: For treatment or symptomatic relief of various gastric disorders including gastric and duodenal ulcers, gastroesophageal reflux disease (GERD), erosive esophagitis, or pathological hypersecretory conditions.

IV (pantoprazole): Short-term treatment (7 to 10 days) of GERD, as an alternative to oral therapy in patients who are unable to continue taking oral pantoprazole. Safety and efficacy of IV pantoprazole as initial treatment for GERD have not been established.

Unlabeled uses: Posterior laryngitis (**omeprazole** 40 mg at bedtime 6 to 24 weeks); enhanced efficacy of pancreatin (for treatment of steatorrhea in cystic fibrosis patients).

Administration and Dosage

OMEPRAZOLE: Take before eating. Do not open, crush, or chew the capsule; swallow whole. In clinical trials, antacids were used concomitantly with omeprazole.

Duodenal ulcer –

Treatment: 20 mg daily for 4 to 8 weeks; most patients heal within 4 weeks, although some may require an additional 4 weeks.

Associated with H. pylori:

Triple therapy (omeprazole/clarithromycin/amoxicillin) – Omeprazole 20 mg plus clarithromycin 500 mg plus amoxicillin 1000 mg each given twice daily for 10 days. If an ulcer is present at the initiation of therapy, continue omeprazole 20 mg for an additional 18 days.

Dual therapy (omeprazole/clarithromycin) – Omeprazole 40 mg once daily plus clarithromycin 500 mg 3 times daily for 14 days. If an ulcer is present at the initiation of therapy, continue omeprazole 20 mg for an additional 14 days.

Gastric ulcer, treatment – 40 mg once a day for 4 to 8 weeks.

Erosive esophagitis –

Treatment: 20 mg daily for 4 to 8 weeks.

Maintenance: 20 mg daily.

GERD –

GERD without esophageal lesions: 20 mg daily for 4 weeks.

GERD with erosive esophagitis: 20 mg daily for 4 to 8 weeks.

Pathological hypersecretory conditions – Individualize dosage. Initial adult dose is 60 mg/day. Doses up to 120 mg 3 times/day have been administered. Administer daily dosages > 80 mg in divided doses.

No dosage adjustment is necessary for patients with renal impairment, hepatic dysfunction, or for the elderly.

LANSOPRAZOLE: Take before meals. For patients who have difficulty swallowing capsules, lansoprazole can be opened and the intact granules contained within can be sprinkled on one tablespoon of applesauce, *Ensure* pudding, cottage cheese, yogurt, or strained pears and swallowed immediately. The delayed-release capsules may be emptied into a small volume of either orange juice or tomato juice (60 mL; ≈ 2 oz), mixed briefly, and swallowed immediately. To ensure complete delivery of the dose, rinse the glass with ≥ 2 volumes of juice (apple, cranberry, grape, orange, pineapple, prune, tomato, or V-8 vegetable juice). Do not chew or crush the granules.

Duodenal ulcer –

Treatment: 15 mg once daily for 4 weeks.

Maintenance: 15 mg once daily to maintain healing of duodenal ulcers.

Associated with H. pylori:

Triple therapy – 30 mg lansoprazole plus 500 mg clarithromycin and 1 g amoxicillin given twice daily for 10 to 14 days.

Dual therapy – 30 mg lansoprazole plus 1 g amoxicillin 3 times daily for 14 days for patients intolerant or resistant to clarithromycin.

Gastric ulcer –

Treatment: 30 mg once daily for ≤ 8 weeks.

Associated with NSAIDs:

Treatment – 30 mg once daily for 8 weeks.

Risk reduction – 15 mg once daily for ≤ 12 weeks.

GERD – 15 mg once daily for ≤ 8 weeks.

Erosive esophagitis –

Treatment: 30 mg/day for up to 8 weeks. For patients who do not heal within 8 weeks (5% to 10%) give an additional 8 weeks of treatment. If there is a recurrence of erosive esophagitis, consider an additional 8-week course.

Maintenance: 15 mg once daily to maintain healing of erosive esophagitis.

Hypersecretory conditions including Zollinger-Ellison syndrome – Individualize dosage. The recommended starting dose is 60 mg/day. Adjust doses to individual patient needs and continue for as long as clinically indicated. Dosages up to 90 mg twice daily have been administered. Administer daily dosages of > 120 mg in divided doses.

Hepatic function impairment – Consider dosage adjustment in patients with severe liver disease.

Nasogastric (NG) tube – For patients who have an NG tube in place, lansoprazole can be opened and the intact granules mixed in 40 mL of apple juice and injected through the NG tube into the stomach. After administering the granules, flush the NG tube with additional apple juice to clear the tube.

RABEPRAZOLE: Swallow tablets whole. Do not chew, crush, or split.

Duodenal ulcer – 20 mg once daily after the morning meal for a period of ≤ 4 weeks. Most patients with duodenal ulcers heal within 4 weeks.

Erosive or ulcerative GERD –

Treatment: 20 mg once daily for 4 to 8 weeks. For those patients not healed after 8 weeks of treatment, consider an additional 8-week course.

Maintenance: 20 mg once daily.

Hypersecretory conditions, including Zollinger-Ellison syndrome – Individualize dosage. Start dosing at 60 mg once daily. Adjust doses to individual patient needs and continue for as long as clinically indicated. Dosing may be divided. Doses ≤ 100 mg/day and 60 mg twice daily have been administered.

Hepatic impairment – Use caution in patients with mild to moderate hepatic impairment.

PANTOPRAZOLE: Swallow tablets whole. Do not chew, crush, or split.

Oral –

Erosive esophagitis associated with GERD:

Treatment – 40 mg once daily for ≤ 8 weeks. For those patients who have not healed after 8 weeks consider an additional 8-week course.

Maintenance – 40 mg once daily.

IV –

Treatment of erosive esophagitis: As an alternative to continued oral therapy, 40 mg pantoprazole once daily by infusion for 7 to 10 days.

Administration – Administer IV pantoprazole admixtures over a period of ≈ 15 minutes at a rate ≤ 3 mg/min (7 mL/min) through a dedicated line, using the in-line filter provided. Do not simultaneously administer IV pantoprazole through the same line with other IV solutions.

Discontinue treatment with IV pantoprazole as soon as the patient is able to resume treatment with pantoprazole delayed-release tablets. Safety and efficacy of IV pantoprazole as a treatment for GERD for > 10 days have not been demonstrated.

ESOMEPRAZOLE: Swallow capsules whole. Take ≥ 1 hour before eating.

Difficulty swallowing – For patients who have difficulty swallowing capsules, 1 tablespoon of applesauce can be added to an empty bowl and the esomeprazole capsule opened and the pellets inside carefully emptied onto the applesauce. The pellets should be mixed with the applesauce and swallowed immediately. The applesauce should not be hot and should be soft enough to swallow without chewing. Do not chew or crush the pellets. Do not store the pellet/applesauce mixture for future use.

In vitro, the pellets have been shown to remain intact when exposed to tap water, orange juice, apple juice, and yogurt.

Erosive esophagitis –

Treatment: 20 to 40 mg once daily for 4 to 8 weeks.

Maintenance: 20 mg once daily.

GERD – 20 mg once daily for 4 weeks.

Duodenal ulcer associated with H. pylori –

Esomeprazole: 40 mg once daily for 10 days.

Amoxicillin: 1000 mg twice daily for 10 days.

Clarithromycin: 500 mg twice daily for 10 days.

Actions

Pharmacology: Proton pump inhibitors do not exhibit anticholinergic or H_2 histamine antagonistic properties, but suppress gastric acid secretion by specific inhibition of the H^+/K^+ ATPase enzyme system at the secretory surface of the gastric parietal cell. Because this enzyme system is the "acid (proton) pump" within the gastric mucosa, these agents have been characterized as gastric acid pump inhibitors; they block the final step of acid production. This effect is dose-related and inhibits basal and stimulated acid secretion regardless of the stimulus.

Pharmacokinetics:

Absorption/Distribution – Proton pump inhibitors are acid-labile and are thus formulated as enteric-coated granules. Absorption is rapid and begins after the granules leave the stomach.

Metabolism/Excretion – These agents are extensively metabolized by the liver. The metabolites have very little or no antisecretory activity. The plasma elimination half-life is < 2 hours while the acid inhibitory effect lasts > 24 hours, apparently because of prolonged binding to the parietal H^+/K^+ ATPase enzyme. When the drug is discontinued, secretory activity returns over 3 to 5 days.

Little unchanged drug is excreted in urine. Approximately 33% of **lansoprazole**, 90% of **rabeprazole**, ≈ 71% of **pantoprazole**, and the majority of **omeprazole** (≈ 77%) is eliminated in urine. The remainder of the dose is excreted in feces. This implies a significant biliary excretion of the metabolites of omeprazole and lansoprazole.

Select Pharmacokinetics of Proton Pump Inhibitors

Drug	Absolute bioavailability (%)	T_{max} (hours)	t½ (hours)	Duration of action (hours)	Clearance (mL/min)	Protein binding (%)
Omeprazole	≈ 30 to 40[1]	0.5 to 3.5	0.5 to 1	≤ 72	500 to 600	≈ 95
Lansoprazole	> 80	≈ 1.7	1.5	> 24	—	97
Rabeprazole	52	2 to 5	1 to 2	> 24	301 to 588	96.3
Pantoprazole	≈ 77	2.4	≈ 1	> 24	127 to 233	≈ 98

[1] The bioavailability of omeprazole increases slightly upon repeat administration.

Races: An increase in AUC of **omeprazole** of ≈ 4-fold was noted in Asian subjects compared with Caucasians. Consider dose adjustment for Asian subjects, particularly where maintenance of healing of erosive esophagitis is indicated.

Contraindications

Hypersensitivity to any component of the formulation; substituted benzimidazoles (**rabeprazole**).

Warnings

Atrophic gastritis: Atrophic gastritis has been noted occasionally in gastric corpus biopsies from patients treated long-term with **omeprazole.**

Hepatic function impairment: In patients with various degrees of chronic hepatic disease, the mean plasma half-life of **lansoprazole**, **rabeprazole**, and **pantoprazole** was prolonged, and the mean AUC increased. Consider dose reduction in severe hepatic disease.

Elderly: Bioavailability of **omeprazole** may be increased. The clearance of **lansoprazole** is decreased in the elderly, with an increase of elimination half-life of ≈ 50% to 100%. Because the mean half-life in the elderly remains between 1.9 and 2.9 hours, repeated once-daily dosing does not result in accumulation of lansoprazole.

Pregnancy: *Category* C (**omeprazole**); *Category B* (**lansoprazole, rabeprazole, pantoprazole**).

Lactation: It is not known whether these agents are excreted in breast milk.

Children: Safety and efficacy in children have not been established.

Precautions

Gastric malignancy: Symptomatic response to therapy with proton pump inhibitors does not preclude gastric malignancy.

Drug Interactions

Drugs that may be affected by proton pump inhibitors include clarithromycin, cyclosporine, ketoconazole, digoxin, benzodiazepines, phenytoin, theophylline, and warfarin. Drugs that affect proton pump inhibitors include clarithromycin and sucralfate.

Proton pump inhibitors cause a profound and long-lasting inhibition of gastric acid secretion; therefore, it is theoretically possible that proton pump inhibitors may interfere with the absorption of drugs where gastric pH is an important determinant of bioavailability (eg, ketoconazole, ampicillin, iron salts, digoxin, cyanocobalamin).

P450 system: **Omeprazole** may interact with other drugs also metabolized via the cytochrome P450 (CYP450) system. There are clinical reports of interaction with other drugs metabolized via the cytochrome P450 system (eg, cyclosporine, disulfiram, benzodiazepines). **Lansoprazole** is metabolized through the cytochrome P450 system via CYP3A and CYP2C19 isoenzymes; however, lansoprazole does not have clinically significant interactions with other drugs metabolized by the cytochrome P450 system. **Rabeprazole** and **pantoprazole** are also metabolized by the cytochrome P450 system, but does not have clinically significant interactions with other drugs metabolized by CYP450. Pantoprazole is metabolized via cytochrome P450 system (CYPC19 and CYP3A4), but does not have clinically relevant interactions with other drugs metabolized by CYP450. In clinical trials, antacids were used concomitantly with these agents.

Drug/Food interactions: C_{max} and AUC are diminished by ≈ 50% if **lansoprazole** is given 30 minutes after food as opposed to in the fasting condition. There is no significant food effect if given before meals.

Adverse Reactions

The most common adverse effects (> 3%) of **omeprazole, lansoprazole**, and **rabeprazole** include headache and diarrhea.

SUCRALFATE

Tablets: 1 g (*Rx*)	Various, *Carafate* (Aventis)
Suspension: 1 g/10 mL (*Rx*)	*Carafate* (Aventis)

Indications

Duodenal ulcer: Short-term treatment (up to 8 weeks) of active duodenal ulcer.

Maintenance therapy (tablets only): Duodenal ulcer patients at reduced dosage after healing of acute ulcers.

Administration and Dosage

Active duodenal ulcer:

Adults – 1 g 4 times daily on an empty stomach (1 hour before meals and at bedtime).

Take antacids as needed for pain relief but not within ½ hour before or after sucralfate.

While healing with sucralfate may occur within the first 2 weeks, continue treatment for 4 to 8 weeks unless healing is demonstrated by X-ray or endoscopic examination.

Maintenance therapy (tablets only):

Adults – 1 g twice daily.

Actions

Pharmacology: Sucralfate does not affect gastric acid output or concentration. It rapidly reacts with hydrochloric acid in the stomach to form a condensed, viscous, adhesive, paste-like substance with the capacity to buffer acid and binds to the surface of gastric and duodenal ulcers.

The barrier formed at the ulcer site protects the ulcer from the potential ulcerogenic properties of pepsin, acid, and bile, thus allowing the ulcer to heal.

Pharmacokinetics: Sucralfate is minimally absorbed from the GI tract following an oral dose. The duration of action depends on the time that the drug is in contact with this site. Binding to the ulcer site has been shown for up to 6 hours. Approximately 95% of the dose remains in the GI tract.

Warnings

Chronic renal failure/dialysis: During sucralfate administration, small amounts of aluminum are absorbed. Concomitant use with other aluminum-containing products may increase the total body burden of aluminum. Patients with chronic renal failure or receiving dialysis have impaired excretion of absorbed aluminum, and aluminum is not dialyzed. Aluminum accumulation and toxicity have occurred.

Pregnancy: Category B.

Lactation: It is not known whether this drug is excreted in breast milk.

Children: Safety and efficacy in children have not been established.

Precautions

Ulcer recurrence: Duodenal ulcer is a chronic recurrent disease. While short-term treatment can completely heal the ulcer, do not expect a successful course to alter posthealing frequency or severity of duodenal ulceration.

Drug Interactions

Drugs that may be affected by sucralfate include aluminum-containing antacids, anticoagulants, diclofenac, digoxin, histamine H_2 antagonists (eg, cimetidine, ranitidine), hydantoins, ketoconazole, levothyroxine, penicillamine, quinidine, quinolones, tetracycline, and theophylline.

Adverse Reactions

Adverse reactions in clinical trials were minor and rarely led to drug discontinuation. Constipation was the most frequent complaint (2%).

SULFASALAZINE

Tablets: 500 mg (*Rx*)	Various, *Azulfidine* (Pharmacia)
Tablets, delayed-release: 500 mg (*Rx*)	*Azulfidine EN-tabs* (Pharmacia)

Sulfasalazine also is indicated for use in rheumatoid arthritis and juvenile rheumatoid arthritis. Refer to the monograph in the CNS chapter.

Indications

Ulcerative colitis: In the treatment of mild to moderate ulcerative colitis and as adjunctive therapy in severe ulcerative colitis; for the prolongation of the remission period between acute attacks of ulcerative colitis.

Rheumatoid arthritis (RA; enteric-coated tablets): In the treatment of patients with RA who have responded inadequately to salicylates or other nonsteroidal anti-inflammatory drugs (NSAIDs).

Juvenile rheumatoid arthritis (JRA; enteric-coated tablets): In the treatment of pediatric patients ≥ 6 years of age with polyarticular-course JRA who have responded inadequately to salicylates or other NSAIDs.

Unlabeled uses: Psoriatic arthritis (2 g/day).

Administration and Dosage

Give the drug in evenly divided doses over each 24-hour period; intervals between nighttime doses should not exceed 8 hours, with administration after meals recommended when feasible. Swallow tablets whole; do not crush or chew. Experience suggests that with daily dosages of ≥ 4 g, the incidence of adverse effects tends to increase.

Some patients may be sensitive to treatment with sulfasalazine. Various desensitization-like regimens have been reported to be effective. These regimens suggest starting with a total daily dose of 50 to 250 mg initially, and doubling it every 4 to 7 days until the desired therapeutic level has been achieved. If the symptoms of sensitivity recur, discontinue sulfasalazine. Do not attempt desensitization in patients who have a history of agranulocytosis, or who have experienced an anaphylactoid reaction while previously receiving sulfasalazine.

Ulcerative colitis:

Initial therapy –

Adults: 3 to 4 g daily in evenly divided doses. It may be advisable to initiate therapy with a lower dosage (eg, 1 to 2 g daily), to reduce possible GI intolerance.

Children ≥ 2 years of age: 40 to 60 mg/kg in each 24-hour period, divided into 3 to 6 doses.

Maintenance therapy –

Adults: 2 g daily.

Children ≥ 2 years of age: 30 mg/kg in each 24-hour period, divided into 4 doses.

It is often necessary to continue medication even when clinical symptoms, including diarrhea, have been controlled. When endoscopic examination confirms satisfactory improvement, reduce dosage to a maintenance level. If diarrhea recurs, increase dosage to previously effective levels.

Actions

Pharmacology: The mode of action of sulfasalazine or its metabolites, 5-aminosalicylic acid (5-ASA) and sulfapyridine (SP), is still under investigation but may be related to the anti-inflammatory or immunomodulatory properties that have been observed in animals and in vitro, to its affinity for connective tissue, or to the relatively high concentration it reaches in serous fluids, the liver, and intestinal walls. In ulcerative colitis, the major therapeutic action may reside in the 5-ASA moiety.

Pharmacokinetics:

Absorption – The absolute bioavailability of oral sulfasalazine is < 15% for parent drug. In the intestine, sulfasalazine is metabolized by intestinal bacteria to SP and 5-ASA. Of the two, SP is relatively well absorbed from the colon and highly metabolized with an estimated bioavailability of 60%. 5-ASA is much less well absorbed with an estimated bioavailability of 10% to 30%. Peak plasma levels of both occur ≈ 10 hours after dosing.

Distribution – Following IV injection, the calculated volume of distribution (Vd_{ss}) for sulfasalazine was ≈ 7.5 L. Sulfasalazine is highly bound to albumin (> 99.3%), while SP is only ≈ 70% bound to albumin.

Metabolism – The observed plasma half-life for IV sulfasalazine is 7.6 hours. The primary route of metabolism of SP is via acetylation to form AcSP. The rate of metabolism of SP to AcSP is dependent on acetylator phenotype. In fast acetylators, the mean plasma half-life of SP is 10.4 hours, while in slow acetylators it is 14.8 hours.

Excretion – Absorbed SP and 5-ASA and their metabolites are primarily eliminated in the urine either as free metabolites or as glucuronide conjugates. The majority of 5-ASA stays within the colonic lumen and is excreted as 5-ASA and acetyl-5-ASA with the feces.

Contraindications

Pediatric patients < 2 years of age; intestinal or urinary obstruction; porphyria, hypersensitivity to sulfasalazine, its metabolites, salicylates, or sulfonamides.

Warnings

Porphyria: Patients with porphyria should not receive sulfonamides as these drugs have been reported to precipitate an acute attack.

GI intolerance: Sulfasalazine enteric-coated tablets are particularly indicated in patients with ulcerative colitis who cannot take uncoated sulfasalazine tablets because of GI intolerance, and in whom there is evidence that this intolerance is not primarily the result of high blood levels of sulfapyridine and its metabolites (eg, patients experiencing nausea and vomiting with the first few doses of the drug, or patients in whom a reduction in dosage does not alleviate the adverse GI effects).

Special risk patients: The presence of clinical signs such as sore throat, fever, pallor, purpura, or jaundice may be indications of serious blood disorders. Use with caution in patients with severe allergy or bronchial asthma.

Deaths: Deaths associated with the administration of sulfasalazine have been reported from hypersensitivity reactions, agranulocytosis, aplastic anemia, other blood dyscrasias, renal and liver damage, irreversible neuromuscular and CNS changes, and fibrosing alveolitis. If toxic or hypersensitivity reactions occur, discontinue sulfasalazine immediately.

Renal/Hepatic function impairment: Only after critical appraisal should sulfasalazine be given to patients with hepatic or renal damage or blood dyscrasias.

Fertility impairment: Oligospermia and infertility have been observed in men treated with sulfasalazine. Withdrawal of the drug appears to reverse these effects.

Elderly: Elderly patients with rheumatoid arthritis showed a prolonged plasma half-life for sulfasalazine, SP, and their metabolites.

Pregnancy: *Category B.*

Lactation: Sulfonamides are excreted in breast milk. In newborns, they compete with bilirubin for binding sites on the plasma proteins and may cause kernicterus.

Children: The safety and efficacy of sulfasalazine in pediatric patients < 2 years of age with ulcerative colitis have not been established.

Precautions

Monitoring: Perform complete blood counts, including differential white cell count and liver function tests before starting sulfasalazine and every second week during the first 3 months of therapy. During the second 3 months, perform the same tests once monthly and, thereafter, once every 3 months and as clinically indicated. Also perform urinalysis and assess renal function periodically during treatment.

The determination of serum sulfapyridine levels may be useful because concentrations > 50 mcg/mL appear to be associated with an increased incidence of adverse reactions.

Ulcerative colitis: Inform patients with this condition that ulcerative colitis rarely remits completely, and that the risk of relapse can be substantially reduced by continued administration of sulfasalazine at a maintenance dosage.

Glucose-6-phosphate dehydrogenase deficiency: Observe patients with glucose-6-phosphate dehydrogenase deficiency closely for signs of hemolytic anemia. This reaction is frequently dose-related.

Undisintegrated tablets: Isolated instances have occurred where sulfasalazine enteric-coated tablets have passed undisintegrated. If this is observed, discontinue the administration of the drug immediately.

Fluid intake: Adequate fluid intake must be maintained in order to prevent crystalluria and stone formation.

Drug Interactions

Drugs that may interact with sulfasalazine include digoxin, sulfonylureas, and folic acid.

Adverse Reactions

Adverse events occurring in ≥ 3% of patients with ulcerative colitis include the following: Anorexia; headache; nausea; vomiting; gastric distress; reversible oligospermia.

TEGASEROD MALEATE

Tablets: 2 and 6 mg (*Rx*) *Zelnorm* (Novartis)

Indications

Irritable bowel syndrome (IBS): For the short-term treatment of women with IBS whose primary bowel symptom is constipation.

The safety and efficacy of tegaserod in men have not been established.

Administration and Dosage

Dose: The recommended dose is 6 mg taken orally before meals twice daily for 4 to 6 weeks. For those patients who respond to therapy at 4 to 6 weeks, an additional 4- to 6-week course may be considered.

The efficacy of tegaserod beyond 12 weeks has not been studied.

Actions

Pharmacology: Tegaserod is a 5-HT_4 receptor partial agonist that binds with high affinity at human 5-HT_4 receptors, whereas it has no appreciable affinity for 5-HT_3 or dopamine receptors. It has moderate affinity for 5-HT_1 receptors. Tegaserod, by acting as an agonist at neuronal 5-HT_4 receptors, triggers the release of further neurotransmitters such as calcitonin gene-related peptide from sensory neurons. The activation of 5-HT_4 receptors in the GI tract stimulates the peristaltic reflex and intestinal secretion, as well as inhibits visceral sensitivity. In vivo studies showed that tegaserod enhanced basal motor activity and normalized impaired motility throughout the GI tract. In addition, studies demonstrated that tegaserod moderated visceral sensitivity during colorectal distention in animals.

Pharmacokinetics:

Absorption – Peak plasma concentrations are reached approximately 1 hour after oral dosing. The absolute bioavailability of tegaserod when administered to fasting subjects is approximately 10%. The pharmacokinetics are dose-proportional over the 2 to 12 mg range given twice daily for 5 days. There was no clinically relevant accumulation of tegaserod in plasma when a 6 mg twice daily dose was given for 5 days.

Distribution – Tegaserod is approximately 98% bound to plasma proteins, predominantly alpha-1-acid glycoprotein. Tegaserod exhibits pronounced distribution into tissues following IV dosing with a volume of distribution at steady state of approximately 368 L.

Metabolism – Tegaserod is metabolized mainly via 2 pathways. The first is a presystemic acid catalyzed hydrolysis in the stomach followed by oxidation and conjugation that produces the main metabolite of tegaserod, 5-methoxyindole-3-carboxylic acid glucuronide. The main metabolite has negligible affinity for 5-HT_4 receptors in vitro. The second metabolic pathway of tegaserod is direct glucuronidation that leads to generation of 3 isomeric N-glucuronides.

Excretion – The plasma clearance of tegaserod is approximately 77 L/h with an estimated terminal half-life ($T_{½}$) of approximately 11 hours following IV dosing. Approximately two-thirds of the orally administered dose of tegaserod is excreted unchanged in the feces, with the remaining one-third excreted in the urine, primarily as the main metabolite.

Special populations –

Renal function impairment: No dosage adjustment is required in patients with mild to moderate renal impairment. Tegaserod is not recommended in patients with severe renal impairment.

Hepatic function impairment: No dosage adjustment is required in patients with mild impairment; however, caution is recommended when using tegaserod in this patient population. Tegaserod has not been studied adequately in patients with moderate and severe hepatic impairment and, therefore, is not recommended in these patients.

Contraindications

Severe renal impairment; moderate or severe hepatic impairment; history of bowel obstruction, symptomatic gallbladder disease, suspected sphincter of Oddi dysfunction, or abdominal adhesions; known hypersensitivity to the drug or any of its excipients.

Warnings

Pregnancy: *Category B.* Use this drug during pregnancy only if clearly needed.

Lactation: Based on the potential for tumorigenicity shown for tegaserod in a mouse carcinogenicity study, decide whether to discontinue nursing or discontinue the drug, taking into account the importance of the drug to the mother.

Children: Safety and efficacy have not been established in children under 18 years of age.

Precautions

Diarrhea: Do not initiate tegaserod in patients who are currently experiencing or frequently experience diarrhea. Discontinue tegaserod immediately in patients with new or sudden worsening of abdominal pain. The majority of tegaserod patients reporting diarrhea had a single episode. In most cases, diarrhea occurred within the first week of treatment. Typically, diarrhea resolved with continued therapy. Patients should consult their physician if they experience severe diarrhea or if the diarrhea is accompanied by severe cramping, abdominal pain, or dizziness.

Abdominal surgeries: An increase in abdominal surgeries was observed on tegaserod (0.3%) vs placebo (0.2%) in Phase 3 clinical studies. The increase was primarily because of a numerical imbalance in cholecystectomies reported in patients treated with tegaserod (0.17%) vs placebo (0.06%). A causal relationship between abdominal surgeries and tegaserod has not been established.

Drug Interactions

Tegaserod interacts with digoxin and oral contraceptives.

Drug/Food interactions: When the drug is administered with food, the bioavailability of tegaserod is reduced 40% to 65% and C_{max} by approximately 20% to 40%. Similar reductions in plasma concentration occur when tegaserod is administered to subjects within 30 minutes prior to a meal or 2.5 hours after a meal.

Adverse Reactions

Adverse reactions in 3% or more of patients include the following: Headache, dizziness, abdominal pain, diarrhea, nausea, vomiting, flatulence, back pain, accidental trauma.

TETRACYCLINES

TETRACYCLINE HCl	
Tablets: 250 and 500 mg (*Rx*)	*Sumycin 250 and 500* (Apothecon)
Capsules: 100, 250 and 500 mg (*Rx*)	Various, *Achromycin V* (Lederle)
Oral suspension: 125 mg/5 mL (*Rx*)	Various, *Achromycin V* (Lederle)
DEMECLOCYCLINE HCl	
Tablets: 150 and 300 mg (*Rx*)	*Declomycin* (Lederle)
Capsules: 50 and 100 mg (*Rx*)	*Declomycin* (Lederle)
DOXYCYCLINE	
Tablets: 50 and 100 mg (as hyclate) (*Rx*)	Various, *Vibra-Tabs* (Pfizer), *Bio-Tab* (Inter. Ethical Labs)
Capsules: 50 and 100 mg (*Rx*)	Various, *Monodox* (Oclassen), *Vibramycin* (Pfizer)
Capsules, coated pellets: 100 mg (as hyclate) (*Rx*)	*Doryx* (Parke-Davis)
Capsules: 50 and 100 mg (as monohydrate) (*Rx*)	*Monodox* (Oclassen)
Powder for oral suspension: 25 mg/5 mL (as monohydrate when reconstituted) (*Rx*)	*Vibramycin* (Pfizer)
Syrup: 50 mg/5 mL (as calcium) (*Rx*)	*Vibramycin* (Pfizer)
Powder for injection: 100 and 200 mg (as hyclate) (*Rx*)	Various, *Vibramycin IV* (Pfizer)
MINOCYCLINE	
Capsules: 50 and 100 mg (*Rx*)	Various, *Dynacin* (Medicis Dermatologics)
Capsules, pellet filled: 50 and 100 mg (*Rx*)	*Minocin* (Lederle)
Oral suspension: 50 mg/5 mL (*Rx*)	*Minocin* (Lederle)
Powder for injection: 100 mg (*Rx*)	*Minocin IV* (Lederle)
OXYTETRACYCLINE	
Capsules: 250 mg (*Rx*)	Various, *Terramycin* (Pfizer)
Injection: 50 and 125 mg/mL (*Rx*)	*Terramycin IM* (Roerig)

Indications

Infections caused by the following microorganisms: Rickettsiae (Rocky Mountain spotted fever, typhus fever and the typhus group, Q fever, rickettsialpox, and tick fevers); *Mycoplasma pneumoniae* (PPLO, Eaton agent); agents of psittacosis and ornithosis; agents of lymphogranuloma venereum and granuloma inguinale; the spirochetal agent of relapsing fever (*Borrelia recurrentis*).

Infections caused by the following gram-negative microorganisms: *Haemophilus ducreyi* (chancroid); *Yersinia pestis* and *Francisella tularensis* (formerly *Pasteurella pestis* and *Pasturella tularensis*); *Bartonella bacilliformis*; *Bacteroides* sp.; *Campylobacter fetus* (formerly *Vibrio fetus*); *Vibrio cholerae* (formerly *Vibrio comma*); *Brucella* sp. (in conjunction with streptomycin).

Infections caused by the following microorganisms, when bacteriologic testing indicates appropriate susceptibility to the drug:

Gram-negative – *Escherichia coli*; *Enterobacter aerogenes* (formerly *Aerobacter aerogenes*); *Shigella* sp.; *Acinetobacter calcoaceticus* (formerly *Mima* and *Herellea* sp.); *Haemophilus influenzae* (respiratory infections); *Klebsiella* sp. (respiratory and urinary infections).

Gram-positive – *Streptococcus* sp. including *S. pneumoniae*. Up to 44% of strains of *S. pyogenes* and 74% of *S. faecalis* are resistant to tetracyclines.

Staphylococcus aureus: *S. aureus*, skin and soft tissue infections. Tetracyclines are not the drugs of choice in the treatment of any type of staphylococcal infection.

Treatment of trachoma: Treatment of trachoma, although the infectious agent is not always eliminated, as judged by immunofluorescence.

When penicillin is contraindicated: When penicillin is contraindicated, tetracyclines are alternatives for treatment of infections caused by: *Neisseria gonorrhoeae*; *Treponema pallidum and T. pertenue* (syphilis and yaws); *Listeria monocytogenes*; *Clostridium* sp.; *Bacillus anthracis*; *Fusobacterium fusiforme* (Vincent's infection); *Actinomyces* sp.; *Neisseria meningitidis* (IV only).

Acute intestinal amebiasis: Tetracyclines may be a useful adjunct to amebicides.

Oral tetracyclines:

Adults – Treatment of uncomplicated urethral, endocervical, or rectal infections caused by *Chlamydia trachomatis*.

Severe acne – Severe acne (where it may be useful as adjunctive therapy).

Inclusion conjunctivitis – Inclusion conjunctivitis (which may be treated with oral tetracyclines or with a combination of oral and topical agents).

Doxycycline, oral – Treatment of uncomplicated gonococcal infections in adults (except for anorectal infections in men); gonococcal arthritis-dermatitis syndrome; acute epididymo-orchitis caused by *N. gonorrhoeae* and *C. trachomatis*; nongonococcal urethritis caused by *C. trachomatis* and *Ureaplasma urealyticum*.

Minocycline, oral – Treatment of asymptomatic carriers of *N. meningitidis* to eliminate meningococci from the nasopharynx. Not indicated for the treatment of meningococcal infection.

Oral minocycline has been successful in *Mycobacterium marinum* infections.

Minocycline also is indicated for the treatment of uncomplicated urethral, endocervical, or rectal infections in adults caused by *U. urealyticum*; uncomplicated gonococcal urethritis in men caused by *N. gonorrhoeae*.

Unlabeled uses: Tetracycline suspension has been used as a mouthwash in the treatment of nonspecific mouth ulcerations, aphthous ulcers, and canker sores. Dosages have ranged from 5 to 10 mL of 125 mg/mL 3 times/day for 5 to 7 days.

Doxycycline has been used to prevent "traveler's diarrhea" commonly caused by enterotoxigenic *Escherichia coli*. In limited trials, this prophylactic (100 mg/day) therapy appears to be superior to placebo.

Lyme disease – Lyme disease (the etiologic agent is a spirochete, *Borrelia burgdorferi*): Oral **tetracycline** 250 mg daily for 10 days is the drug of choice for stage I disease in adults; **doxycycline** has also been recommended for early disease. Both agents have been recommended for stage II disease, and they are being evaluated for treatment of stage III disease. However, the efficacy of tetracycline at the recommended dose for early Lyme disease has been questioned.

Administration and Dosage

Avoid rapid IV administration. Thrombophlebitis may result from prolonged IV therapy.

Continue therapy at least 24 to 48 hours after symptoms and fever subside. Treat all infections caused by group A β-hemolytic streptococci for at least 10 days.

TETRACYLINE HCl:

Adults –

Usual dose: 1 to 2 g/day in 2 or 4 equal doses.

Children (> 8 years of age) – Daily dose is 10 to 20 mg/lb (25 to 50 mg/kg in 4 equal doses.

Brucellosis – 500 mg 4 times/day for 3 weeks, accompanied by 1 g streptomycin IM twice/day the first week, and once daily the second week.

Syphilis – 30 to 40 g in equally divided doses over 10 to 15 days. Perform close follow-up and laboratory tests.

Gonorrhea – 1.5 g initially, then 500 mg every 6 hours, to a total of 9 g.

Gonorrhea in patients sensitive to penicillin – Initially, 1.5 g; follow with 500 mg every 6 hours for 4 days to a total of 9 g.

Uncomplicated urethral, endocervical, or rectal infections caused by Chlamydia trachomatis – 500 mg 4 times/day for at least 7 days.

Severe acne (long-term therapy) – Initially, 1 g/day in divided doses. For maintenance, give 125 to 500 mg/day.

CDC-recommended treatment schedules for sexually transmitted diseases –

Chlamydia trachomatis – Uncomplicated urethral, endocervical, or rectal infections in adults: 500 mg 4 times/day for 7 days.

Gonococcal infections – Uncomplicated urethral, endocervical, or rectal infections in adults: 3 g amoxicillin, 3.5 g oral ampicillin, 4.8 million units IM aqueous procaine penicillin G or 250 mg IM ceftriaxone. Each (except ceftriaxone) should be accompanied by 1 g oral probenecid. Follow with 500 mg tetracycline 4 times/day for 7 days.

In adults allergic to penicillins, cephalosporins, or probenecid – 500 mg 4 times/day for 7 days.

Penicillinase-producing Neisseria gonorrheae (PPNG): 2 g IM spectinomycin or 250 mg IM ceftriaxone. Follow with 500 mg tetracycline 4 times/day for 7 days.

Children – 40 mg/kg/day in 4 divided doses for 5 days.

In PPNG-endemic and -hyperendemic areas: 250 mg IM ceftriaxone plus 100 mg oral doxycycline twice daily for 7 days or 500 mg oral tetracycline 4 times/day for 7 days. If tetracyclines are contraindicated or not tolerated, follow the single-dose regimen with erythromycin.

Disseminated gonococcal infections in patients allergic to penicillins or cephalosporins: 500 mg 4 times/day for ≥ 7 days

Lymphogranuloma venereum – Genital, inguinal, or anorectal: 500 mg 4 times/day for ≥ 2 weeks.

Nongonococcal urethritis: 500 mg 4 times/day for 7 days.

Acute pelvic inflammatory disease – Ambulatory treatment: 2 g IM cefoxitin, 3 g amoxicillin, 3.5 g oral ampicillin, 4.8 million units IM aqueous procaine penicillin G at 2 sites or 250 mg IM ceftriaxone. Each (except for ceftriaxone) should be accompanied by 1 g oral probenecid. Follow with 500 mg tetracycline 4 times/day. (However, doxycycline is preferred.)

Children > 7 years of age – 150 mg/kg/day IV cefuroxime or 100 mg/kg/day IV ceftriaxone followed by 30 mg/kg/day IV tetracycline in 3 doses, continued for ≥ 4 days. Thereafter, continue tetracycline orally to complete ≥ 14 days of therapy.

Syphilis (penicillin-allergic patients):

Early – 500 mg 4 times/day for 15 days.

More than 1 year's duration – 500 mg 4 times/day for 30 days.

Sexually transmitted epididymo-orchitis: 3 g oral amoxicillin, 3.5 g oral ampicillin, 4.8 million units IM aqueous procaine penicillin G at 2 sites (each with 1 g oral probenecid), 2 g IM spectinomycin or 250 mg ceftriaxone followed by 500 mg tetracycline 4 times/day for 10 days.

Urethral syndrome in women: 500 mg 4 times/day for 7 days.

Rape victims – Prophylaxis: 500 mg 4 times/day for 7 days.

DEMECLOCYCLINE HCl:

Adults –

Daily dose: 4 divided doses of 150 mg each or 2 divided doses of 300 mg each.

Children (over 8 years of age) –

Usual daily dose: 3 to 6 mg/lb (6 to 12 mg/kg), depending upon the severity of the disease, divided into 3 or 4 doses.

Gonorrhea patients sensitive to penicillin – Initially, 600 mg; follow with 300 mg every 12 hours for 4 days to a total of 3 g.

DOXYCYCLINE:

Oral –

Adults:

Usual dose – 200 mg on the first day of treatment (100 mg every 12 hours); follow with a maintenance dose of 100 mg/day. The maintenance dose may be administered as a single dose or as 50 mg every 12 hours.

More severe infections (particularly chronic urinary tract infections) – 100 mg every 12 hours.

Children (> 8 years of age):

≤ 100 lbs (< 45 kg) – 2 mg/lb (4.4 mg/kg) divided into 2 doses on the first day of treatment; follow with 1 mg/lb (2.2 mg/kg) given as a single daily dose or divided into 2 doses on subsequent days.

More severe infections – Up to 2 mg/lb (4.4 mg/kg) may be used. For children > 100 lbs (45 kg), use the usual adult dose.

Acute gonococcal infection: 200 mg immediately, then 100 mg at bedtime on the first day. Follow by 100 mg 2 times/day for 3 days.

Single visit dose – Immediately give 300 mg; follow with 300 mg in 1 hour, which may be administered with food, milk, or carbonated beverage.

Primary and secondary syphilis: 300 mg/day in divided doses for ≥ 10 days.

Uncomplicated urethral, endocervical, or rectal infections in adults caused by Chlamydia trachomatis: 100 mg twice daily for ≥ 7 days.

Endometritis, salpingitis, parametritis, or peritonitis: Give 100 mg doxycycline IV, twice/day and 2 g cefoxitin IV 4 times/day. Continue IV administration for ≥ 4 days and for ≥ 48 hours after patient improves. Then continue oral doxycycline (100 mg) twice daily to complete 10 to 14 days total therapy.

Parenteral – Do not inject IM or SC. The duration of IV infusion may vary with the dose (100 to 200 mg/day), but is usually 1 to 4 hours. A recommended minimum infusion time for 100 mg of a 0.5 mg/mL solution is 1 hour.

Adults: The usual dosage is 200 mg IV on the first day of treatment, administered in 1- or 2-hour infusions. Subsequent daily dosage is 100 to 200 mg, depending upon the severity of infection, with 200 mg administered in 1 or 2 infusions.

Primary and secondary syphilis – 300 mg daily for ≥ 10 days.

Children (> 8 years): ≥ 100 lbs (45 kg), give 2 mg/lb (4.4 mg/kg) on the first day of treatment, in 1 or 2 infusions. Subsequent daily dosage is 1 to 2 mg/lb (2.2 to 4.4 mg/kg) given as 1 or 2 infusions, depending on the severity of the infection. For children > 100 lbs (45 kg), use the usual adult dose.

Children (< 8 years): Safety of IV use has not been established.

CDC-recommended treatment schedules for sexually transmitted diseases –

Chlamydia trachomatis – Uncomplicated urethral, endocervical, or rectal infections in adults: 100 mg 2 times/day for 7 days.

Gonococcal infections:

Uncomplicated urethral, endocervical, or rectal infections in adults – 3 g oral amoxicillin, 3.5 g oral ampicillin, 4.8 million units IM aqueous procaine penicillin G or 250 mg IM ceftriaxone. Each (except for ceftriaxone) should be accompanied by 1 g oral probenecid. Follow with 100 mg doxycycline twice daily for 7 days.

In adults allergic to penicillins, cephalosporins, or probenecid: 100 mg twice daily for 7 days.

In PPNG-endemic and -hyperendemic areas: 250 mg IM ceftriaxone plus 100 mg oral doxycycline twice daily for 7 days. If tetracyclines are contraindicated or not tolerated, follow the single-dose regimen with erythromycin.

PPNG: 2 g IM spectinomycin or 250 mg IM ceftriaxone. Follow with 100 mg doxycycline, twice daily for 7 days.

Disseminated gonococcal infections in patients allergic to penicillins or cephalosporins: 100 mg, twice daily for ≥ 7 days.

Lymphogranuloma venereum:

Genital, inguinal, or anorectal – 100 mg twice daily for ≥ 2 weeks.

Nongonococcal urethritis: 100 mg twice daily for 7 days.

Acute pelvic inflammatory disease:

Ambulatory treatment – 250 mg single IM dose of ceftriaxone plus 100 mg oral doxycycline twice daily for 10 to 14 days. Other effective third-generation cephalosporins may be substituted in the appropriate doses for ceftriaxone.

Inpatient treatment – 100 mg IV doxycycline twice daily, plus 2 g IV cefoxitin 4 times/day. Continue drugs IV for ≥ 4 days and ≥ 48 hours after patient improves. Then continue doxycycline 100 mg orally twice daily to complete 10 to 14 days of total therapy.

Sexually transmitted epididymo-orchitis: 3 g oral amoxicillin, 3.5 g oral ampicillin, 4.8 million units IM aqueous procaine penicillin G at 2 sites (each with 1 g oral probenecid), 2 g IM spectinomycin or 250 mg IM ceftriaxone followed by 100 mg doxycycline twice daily for 7 days.

Rape victims prophylaxis: 100 mg twice daily for 7 days.

MINOCYCLINE:

Oral –

Usual dosage:

Adults – 200 mg initially, followed by 100 mg every 12 hours. If more frequent doses are preferred, give 100 or 200 mg initially; follow with 50 mg 4 times/day.

Children (over 8 years of age) – Initially, 4 mg/kg; follow with 2 mg/kg every 12 hours.

Syphilis: Administer usual dose over a period of 10 to 15 days. Close follow-up, including laboratory tests, is recommended.

Uncomplicated urethral, endocervical, or rectal infections in adults caused by Chlamydia trachomatis: 100 mg 2 times/day for ≥ 7 days.

Uncomplicated gonococcal urethritis in men: 100 mg 2 times/day for 5 days.

Mycobacterium marinum infections: Although optimal doses are not established, 100 mg twice daily for 6 to 8 weeks has been successful in a limited number of cases.

Parenteral –

Adults: 200 mg followed by 100 mg every 12 hours; do not exceed 400 mg in 24 hours.

Children (over 8 years of age): Usual pediatric dose is 4 mg/kg, followed by 2 mg/kg every 12 hours.

OXYTETRACYCLINE:

Oral – See Tetracycline HCl.

Parenteral –

Adults: The usual daily dose is 250 mg administered once every 24 hours or 300 mg given in divided doses at 8- to 12-hour intervals.

Children (> 8 years of age): 15 to 25 mg/kg, up to a maximum of 250 mg/single daily injection. Dosage may be divided and given at 8 to 12 hour intervals.

Actions

Pharmacology: The tetracyclines are bacteriostatic. They exert their antimicrobial effect by inhibition of protein synthesis.

Pharmacokinetics:

Tetracycline Pharmacokinetic Variables and Dosage Regimens

Tetracyclines	Serum protein binding (%)	Normal serum half-life (hrs)	% excreted unchanged in urine	Usual oral adult maintenance dosage	Lipid solubility
Tetracycline	65	16 to 12	60	250 mg q 6 h or 500 mg q 6 to 12 h	Intermediate
Demeclocycline	65 to 91	12 to 16	39	150 mg q 6 h or 300 mg q 12 h	Intermediate
Doxycycline	80 to 95	15 to 25	30 to 42	150 mg q 12 h or 100 mg q 24 h	High
Minocycline	70 to 80	11 to 18	16 to 12	100 mg q 12 h	High
Oxytetracycline	20 to 40	16 to 12	70	250 to 500 mg q 6 h	Low

Contraindications

Hypersensitivity to any of the tetracyclines.

Warnings

Photosensitivity: Photosensitivity manifested by an exaggerated sunburn reaction has been observed in some individuals taking tetracyclines. Advise patients who are apt to be exposed to direct sunlight or ultraviolet light that this reaction can occur with tetracycline drugs, and discontinue treatment at the first evidence of skin erythema.

Phototoxic reactions are most frequent with demeclocycline, and occur less frequently with the other tetracyclines; minocycline is least likely to cause phototoxic reactions.

Parenteral therapy: Reserve for situations in which oral therapy is not indicated. Institute oral therapy as soon as possible. If given IV over prolonged periods, thrombophlebitis may result. IM use produces lower blood levels than recommended oral dosages.

Nephrogenic diabetes insipidus: Administration of **demeclocycline** has resulted in appearance of the diabetes insipidus syndrome (polyuria, polydipsia, and weakness) in some patients on long-term therapy.

Hazardous tasks: Lightheadedness, dizziness or vertigo may occur with **minocycline.** Patients should observe caution while driving or performing other tasks requiring alertness.

Renal function impairment: If renal impairment exists, even usual doses may lead to excessive systemic accumulation of the tetracyclines (with the exception of doxycycline and minocycline) and possible liver toxicity. Use lower than usual doses.

Hepatic function impairment: Doses > 2 g/day IV can be extremely dangerous. In the presence of renal dysfunction, and particularly in pregnancy, IV tetracycline > 2 g/day has been associated with death secondary to liver failure.

Pregnancy: Category D (**doxycycline**). Do not use during pregnancy. They readily cross the placenta; concentrations of oxytetracycline in cord blood are ≈ 50% of those of the mother. Tetracyclines are found in fetal tissues and can have toxic effects on the developing fetus (retardation of skeletal development).

Lactation: Tetracyclines are excreted in breast milk. A dosage of 2 g/day for 3 days has achieved a milk:plasma ratio of 0.6 to 0.8.

Children: Tetracyclines generally should not be used in children < 8 years of age unless other drugs are not likely to be effective or are contraindicated.

Teeth – The use of tetracyclines during the period of tooth development (from the last half of pregnancy through the eighth year of life) may cause permanent discoloration (yellow-gray-brown) of deciduous and permanent teeth. Doxycycline and oxytetracycline may be less likely to affect teeth.

Bone – Tetracycline forms a stable calcium complex in any bone-forming tissue. Decreased fibula growth rate occurred in premature infants given 25 mg/kg oral tetracycline every 6 hours.

Precautions

Pseudotumor cerebri: Pseudotumor cerebri (benign intracranial hypertension) in adults has been associated with tetracycline use.

Outdated products: Under no circumstances should outdated tetracyclines be administered; the degradation products of tetracyclines are highly nephrotoxic and have, on occasion, produced a Fanconi-like syndrome.

Drug Interactions

Drugs that may affect tetracyclines include antacids containing aluminum, calcium, zinc, magnesium, bismuth salts, divalent and trivalent cations; barbiturates; carbamazepine; hydantoins; cimetidine; oral iron salts; methoxyflurane; and sodium bicarbonate.

Drugs that may be affected by tetracyclines include oral anticoagulants, digoxin, insulin, lithium, methoxyflurane, oral contraceptives, and penicillins.

Drug/Food interactions: Food and some dairy products interfere with absorption of tetracyclines. Administer oral tetracycline 1 hour before or 2 hours after meals. Doxycycline has a low affinity for calcium binding. GI absorption of minocycline and doxycycline is not significantly affected by food or dairy products.

Adverse Reactions

CNS: Lightheadedness, dizziness, or vertigo has been reported with **minocycline**.

Dermatologic: Maculopapular and erythematous rashes.

GI:

Oral and parenteral – Anorexia; nausea; vomiting; diarrhea; epigastric distress; bulky loose stools; stomatitis; sore throat; glossitis; hoarseness.

Oral – Esophageal ulcers, most commonly in patients with an esophageal obstructive element or hiatal hernia.

Hematologic: Hemolytic anemia; thrombocytopenia; thrombocytopenic purpura; neutropenia; eosinophilia.

Hepatic: Fatty liver; increases in liver enzymes.

Hypersensitivity: Urticaria; angioneurotic edema; anaphylaxis; anaphylactoid purpura; pericarditis; exacerbated systemic lupus erythematosus; polyarthralgia; serum sickness-like reactions (eg, fever, rash, arthralgia).

Miscellaneous: Pseudotumor cerebri (adults); bulging fontanels (infants). Nephrogenic diabetes insipidus has been reported with **demeclocycline**.

TRIMETHOPRIM AND SULFAMETHOXAZOLE (Co-Trimoxazole; TMP-SMZ)

Tablets: 80 mg trimethoprim and 400 mg sulfamethoxazole (*Rx*)	Various, *Bactrim* (Roche), *Septra* (GlaxoSmith-Kline)
Tablets, double strength: 160 mg trimethoprim and 800 mg sulfamethoxazole (*Rx*)	Various, *Bactrim DS* (Roche), *Septra DS* (Glaxo-SmithKline)
Oral suspension: 40 mg trimethoprim and 200 mg sulfamethoxazole/5 mL (*Rx*)	Various, *Bactrim Pediatric* (Roche), *Septra* (Glaxo-SmithKline)
Injection: 80 mg trimethoprim and 400 mg sulfamethoxazol/5 mL (*Rx*)	Various, *Bactrim IV* (Roche), *Septra IV* (Glaxo-SmithKline)

Indications

Oral and parenteral:

Urinary tract infections (UTIs) – Urinary tract infections (UTIs) caused by susceptible strains of *Escherichia coli*, *Klebsiella* and *Enterobacter* sp., *Morganella morganii*, *Proteus mirabilis*, and *Proteus vulgaris*.

Shigellosis – Shigellosis enteritis caused by susceptible strains of *Shigella flexneri* and *Shigella sonnei* in children and adults.

Pneumocystis carinii pneumonia (PCP) – Treatment in children and adults.

Oral:

Pneumocystis carinii pneumonia – Prophylaxis in individuals who are immunosuppressed and considered to be at increased risk.

Acute otitis media in children – Acute otitis media in children due to susceptible strains of *Haemophilus influenzae* or *Streptococcus pneumoniae*. There are limited data on the safety of repeated use in children < 2 years of age. Not indicated for prophylactic use or prolonged administration.

Acute exacerbations of chronic bronchitis in adults – Acute exacerbations of chronic bronchitis in adults caused by susceptible strains of *H. influenzae* and *S. pneumoniae*.

Travelers' diarrhea in adults – Travelers' diarrhea in adults caused by susceptible strains of enterotoxigenic *E. coli*.

Unlabeled uses: TMP 40 mg and SMZ 200 mg daily at bedtime, a minimum of 3 times weekly or postcoitally has been used to prevent recurrent UTIs in females.

Treatment of acute and chronic prostatitis – 160 mg TMP/800 mg SMZ twice daily has been used for chronic bacterial prostatitis for up to 12 weeks.

Administration and Dosage

Administration and Dosage of TMP-SMZ

Organisms/Infections	Dosage	
Urinary tract infections, shigellosis and acute otitis media:		
Adults:	160 mg TMP/800 mg SMZ every 12 hours for 10 to 14 days (5 days for shigellosis).	
Children (≥ 2 months of age):	8 mg/kg TMP/40 mg/kg SMZ per day given in 2 divided doses every 12 hours for 10 days (5 days for shigellosis).	
Guideline for proper dosage:	Dose every 12 hours:	
Weight (kg)	Teaspoonfuls	Tablets
10	1 (5 mL)	-
20	2 (10 mL)	1
30	3 (15 mL)	1½
40	4 (20 mL)	2 (or 1 double strength tablet)
Patients with impaired renal function Ccr (mL/min):	Recommended dosage regimen:	
> 30	Usual regimen	
15 to 30	½ usual regimen	
< 15	Not recommended	
IV: Adults and children > 2 months with normal renal function for severe UTIs and shigellosis.	8 to 10 mg/kg/day (based on TMP) in 2 to 4 divided doses every 6, 8 or 12 hours for up to 14 days for severe UTIs and 5 days for shigellosis.	

Administration and Dosage of TMP-SMZ		
Organisms/Infections	Dosage	
Travelers' diarrhea in adults:	160 mg TMP/800 mg SMZ every 12 hrs for 5 days.	
Acute exacerbations of chronic bronchitis in adults:	160 mg TMP/800 mg SMZ every 12 hrs for 14 days.	
Pneumocystis carinii pneumonia:		
Treatment:	15 to 20 mg/kg TMP/100 mg/kg SMZ per day in divided doses every 6 hours for 14 to 21 days.	
Guideline for proper dosage in children	Dose every 6 hours:	
Weight (kg)	Teaspoonfuls	Tablets
8	1 (5 mL)	-
16	2 (10 mL)	1
24	3 (15 mL)	1½
32	4 (20 mL)	2 (or 1 double strength tablet)
IV for adults and children > 2 months:	15 to 20 mg/kg/day (based on TMP) in 3 or 4 divided doses every 6 to 8 hours for up to 14 days.	
Prophylaxis:		
Adults:	160 mg TMP/800 mg SMZ given orally every 24 hours.	
Children:	150 mg/m^2 TMP/ 750 mg/m^2 SMZ per day given orally in equally divided doses twice a day, on 3 consecutive days per week. The total daily dose should not exceed 320 mg TMP/1600 mg SMZ.	
Guideline for proper dosage in children	Dose every 12 hours	
Body surface area (m^2)	Teaspoonfuls	Tablets
0.26	½ (2.5 mL)	-
0.53	1 (5 mL)	½
1.06	2 (10 mL)	1

Parenteral:

IV – Administer over 60 to 90 minutes. Avoid rapid infusion or bolus injection. Do not give IM.

Actions

Pharmacology: SMZ inhibits bacterial synthesis of dihydrofolic acid by competing with para-aminobenzoic acid. TMP blocks the production of tetrahydrofolic acid by inhibiting the enzyme dihydrofolate reductase.

Pharmacokinetics:

Absorption/Distribution – TMP-SMZ is rapidly and completely absorbed following oral administration. Approximately 44% of TMP and 70% of SMZ are protein bound. Following oral administration, the half-lives of TMP (8 to 11 hours) and SMZ (10 to 12 hours) are similar. Following IV administration, the mean plasma half-life was 11.3 hours for TMP and 12.8 hours for SMZ.

Metabolism/Excretion – TMP is metabolized to a small extent; SMZ undergoes biotransformation to inactive compounds.

Urine concentrations are considerably higher than serum concentrations.

Contraindications

Hypersensitivity to TMP or SMZ; megaloblastic anemia caused by folate deficiency; pregnancy at term and lactation; infants < 2 months of age.

The sulfonamides are chemically similar to some goitrogens, diuretics (acetazolamide and the thiazides) and oral hypoglycemic agents. Goiter production, diuresis, and hypoglycemia occur rarely in patients receiving sulfonamides. Cross-sensitivity may exist with these agents.

Warnings

Streptococcal pharyngitis: Do not use to treat streptococcal pharyngitis.

Hematologic effects: Sulfonamide-associated deaths, although rare, have occurred from hypersensitivity of the respiratory tract, Stevens-Johnson syndrome, toxic epidermal necrolysis, fulminant hepatic necrosis, agranulocytosis, aplastic anemia, and other blood dyscrasias.

IV use at high doses or for extended periods of time may cause bone marrow depression manifested as thrombocytopenia, leukopenia, or megaloblastic anemia.

PCP in patients with Acquired Immunodeficiency Syndrome (AIDS): AIDS patients may not tolerate or respond to TMP-SMZ.

Renal/Hepatic function impairment: Use with caution. Maintain adequate fluid intake to prevent crystalluria and stone formation. Patients with severely impaired renal function exhibit an increase in the half-lives of both TMP and SMZ, requiring dosage regimen adjustment.

Elderly: There may be an increased risk of severe adverse reactions, particularly when complicating conditions exist.

Pregnancy: Category C.

Lactation: TMP-SMZ is not recommended in the nursing period because sulfonamides are excreted in breast milk and may cause kernicterus. Premature infants and infants with hyperbilirubinemia or G-6-PD deficiency are also at risk for adverse effects.

Children: Not recommended for infants < 2 months of age. See Indications.

Precautions

Extravascular infiltration: If local irritation and inflammation caused by extravascular infiltration of the infusion occurs, discontinue the infusion and restart at another site.

Benzyl alcohol: Benzyl alcohol, contained in some of these products as a preservative, has been associated with a fatal "gasping syndrome" in premature infants.

Special risk: Use with caution in patients with possible folate deficiency, severe allergy or bronchial asthma. In G-6-PD deficient individuals, hemolysis may occur; it is frequently dose-related.

Drug Interactions

Drugs that may be affected by TMP-SMZ include anticoagulants, cyclosporine, dapsone, diuretics, hydantoins, methotrexate, sulfonylureas, and zidovudine. Drugs that may affect TMP-SMZ include dapsone.

Adverse Reactions

Adverse reactions may include GI disturbances; allergic skin reactions; agranulocytosis; aplastic, hemolytic or megaloblastic anemia; thrombocytopenia; leukopenia; neutropenia; hypoprothrombinemia; eosinophilia; methemoglobinemia; hyperkalemia; hyponatremia; erythema multiforme; Stevens-Johnson syndrome; generalized skin eruptions; rash; toxic epidermal necrolysis; urticaria; pruritus; exfoliative dermatitis; anaphylactoid reactions; photosensitization; allergic myocarditis; angioedema; drug fever; chills; systemic lupus erythematosus; generalized allergic reactions; glossitis; anorexia; stomatitis; pancreatitis; elevation of serum transaminase and bilirubin; headache; mental depression; convulsions; ataxia; hallucinations; tinnitus; vertigo; insomnia; apathy; fatigue; weakness; nervousness; peripheral neuritis; renal failure; interstitial nephritis; BUN and serum creatinine elevation; toxic nephrosis with oliguria and anuria; crystalluria; arthralgia; myalgia.

URSODIOL

Capsules: 300 mg — *Actigall* (Watson)

Warning:
Gallbladder stone dissolution with ursodiol treatment requires months of therapy. Complete dissolution does not occur in all patients and recurrence of stones within 5 years has been observed in up to 50% of patients who do dissolve their stones on bile acid therapy. Carefully select patients for therapy with ursodiol, and consider alternative therapies.

Indications

Gallstone disolution: Dissolution of gallstones in patients with radiolucent, noncalcified, gallbladder stones < 20 mm in greatest diameter in whom elective cholecystectomy would be undertaken except for the presence of increased surgical risk due to systemic disease, advanced age, idiosyncratic reaction to general anesthesia, or for those patients who refuse surgery.

Administration and Dosage

Radiolucent gallbladder stones: 8 to 10 mg/kg/day given in 2 or 3 divided doses.

Obtain ultrasound images of the gallbladder at 6-month intervals for the first year of therapy to monitor gallstone response. If gallstones appear to have dissolved, continue therapy and confirm dissolution on a repeat ultrasound within 1 to 3 months. Most patients who eventually achieve complete stone dissolution will show partial or complete dissolution at the first on-treatment reevaluation. If partial stone dissolution is not seen by 12 months, likelihood of success is greatly reduced.

Actions

Pharmacology: Ursodiol suppresses hepatic synthesis and cholesterol secretion, and also inhibits intestinal absorption of cholesterol. It has little inhibitory effect on synthesis and secretion into bile of endogenous bile acids and does not appear to affect phospholipid secretion into bile. With repeated dosing, bile ursodeoxycholic acid concentrations reach steady state in about 3 weeks.

Pharmacokinetics: About 90% of a therapeutic dose of ursodiol is absorbed in the small bowel after oral administration. Small quantities of ursodiol appear in the systemic circulation and very small amounts are excreted into urine.

Contraindications

Presence of calcified cholesterol stones, radiopaque stones, or radiolucent bile pigment stones (ursodiol will not dissolve these stones; hence, patients with such stones are not candidates for ursodiol); patients with compelling reasons for cholecystectomy including unremitting acute cholecystitis, cholangitis, biliary obstruction, gallstone pancreatitis, or biliary-gastrointestinal fistula; allergy to bile acids; chronic liver disease.

Warnings

Length of therapy: Safety of use of ursodiol beyond 24 months is not established.

Gallbladder nonvisualization: Nonvisualizing gallbladder by oral cholecystogram prior to the initiation of therapy is not a contraindication to ursodiol therapy. However, gallbladder nonvisualization developing during ursodiol treatment predicts failure of complete stone dissolution and therapy should be discontinued.

Pregnancy: Category B. Do not use the drug during pregnancy.

Lactation: It is not known whether ursodiol is excreted in breast milk. Exercise caution when ursodiol is administered to a nursing mother.

Children: Safety and efficacy for use in children have not been established.

Precautions

Hepatic effects: Ursodiol therapy has not been associated with liver damage. Lithocholic acid, a naturally occurring bile acid and metabolite of ursodiol, is known to be a liver-toxic metabolite. Measure AST and ALT at the initiation of therapy, after 1 and 3 months of therapy, and every 6 months thereafter.

Frequently monitor patients with significant abnormalities in liver tests at any point; evaluate carefully for worsening gallstone disease which, in the controlled clinical trials, has been the only identified cause of significant liver test abnormality. Discontinue therapy with ursodiol if increased levels persist.

Drug Interactions

Ursodiol interacts with antacids, bile acid sequestrants, clofibrate, estrogens, and oral contraceptives.

Adverse Reactions

Dermatologic: Pruritus; rash; urticaria; dry skin; sweating; hair thinning. One patient with preexisting psoriasis apparently developed exacerbation of itching which remitted on withdrawal of the drug.

GI: Nausea; vomiting; dyspepsia; metallic taste; abdominal pain; biliary pain; cholecystitis; constipation; stomatitis; flatulence. Doses of 8 to 10 mg/kg/day rarely cause diarrhea (< 1%); in one study, incidence of mild, transient diarrhea was 6%.

Miscellaneous: Headache; fatigue; anxiety; depression; sleep disorder; arthralgia; myalgia; back pain; cough; rhinitis.

VANCOMYCIN

Pulvules: 125 mg and 250 mg (Rx)	*Vancocin* (Lilly)
Powder for oral solution: 1 and 10 g (Rx)	*Vancomycin HCl* (ESI Lederle), *Vancocin* (Lilly)
Powder for injection: 500 mg, 1, 5, and 10 g (Rx)	Various, *Vancocin* (Lilly), *Vancoled* (Lederle)

Indications

Parenteral: Serious or severe infections not treatable with other antimicrobials, including the penicillins and cephalosporins.

Severe staphylococcal infections – Severe staphylococcal infections (including methicillin-resistant staphylococci) in patients who cannot receive or who have failed to respond to penicillins and cephalosporins, or who have infections with resistant staphylococci. Infections may include endocarditis, bone infections, lower respiratory tract infections, septicemia, and skin and skin structure infections.

Endocarditis –

Staphylococcal: Vancomycin is effective alone.

Streptococcal: Vancomycin is effective alone or in combination with an aminoglycoside for endocarditis caused by S. *viridans* or S. *bovis*. It is only effective in combination with an aminoglycoside for endocarditis caused by enterococci (eg, S. *faecalis*).

Diphtheroid: Vancomycin is effective for diphtheroid endocarditis, and has been used successfully with rifampin, an aminoglycoside, or both in early onset prosthetic valve endocarditis caused by *Staphylococcus epidermidis* or diphtheroids.

Prophylactic: Although no controlled clinical efficacy studies have been conducted, IV vancomycin has been suggested for prophylaxis against bacterial endocarditis in penicillin-allergic patients who have congenital heart disease or rheumatic or other acquired or valvular heart disease when these patients undergo dental procedures or surgical procedures of the upper respiratory tract.

Pseudomembranous colitis/staphylococcal enterocolitis caused by Clostridium difficile – The parenteral form may be administered orally; parenteral use alone is unproven. The oral use of parenteral vancomycin is not effective for other infections.

Oral: Staphylococcal enterocolitis and antibiotic-associated pseudomembranous colitis produced by C. *difficile*. The parenteral product may also be given orally for these infections. Oral vancomycin is *not* effective for other types of infection.

Administration and Dosage

Complete full course of therapy; do not discontinue therapy without notifying physician.

Oral:

Adults – 500 mg to 2 g/day given in 3 or 4 divided doses for 7 to 10 days.

Alternatively, dosages of 125 mg 3 or 4 times daily for C. *difficile* colitis may be as effective as the 500 mg dose regimen.

Children – 40 mg/kg/day in 3 or 4 divided doses for 7 to 10 days. Do not exceed 2 g/day.

Neonates – 10 mg/kg/day in divided doses.

Parenteral: Administer each dose over at least 60 minutes. Intermittent infusion is the preferred administration method.

Adults – 500 mg IV every 6 hours or 1 g every 12 hours.

Children – 10 mg/kg/dose given every 6 hours.

Infants and neonates – Initial dose of 15 mg/kg, followed by 10 mg/kg every 12 hours for neonates in the first week of life and every 8 hours thereafter up to the age of 1 month.

Prevention of bacterial endocarditis:

GU/GI procedures (high-risk, penicillin-allergic patients) – 1 g IV over 1 to 2 hours (children, 20 mg/kg) plus gentamicin 1.5 mg/kg IV or IM for both adult (not to exceed 120 mg) and children. Complete injection or infusion within 30 minutes of starting procedure.

(Moderate-risk, penicillin-allergic patients) – 1 g IV over 1 to 2 hours (children 20 mg/kg). Complete infusion within 30 minutes of starting procedure.

Renal function impairment: Adjust dosage; check serum levels regularly. In premature infants and the elderly, dosage reduction may be necessary caused by decreasing renal function.

For most patients, if Ccr can be measured or estimated accurately, the dosage may be calculated by using the following table.

Vancomycin Dosage in Impaired Renal Function	
Ccr (mL/min)	Dose (mg/24 hr)
100	1545
90	1390
80	1235
70	1080
60	925
50	770
40	620
30	465
20	310
10	155

The table is not valid for functionally anephric patients on dialysis. For such patients, give a loading dose of 15 mg/kg to achieve therapeutic serum levels promptly and a maintenance dose of 1.9 mg/kg/24 hr. In patients with marked renal impairment, it may be more convenient to give maintenance doses of 250 to 1000 mg once every several days rather than administering the drug on a daily basis. In anuria a dose of 1000 mg every 7 to 10 days has been recommended.

Actions

Pharmacology: Vancomycin is a tricyclic glycopeptide antibiotic that inhibits cell-wall biosynthesis. It also alters bacterial-cell-membrane permeability and RNA synthesis.

Pharmacokinetics:

Absorption/Distribution – Systemic absorption of oral vancomycin is generally poor.

Metabolism/Excretion – In the first 24 hours, ≈ 75% of a dose is excreted in urine by glomerular filtration. Elimination half-life is 4 to 6 hours in adults and 2 to 3 hours in children. About 60% of an intraperitoneal dose administered during peritoneal dialysis is absorbed systemically in 6 hours. Accumulation occurs in renal failure. Serum half-life in anephric patients is ≈ 7.5 days. Vancomycin is not significantly removed by hemodialysis or continuous ambulatory peritoneal dialysis, although there have been reports of increased clearance with hemoperfusion and hemofiltration.

Contraindications

Hypersensitivity to vancomycin.

Warnings

Ototoxicity: Ototoxicity has occurred in patients receiving vancomycin. It may be transient or permanent. It has occurred mostly in patients who have been given excessive doses, who have an underlying hearing loss, or who are receiving concomitant therapy with another ototoxic agent.

Hypotension: Rapid bolus administration may be associated with exaggerated hypotension, including shock, and rarely, cardiac arrest. To avoid hypotension, administer in a dilute solution over ≥ 60 minutes. Stopping the infusion usually results in prompt cessation of these reactions. Frequently monitor blood pressure and heart rate.

Pseudomembranous colitis: In rare instances, pseudomembranous colitis has occurred because of *C. difficile* developing in patients who received IV vancomycin.

Reversible neutropenia: Reversible neutropenia has occurred in patients receiving vancomycin.

Tissue irritation: Vancomycin is irritating to tissue and must be given by a secure IV route of administration. Pain, tenderness, and necrosis occur with IM injection or inadvertent extravasation.

Reports have revealed that administration of sterile vancomycin by the intraperitoneal route during continuous ambulatory peritoneal dialysis (CAPD) has resulted in a syndrome of chemical peritonitis. This syndrome has ranged from a cloudy dialysate alone to a cloudy dialysate accompanied by variable degrees of abdominal pain and fever. This syndrome appears to be short-lived after discontinuation of intraperitoneal vancomycin.

Nephrotoxicity: The risk of toxicity may be appreciably increased by high serum concentrations or prolonged therapy. Factors that may increase the risk of nephrotoxicity include use in elderly and neonatal patients and concomitant use with other nephrotoxic drugs.

Renal function impairment: Because of its nephrotoxicity, use carefully in renal insufficiency.

Pregnancy: *Category* C; *Category B* (pulvules only).

Lactation: Vancomycin is excreted in breast milk.

Children: In premature and full-term neonates it may be appropriate to confirm desired vancomycin serum concentrations.

Precautions

Monitoring: Perform auditory function serial tests and monitor serum levels. When monitoring vancomycin serum levels, draw a peak concentration 1.5 to 2.5 hours after the completion of a 1-hour infusion and a trough concentration within 1 hour of the next scheduled dose. Peak levels are generally expected to be in the 30 to 40 mg/mL range and trough levels in the 10 to 15 mg/mL range.

Systemic absorption: Clinically significant serum concentrations may occur in some patients who have taken multiple oral doses for active C. *difficile*-induced pseudomembranous colitis or who have inflammatory disorders of the intestinal mucosa; the risk is greater with the presence of renal impairment.

Red Man (or Redneck) syndrome: Red Man (or Redneck) syndrome is usually stimulated by a too-rapid IV infusion (dose given over a few minutes), but it has been reported rarely when given as recommended and following oral or intraperitoneal administration. The onset may occur anytime within a few minutes of starting an IV infusion to a short time after infusion completion. The rash generally resolves several hours after termination of administration.

Drug Interactions

Drugs that may interact with vancomycin include aminoglycosides, anesthetics, neurotoxic/nephrotoxic agents, and nondepolarizing muscle relaxants.

Adverse Reactions

Adverse reactions may include renal impairment; hearing loss; neutropenia; vertigo; dizziness; anaphylaxis; drug fever; nausea; chills; eosinophilia; rashes; hypotension; wheezing; dyspnea; urticaria; inflammation at injection site; Red Man (or Redneck) syndrome; chemical peritonitis has been reported following intraperitoneal administration of vancomycin.

VASOPRESSIN

Injection: 20 pressor units/mL	Various, *Pitressin* (Monarch)

Indications

Treatment of diabetes insipidus.

Prevention and treatment of abdominal distention.

To dispel interfering gas shadows in abdominal roentgenography.

Unlabeled uses: Vasopressin has been used to control acute variceal hemorrhage.

Administration and Dosage

May be given IM or SC.

Usual dose: 5 to 10 units usually elicit full physiologic response. Give IM at 3- or 4-hour intervals as needed. Reduce dosage proportionately for children.

Diabetes insipidus:

Intranasal – The injection solution may be administered intranasally on cotton pledgets, by nasal spray, or dropper. Individualize dosage.

Parenteral – 5 to 10 units 2 or 3 times/day as needed.

Abdominal distention: To prevent or relieve postoperative distention, give 5 units initially; increase to 10 units at subsequent injections, if necessary. Give IM at 3- or 4-hour intervals. Reduce dosage proportionately for children.

Abdominal roentgenography: Administer 2 injections of 10 units each. Give 2 hours and ½ hour, respectively, before films are exposed. An enema may be given prior to first dose.

Actions

Pharmacology: The antidiuretic action of vasopressin is attributed to increasing reabsorption of water by the renal tubules. Vasopressin can cause contraction of smooth muscle of the GI tract and of all parts of the vascular bed. The direct effect on the contractile elements is neither antagonized by adrenergic blocking agents nor prevented by vascular denervation.

Pharmacokinetics: Following IM or SC injection, the duration of antidiuretic activity for vasopressin is 2 to 8 hours. Most is metabolized and rapidly destroyed in liver and kidneys. Vasopressin has a plasma half-life of ≈ 10 to 20 minutes. After 4 hours, ≈ 5% of an SC dose is excreted unchanged in urine.

Contraindications

Anaphylaxis or hypersensitivity to vasopressin or its components.

Warnings

Vascular disease: Use with extreme caution because even small doses may precipitate anginal pain; with larger doses, consider the possibility of MI.

Water intoxication: Early signs of drowsiness, listlessness, and headaches precede terminal coma and convulsions.

Vasoconstriction/Necrosis: May result if vasopressin extravasates during IV infusion.

Chronic nephritis: Contraindicates use until reasonable nitrogen blood levels have been attained.

Pregnancy: Category C.

Lactation: Exercise caution when administering to a nursing woman.

Precautions

Monitoring: Electrocardiograms and fluid and electrolyte status determinations are recommended at intervals during therapy.

Special risk patients: Use vasopressin cautiously in the presence of epilepsy, migraine, asthma, heart failure, or any state in which a rapid increase in extracellular water may result in further compromise.

Drug Interactions

Vasopressin may interact with carbamazepine, chlorpropamide, clofibrate, urea, fludrocotisone, tricyclic antidepressants, demeclocycline, norepinephrine, lithium, heparin, alcohol, and glanglionic blocking agents.

Adverse Reactions

Cardiac arrest, circumoral pallor, arrhythmias, decreased cardiac output, angina, myocardial ischemia, peripheral vasoconstriction, gangrene; tremor, vertigo, "pounding" in head; sweating, urticaria, cutaneous gangrene; abdominal cramps, nausea, vomiting, passage of gas; anaphylaxis (cardiac arrest or shock), bronchial constriction.

APPENDIX

DRUGS THAT REQUIRE HEPATIC MONITORING[1]

Generic	Brand
Antibiotic/Antifungal agents	
Griseofulvin	*Fulvicin P/G*
Itraconazole	*Sporanox*
Ketoconazole	*Nizoral*
Terbinafine	*Lamisil*
Arthritis agents	
Oral gold	*Auranofin*
Methotrexate	*Rheumatrex*
Rofecoxib	*Vioxx*
Diclofenac	*Voltaren*
Nabumetone	*Relafen*
Valdecoxib	*Bextra*
Meloxicam	*Mobic*
Leflunomide	*Arava*
Cardiovascular agents	
Atorvastatin	*Lipitor*
Fluvastatin	*Lescol*
Lovastatin	*Mevacor*
Pravastatin	*Pravachol*
Simvastatin	*Zocor*
Gemfibrozil	*Lopid*
Fenofibrate	*Tricor*
Niacin	*Niaspan*
Amiodarone	*Cordarone*
Chemotherapy agents	
Tretinoin	*Vesanoid*
Gemtuzumab	*Mylotarg*
Imatinib	*Gleevec*
Flutamide	*Eulexin*
CNS agents	
Carbamazepine	*Tegretol*
Felbamate	*Felbatol*
Valproic acid	*Depakote*
Ethotoin	*Peganone*

continued

DRUGS THAT REQUIRE HEPATIC MONITORING[1]—*continued*

Generic	Brand
Ethosuximide	*Zarontin*
Methsuximide	*Celontin*
Oxcarbazepine	*Trileptal*
Pemoline	*Cylert*
Nefazodone	*Serzone*
Tacrine	*Cognex*
Tolcapone	*Tasmar*
Riluzole	*Rilutek*
Tizanidine	*Zanaflex*
Diabetic agents	
Pioglitazone	*Actos*
Rosiglitazone	*Avandia*
HIV agents	
Ritonavir	*Norvir*
Indinavir	*Crixivan*
Lamivudine	*Epivir*
Nevirapine	*Viramune*
Efavirenz	*Sustiva*
Tuberculosis agents	
Isoniazid	*Nydrazid*
Rifampin	*Rifadin*
Pyrazinamide	
Dapsone	
Miscellaneous agents	
Ribavirin/Interferon alfa	*Rebetron*
Ribavirin	*Rebetol*
Tazarotene	*Tazorac gel*
Testosterone	*Androgel*
Bosentan	*Tracleer*
Succimer	*Chemet*
Azathioprine	*Imuran*
Acetaminophen	*Tylenol*
Pentamidine	*Pentam*
Albendazole	*Albenza*

[1] Tice SA & Parry D. Hospital Pharmacy
http://www.factsandcomparisons.com/assets/hospitalpharm/feb2002_HepSp.pdf

INHIBITORS, INDUCERS, AND SUBSTRATES OF CYTOCHROME P450 ENZYMES

Inhibitors, Inducers, and Substrates of Cytochrome P450 Enzymes[1-18]				
CYP Enzyme	Inhibitor	Inducer	Substrate	
1A2	Anastrozole Cimetidine Ciprofloxacin Diethyldithiocarbamate Enoxacin Erythromycin Fluvoxamine Grapefruit Juice (?) Mexiletine Mibefradil Mirtazapine (weak) Norfloxacin Propranolol Ritonavir Tacrine	Charbroiled food Cigarette smoke Omeprazole Phenobarbital Primidone Rifampin	Acetaminophen Caffeine Clozapine (major) Cyclobenzaprine Diazepam Fluvoxamine Haloperidol Isotretinoin Methadone Mexiletine (minor) Mirtazapine Naproxen Olanzapine Ondansetron Phenacetin Propafenone Propranolol Riluzole	Ritonavir Ropivacaine Tacrine Tamoxifen Testosterone Theophylline (major) TCAs (demethylation) Amitriptyline Clomipramine Desipramine Imipramine Nortriptyline Verapamil R-Warfarin Zileuton Zolpidem
2A6	Diethyldithiocarbamate Ketoconazole Methoxsalen Miconazole Pilocarpine Ritonavir		Ritonavir Tamoxifen	
2B6	Diethyldithiocarbamate Orphenadrine	Phenobarbital Phenytoin Primidone	Cyclophosphamide Ifosfamide Tamoxifen	
2C8-10	Amiodarone (2C9) Anastrozole (2C8/2C9) Chloramphenicol (2C9) Cimetidine (2C9) Diclofenac (2C9) Diethyldithiocarbamate (2C8) Disulfiram (2C9) Fluconazole (2C9) Fluoxetine (2C9) Flurbiprofen (2C9) Fluvastatin (2C9) Fluvoxamine (2C9) Ketoprofen (2C9) Metronidazole (2C9) Miconazole (2C9) Omeprazole (2C8) Phenylbutazone (2C9) Ritonavir (2C9) Sertraline (suspected) Sulfonamides (2C9) Sulfadiazine (2C9) Sulfamethizole (2C9) Sulfamethoxazole (2C9) Sulfinpyrazone (2C9) Trimethoprim (2C9) Zafirlukast (2C9)	Carbamazepine (2C9) Ethanol (2C9) Phenobarbital (2C8) Phenytoin (2C9) Primidone (2C8) Rifampin (2C9)	Barbiturates Hexobarbital (2C9) Mephobarbital (2C9) Benzphetamine (2C8) Carvedilol (2C9) Dapsone (2C9) Diazepam (2C8) Diclofenac (2C8/2C9) Dronabinol (2C9) Fluoxetine (2C9) Flurbiprofen (2C9) Glimepiride (2C9) Ibuprofen (2C9) Indomethacin (2C9) Isotretinoin (2C8) Losartan (2C9) Mefenamic Acid (2C9) Mephenytoin (2C9) Mirtazapine (2C9) Montelukast (2C9) Naproxen (2C9) Omeprazole (2C8) Paclitaxel (2C8; major) Phenytoin (2C9) Piroxicam (2C9) Retinoic acid (2C8) Ritonavir (2C9) Suprofen (2C9) Terbinafine (2C9) Tetrahydrocannabinol (2C9)	Tolbutamide (2C8/2C9) Torsemide (2C9) TCAs Amitriptyline (2C9) Imipramine (2C9) S-Warfarin (2C9) Zafirlukast (2C9) Zileuton (2C9)

INHIBITORS, INDUCERS, AND SUBSTRATES OF CYTOCHROME P450 ENZYMES—*continued*

Inhibitors, Inducers, and Substrates of Cytochrome P450 Enzymes[1-18]

CYP Enzyme	Inhibitor	Inducer	Substrate	
2C18-19	Cimetidine (2C18) Felbamate (2C19) Fluoxetine (2C19) Fluvoxamine (2C19) Omeprazole (2C19) Ritonavir (2C19) Tolbutamide (2C19) Topiramate (2C19) Tranylcypromine (2C19)	Rifampin (2C19)	Carisoprodol (2C19) Citalopram (2C19) Desmethyldiazepam (2C19) Diazepam (2C19) Divalproex Sodium (2C19) Hexobarbital (2C19) Lansoprazole (2C19) Mephenytoin (2C19) S-Mephenytoin (2C19) Naproxen (2C18) Omeprazole (2C19)	Piroxicam (2C18) Propranolol (2C19) Retinoic Acid (2C18) Ritonavir (2C19) S-Tetrahydrocannabinol (2C18) Tolbutamide (2C19) TCAs Clomipramine (2C19) Imipramine (2C19) Valproic Acid (2C19) S-Warfarin (2C18)
2D6	Amiodarone Chloroquine Cimetidine Codeine Delavirdine Dextropropoxyphene Doxorubicin Fluoxetine Fluphenazine Fluvoxamine Haloperidol Lomustine Methadone Mibefradil Mirtazapine (weak) Norfluoxetine Norfluvoxamine Paroxetine Perphenazine Primaquine Propafenone Propranolol Quinidine Ranitidine Ritonavir Sertraline (suspected) Thioridazine Venlafaxine Vinblastine Vinorelbine Yohimbine	Not affected by common inducers	Carvedilol Chloroquine (possible) Chlorpromazine Clozapine Codeine Cyclobenzaprine Debrisoquin Delavirdine Dexfenfluramine Dextromethorphan Dolasetron Donepezil Encainide Flecainide Fluoxetine Fluphenazine Halofantrine Haloperidol Hydrocodone Hydroxyamphetamine Labetalol Maprotiline Methamphetamine Metoprolol Mexiletine (major) Mirtazapine Morphine Olanzapine (minor) Ondansetron Oxamniquine	Oxycodone Paroxetine Pentazocine Perphenazine Phenformin Primaquine (possible) Propafenone Propoxyphene Propranolol (minor) Risperidone Ritonavir Ropivacaine Selegiline Sertraline Sparteine Tamoxifen Thioridazine Timolol Tolterodine (major) Tramadol Trazodone TCAs (hydroxylation) Amitriptyline Clomipramine Desipramine Imipramine Nortriptyline Trimipramine Venlafaxine Zolpidem
2E1	Diethyldithiocarbamate Disulfiram Ritonavir	Ethanol Isoniazid	Acetaminophen Chlorzoxazone Dapsone Enflurane Ethanol (minor) Halothane Isoflurane	Isoniazid Methoxyflurane Ondansetron Ritonavir Sevoflurane Tamoxifen Theophylline
3A3	Cimetidine Nefazodone (suspected) Ranitidine		Erythromycin Midazolam	

INHIBITORS, INDUCERS, AND SUBSTRATES OF CYTOCHROME P450 ENZYMES—*continued*

Inhibitors, Inducers, and Substrates of Cytochrome P450 Enzymes[1-18]

CYP Enzyme	Inhibitor	Inducer	Substrate	
3A4	Anastrozole	Carbamazepine	Acetaminophen	Miconazole
	Cimetidine	Glucocorticoids	Alfentanil	Midazolam
	Clarithromycin	Dexamethasone	Alprazolam	Mifepristone
	Clotrimazole	Prednisone	Amiodarone	Mirtazapine
	Danazol	Macrolide Anti-	Amlodipine	Montelukast
	Delavirdine	biotics	Astemizole	Navelbine
	Diethyldithiocarba-	Phenobarbital	Atorvastatin	Nefazodone
	mate	Phenylbutazone	Benzphetamine	Nelfinavir
	Diltiazem	Phenytoin	Bromocriptine	Nevirapine
	Erythromycin	Primidone	Busulfan	Nicardipine
	Fluconazole	Rifabutin	Carbamazepine	Nifedipine
	Fluoxetine	Rifampin	Cerivastatin	Nimodipine
	Fluvoxamine	Sulfinpyrazone	Chlorpromazine	Nisoldipine
	Grapefruit Juice		Citalopram	Nitrendipine
	Indinavir		Clarithromycin	Omeprazole
	Itraconazole		Clindamycin	Ondansetron
	Ketoconazole		Clonazepam	Paclitaxel (minor)
	Metronidazole		Cocaine	Pimozide
	Mibefradil		Codeine	Progesterone
	Miconazole		Cyclobenzaprine	Propafenone
	Mirtazapine (weak)		Cyclophosphamide	Quinidine
	Nefazodone		Cyclosporine	Quinine
	Nelfinavir		Dapsone	Ritonavir
	Nevirapine		Delavirdine	Salmeterol
	Norfloxacin		Dexamethasone	Saquinavir
	Norfluoxetine		Dextromethorphan	Sertraline
	Paroxetine		Diazepam	Sibutramine
	Propranolol		Diltiazem	Simvastatin
	Quinine		Disopyramide	Sufentanil
	Quinidine		Dolasetron	Tacrolimus
	Ranitidine		Donepezil	Tamoxifen
	Ritonavir		Doxorubicin	Teniposide
	Saquinavir		Dronabinol	Terfenadine
	Sertraline		Erythromycin	Testosterone
	Troleandomycin		Ethinyl Estradiol	Theophylline (minor)
	Zafirlukast		Ethosuximide	Tiagabine
			Etoposide	Tolterodine
			Felodipine	Tretinoin
			Fentanyl	Triazolam
			Granisetron	TCAs (demethylation)
			Halofantrine	Amitriptyline
			Hydrocortisone	Clomipramine
			Ifosfamide	Imipramine
			Indinavir	Troleandomycin
			Isradipine	Venlafaxine
			Itraconazole (?)	Verapamil
			Ketoconazole	Vinblastine
			Lansoprazole	Vincristine
			Lidocaine	R-Warfarin
			Loratadine	Yohimbine
			Losartan	Zileuton
			Lovastatin	Zolpidem (major)
			Mibefradil	
3A5-7	Clotrimazole	Phenobarbital	Ethinyl Estradiol	Terfenadine
	Ketoconazole	Phenytoin	Lovastatin (3A5)	Testosterone
	Metronidazole	Primidone	Midazolam (3A5)	Triazolam
	Miconazole	Rifampin	Nifedipine (3A5)	Vinblastine
	Troleandomycin		Quinidine	Vincristine

(?) = Effect uncertain or minimal.

GASTROINTESTINAL DRUGS WITH BLACK BOX WARNINGS

Generic name	Black box synopsis[1]	Classification	Monitoring recommendations related to black box data[2]
GASTROINTESTINAL AGENTS			
Alosetron	*GI*: Serious adverse events, some fatal, have been reported with use, including ischemic colitis and serious complications of constipation. *Restricted prescribing program* *Indication*: Only for women with severe diarrhea in predominant irritable bowel syndrome refractory to conventional therapy. *Patient signed Patient–Physician Agreement* *Discontinue immediately upon signs of constipation or symptoms of ischemic colitis.*	• GI • Restricted program • Indication • Patient agreement	• Removed from US market in November 2000 and remarketed under restricted dispensing program in June 2002.
Cisapride	*Cardiovascular*: Serious cardiac arrhythmias including ventricular tachycardia, ventricular fibrillation, torsades de pointes, and QT prolongation. Risk factors include concurrent therapy with drugs known to cause QT prolongation and depleted serum electrolytes. *Drug interactions*: Contraindicated with numerous drugs including those known to cause QT prolongation (tricyclics, certain antipsychotics) or CYP450 3A4 inhibitors (fluconazole, ketoconazole, itraconazole). See package insert. *Do not exceed recommended doses.*	• Cardiovascular • Drug interactions • Dosage restriction • Restricted distribution program	• 12 ECG lead prior to administration • Do not initiate therapy if $QT_C > 450$ msec • Serum electrolytes and creatinine assessed prior to therapy and whenever condition develops that may affect electrolyte balance or renal function. • If syncope or rapid or irregular heartbeat develops, stop drug. • Drug withdrawn in 2000 and is available only via restricted distribution and registration program.

continued

GASTROINTESTINAL DRUGS WITH BLACK BOX WARNINGS—*continued*

Generic name	Black box synopsis[1]	Classification	Monitoring recommendations related to black box data[2]
GASTROINTESTINAL AGENTS			
Infliximab	*Tuberculosis, invasive fungal infections, and opportunistic infections*: Have been reported with use. May be fatal.	• Infection	• Evaluate patients for latent tuberculosis with tuberculin skin test. • Treatment of latent infection should be initiated prior to infliximab therapy. • FDA Safety Alert 10/01
Misoprostol	*Abortion, premature birth, birth defects, and uterine rupture*: Reported when administered in pregnant women to induce labor or abortion beyond 8th wk of pregnancy. *Should not be taken by pregnant women for risk reduction of NSAID ulcers*. *Patient counseling* of abortifacient properties.	• Abortifacient properties	• Prescribed for NSAID ulcer reduction in women if negative serum pregnancy test within 2 wk prior to therapy and if capable of contraception compliance. • Requires written and oral patient counseling • Begin therapy only on second or third day of the next normal menstrual period.

1. Synopsis information presents a summary of black box data from the product information. Patient care decisions should not be made without reviewing the most recent product information insert.
2. Monitoring recommendations pertain only to the data that is presented in the black box. Some drugs may require additional monitoring for other safety issues. Always check the most recent and complete product information prior to making patient care decisions.

DRUGS WITH BLACK BOX WARNINGS RELATED TO HEPATOTOXICITY OR GI TOXICITIES

Generic name	Black box synopsis[1]	Organ system/ Other	Monitoring recommendations related to black box data[2]
Abacavir	*Fatal hypersensitivity reactions:* Associated with therapy. Drug should not be restarted after suspected reaction. Severe or fatal reaction may occur within hrs after reintroduction of drug in patients with unrecognized symptoms of hypersensitivity. *Lactic acidosis and Hepatomegaly:* Reported with steatosis (including fatal cases) reported with the use of nucleoside analog alone or in combination.	• Hypersensitivity • Hepatotoxicity • Lactic acidosis	• Patients developing signs or symptoms of hypersensitivity should stop drug immediately. If hypersensitivity reaction cannot be ruled out, permanently discontinue the drug to prevent life-threatening reaction. Do not restart after suspected reaction.
Alosetron	*GI:* Serious adverse events, some fatal, have been reported with use, including ischemic colitis and serious complications of constipation. *Restricted Prescribing Program* *Indication:* Only for women with severe diarrhea in predominant irritable bowel syndrome refractory to conventional therapy *Patient signed Patient-Physician Agreement* *Discontinue immediately upon signs of constipation or symptoms of ischemic colitis.*	• GI • Restricted program • Indication • Patient agreement	• Removed from US market in November 2000 and remarketed under restricted dispensing program in June 2002.

continued

DRUGS WITH BLACK BOX WARNINGS RELATED TO HEPATOTOXICITY OR GI TOXICITIES—*continued*

Generic name	Black box synopsis[1]	Organ system/ Other	Monitoring recommendations related to black box data[2]
Amiodarone	*Life threatening arrhythmias:* Only indication *Potentially pulmonary fatal toxicities:* Include hypersensitivity pneumonitis or interstitial /alveolar pneumonitis *Liver disease:* Can occur *Proarrhythmic effects*	• Indication • Respiratory • Hepatotoxicity • Cardiovascular	
Anabolic steroids	*Hepatotoxicity:* Peliosis hepatis, liver cell tumors. *Lipid changes:* Lipid changes known to increase risk of atherosclerosis or coronary artery disease have occurred with androgens and anabolic steroids.	• Hepatotoxicity • Lipid changes	
Clindamycin	*Pseudomembranous colitis:* May range from mild to life-threatening. Because of association with severe colitis, reserve clindamycin for serious infections only.	• GI	• Consider colitis in patient who presents with diarrhea during or several wk after therapy completely.

continued

DRUGS WITH BLACK BOX WARNINGS RELATED TO HEPATOTOXICITY OR GI TOXICITIES—*continued*

Generic name	Black box synopsis[1]	Organ system/ Other	Monitoring recommendations related to black box data[2]
Dacarbazine	*Experienced physician* *Special handling procedures:* Avoid inhalation or contact with skin/mucous membranes. Extremely corrosive. *Avoid extravasation* *Hemopoietic depression* *Hepatic necrosis*	• Experience • Handling • Precautions • Extravasation • Hematological • Hepatotoxicity	
Dactinomycin	*Experienced physician* *Hemapoietic depression* *Hepatic necrosis* *Avoid extravasation* *Carcinogenic, teratogenic* *Assessment of Benefit/risk ratio*	• Experience • Hematological • Hepatotoxicity • Carcinogenecity • Teratogenecity	
Dantrolene	*Hepatotoxicity:* Symptomatic (fatal and nonfatal) hepatitis is dose related. Incidence is lower with doses up to 400 mg/day compared with ≥ 800 mg/day. Overt hepatitis is most frequent during third and twelfth months. Risk higher in females, patients > 35 yr, and concurrent therapy.	• Hepatotoxicity	• Use lowest possible effective dose. • If no benefit observed after 45 days of therapy, discontinue drug. • Monitor hepatic function, including frequent determinations of AST or ALT.

continued

DRUGS WITH BLACK BOX WARNINGS RELATED TO HEPATOTOXICITY OR GI TOXICITIES—*continued*

Generic name	Black box synopsis[1]	Organ system/ Other	Monitoring recommendations related to black box data[2]
Didanosine	*Pancreatitis:* Fatal and nonfatal cases have occurred with monotherapy or in combination. *Hepatotoxicity:* With steatosis (including fatal cases) have been reported with nucleoside analogs alone or in combination. *Lactic acidosis:* Reported in pregnant women who have received didanosine and stavudine with other antiretroviral agents. Use the combination with caution in pregnant women.	• Hepatotoxicity • Lactic acidosis • Pancreatitis	• Patients with prodromal symptoms of hepatitis should seek medical attention immediately and promptly discontinue drug.
Gemtuzumab	*Experience/Hospital setting:* Should be used by experienced personnel in the treatment of acute leukemia in facility with appropriate equipment to monitor and treat leukemia patients. *Use as single agent:* No studies demonstrating efficacy/safety in conjunction with other agents. *Myelosuppression:* Severe cases may occur at recommended doses.	• Experience/ Equipped facility • Administration • Hematological • Hepatotoxicity	• Interrupt infusion in patients experiencing dyspnea or clinically significant hypotension. Monitor until complete resolution of symptoms. • Discontinue treatment in patients who develop anaphylaxis, pulmonary edema, or adult respiratory distress syndrome. • Monitor for hepatotoxicity signs (eg, rapid weight gain, right upper quadrant pain, hepatomegaly, ascites, increases in LFTs/bilirubin).

continued

DRUGS WITH BLACK BOX WARNINGS RELATED TO HEPATOTOXICITY OR GI TOXICITIES—*continued*

Generic name	Black box synopsis[1]	Organ system/ Other	Monitoring recommendations related to black box data[2]
Gemtuzumab *(cont.)*	*Hypersensitivity/Anaphylaxis:* Severe cases, including pulmonary events, may occur. Patients with high peripheral blast counts may be at greater risk for pulmonary events or tumor lysis syndrome. Consider leukoreduction prior to administration. *Hepatotoxicity:* Severe hepatic veno-occlusive disease has been reported with use. Increased risk in patients with hematopoietic stem-cell transplants, underlying liver disease or abnormal liver function, and in patients receiving adjunctive chemotherapy.		
Isoniazid	*Hepatitis:* Severe and sometimes fatal hepatitis may occur during and many months after treatment. Risk is related to age and increased with daily alcohol consumption. Patients should be instructed about signs and symptoms of hepatitis. If reinitiated, start in small and gradual doses. Not for use in patients with active liver disease.	• Hepatotoxicity	• Careful monitoring and monthly interviews. • Discontinue abruptly if symptoms appear.

continued

DRUGS WITH BLACK BOX WARNINGS RELATED TO HEPATOTOXICITY OR GI TOXICITIES—*continued*

Generic name	Black box synopsis[1]	Organ system/ Other	Monitoring recommendations related to black box data[2]
Irinotecan	*Experienced physician/Equipped facilities* *Diarrhea:* Early and late forms of severe diarrhea. May be life-threatening (see monitoring). *Myelosuppression*	• Experience • GI toxicity • Hematological	• Early diarrhea may be ameliorated by atropine. • Treat late diarrhea promptly with loperamide. • Carefully monitor patients with diarrhea. Give fluids and electrolyte replacement if dehydration occurs. Administer antibiotics if ileus, fever, or neutropenia develops.
Ketoconazole (oral)	*Hepatotoxicity:* Including fatalities. *Drug interactions:* Severe cardiovascular events when coadministered with cisapride.	• Hepatotoxicity • Drug interactions	• LFTs and bilirubin at baseline and frequent intervals during therapy.
Ketorolac	*Therapy duration:* Limited to 5 days *Management of moderate to severe acute pain:* That requires analgesia at the opioid level. Not for chronic pain syndromes. *Tablet administration:* Only indicated as continuation of injection therapy. *Total daily dose:* Oral (40 mg), injectable (120 mg) *Dosage adjustment* required in patients ≥ 65 yr, ≤ 50 kg, moderately elevated serum creatinine. Maximum dose in these patients ≤ 60 mg/day	• Dosage limits • Duration limits • Indication • GI toxicity • Nephrotoxicity • Hepatotoxicity • Hematological • Drug interactions	

continued

DRUGS WITH BLACK BOX WARNINGS RELATED TO HEPATOTOXICITY OR GI TOXICITIES—*continued*

Generic name	Black box synopsis[1]	Organ system/ Other	Monitoring recommendations related to black box data[2]
Ketorolac *(cont.)*	*GI effects*: Peptic ulcers, GI bleeding and/or perforation. Contraindicated in patients with active or history of these states. *Renal effects*: Contraindicated in patients with advanced renal impairment or at risk of renal failure due to volume depletion. *Bleeding risk*: Due to platelet inhibition. Contraindicated as pre-op or intra-op analgesic and in patients at high risk of bleeding. *Hypersensitivity* has been reported in patients with ASA/NSAID allergies. *Inthrathecal/Epidural administration* contraindicated due to alcohol content. *Use in labor/delivery and nursing contraindicated.* *Concurrent use with NSAIDs contraindicated.*		
Lamivudine	*Lactic acidosis and hepatomegaly*: Reported with steatosis (including fatal cases) reported with the use of nucleoside analogs alone or in combination.	• Hepatotoxicity • Lactic acidosis • Dosing formulations	• Patients with prodromal symptoms of hepatitis should seek medical attention immediately and promptly discontinue drug.

continued

DRUGS WITH BLACK BOX WARNINGS RELATED TO HEPATOTOXICITY OR GI TOXICITIES—*continued*

Generic name	Black box synopsis[1]	Organ system/ Other	Monitoring recommendations related to black box data[2]
Lamivudine (*cont.*)	*Dosing Formulation: Epivir* tablets and oral solution are used to treat HIV infection and contain a higher dose of lamivudine than *Epivir-HBV*, which is used to treat chronic hepatitis B infection. HIV patients should receive only *Epivir* formulations.		
Nefazodone	*Hepatic Failure* (life-threatening) reported with use. *Patient instructions for signs of liver dysfunction*	• Hepatotoxicity	• Withdraw therapy if serum AST or serum ALT $\geq$ 3 times upper limit of normal
Nevirapine	*Hepatotoxicity*: Severe, life-threatening, and in some cases, fatal, including fulminant and cholestatic hepatitis, necrosis, and failure. *Dermal reactions*: Severe, life-threatening skin reactions (sometimes fatal) have occurred during therapy. Cases include Stevens-Johnson syndrome, toxic epidermal necrolysis, and hypersensitivity reactions. *Patient Monitoring*: Close monitoring for first 12 wk to detect signs and symptoms of skin/hepatic reactions. *Dosing*: 14-day initiation period (200 mg/day) must be strictly followed.	• Hepatotoxicity • Dermal reactions • Patient monitoring • Initial dosing • Resistance	• Patients should be closely monitored at baseline and for first 12 wks for signs of potentially life-threatening liver or skin reactions. Optimal frequency of monitoring not defined. • Patients with prodromal symptoms of hepatitis should seek medical attention immediately and promptly discontinue drug. • Patients developing signs or symptoms of severe skin reactions or hypersensitivity reactions should discontinue drug immediately

continued

DRUGS WITH BLACK BOX WARNINGS RELATED TO HEPATOTOXICITY OR GI TOXICITIES—*continued*

Generic name	Black box synopsis[1]	Organ system/ Other	Monitoring recommendations related to black box data[2]
Nevirapine (*cont.*)	*Resistance:* Resistance proven with monotherapy. Nevirapine should always be administered in combination therapy with other antiretrovirals.		
Pemoline	*Life-threatening hepatotoxicity:* Limits use as first line agent in ADHD. May have long latency period. *Written informed consent:* From patient prior to initiation.	• Hepatotoxicity • Patient consent	• Unresponsive patients removed from therapy at 3 wk. • Initiate only in patients with normal baseline LFTs and without liver disease. • Serum ALT at baseline and every 2 wk. • Informed consent recommended. • Discontinue if serum ALT increases are clinically significant or any increase ≥ 2 times upper limit of normal.
Pentostatin	*Experienced physician.* *Do not exceed recommended doses.* *Nephrotoxicity, hepatotoxicity,* CNS, *pulmonary toxicity:* Dose-related. *Do not use with concurrent fludarabine:* Increased risk of pulmonary toxicity.	• Experience • Dosage • Nephrotoxicity • Hepatotoxicity • CNS • Respiratory	
Sirolimus	*Experienced physicians/equipped facility* *Increased susceptibility to infection* *Increased risk of lymphoma*	• Experience • Equipped facility • Infection	

continued

DRUGS WITH BLACK BOX WARNINGS RELATED TO HEPATOTOXICITY OR GI TOXICITIES—*continued*

Generic name	Black box synopsis[1]	Organ system/ Other	Monitoring recommendations related to black box data[2]
Sirolimus (*cont.*)	*Hepatic artery thrombosis*: Reported in liver transplant patients who received drug in combination with cyclosporine or tacrolimus. Most cases occurred 30 days posttransplantation. *Use in liver transplant patients*: Not recommended.	• Cancer • Hepatic thrombosis	
Stavudine	*Pancreatitis*: Fatal and nonfatal cases have occurred with monotherapy or in combination with didanosine with or without hydroxyurea. *Hepatotoxicity*: With steatosis (including fatal cases) has been reported with nucleoside analogs alone or in combination. *Lactic acidosis*: Reported in pregnant women who have received didanosine and stavudine with other antiretroviral agents. Use the combination with caution in pregnant women.	• Pancreatitis • Hepatotoxicity • Lactic acidosis	• Patients with prodromal symptoms of hepatitis should seek medical attention immediately and promptly discontinue drug.
Streptozocin	*Experienced physician/Equipped facility* *Nephrotoxicity*: Dose related and cumulative. May be fatal. *Severe nausea and vomiting, diarrhea* *Liver dysfunction, hematological changes*	• Experience • Equipped facility • Nephrotoxicity • GI • Hepatotoxicity	• Serial urinalysis, BUN, plasma creatinine, serum electrolytes and Ccr at baseline and at least weekly during and for 4 wk after drug administration.

continued

DRUGS WITH BLACK BOX WARNINGS RELATED TO HEPATOTOXICITY OR GI TOXICITIES—*continued*

Generic name	Black box synopsis[1]	Organ system/ Other	Monitoring recommendations related to black box data[2]
Terbinafine (oral)	*Hepatotoxicity*: Rare cases of severe and fatal liver failure. Not recommended for patients with chronic or active liver disease. May occur in patients without pre-existing liver disease	• Hepatotoxicity	• Baseline ALT and AST prior to treatment. • Obtain nail specimens for laboratory testing prior to prescribing the medications for onychomycosis to confirm the diagnosis.
Tolcapone	*Hepatotoxicity*: May be fatal. Do not initiate therapy or withdraw therapy if patient exhibits clinical evidence of liver disease or ALT or AST values are greater than upper limit of normal	• Hepatotoxicity	• If no benefit observed after 3 weeks of therapy, discontinue drug. • Baseline AST and ALT and every 2 wks for first year, every 4 wk for next 6 months, and every 8 wk thereafter. Monitor liver enzymes before increasing dose to 200 mg 3 times/day and reinitiate monitoring frequency. • If hepatocellular injury occurs, withdraw therapy and do not restart.
Trovafloxacin	*Hepatotoxicity*: Severe leading to transplantation and death. Risk increased with > 2 wk duration. Use only in life-threatening infections.	• Hepatotoxicity	
Valproic acid and derivatives	*Hepatotoxicity*: Increased risk in children < 2 yr with multiple anticonvulsants, congenital metabolic disorders, severe seizure disorders, mental retardation, or organic brain syndrome. *Onset*: Typically first 6 months. *Teratogenicity*: Neural tube defects.	• Hepatotoxicity • Teratogenecity • Pancreatitis	• *Hepatotoxicity*: Symptoms and LFTs at baseline and frequent intervals, especially within first 6 months. • *Pancreatitis*: Patients should be informed of warning signs.

continued

DRUGS WITH BLACK BOX WARNINGS RELATED TO HEPATOTOXICITY OR GI TOXICITIES—*continued*

Generic name	Black box synopsis[1]	Organ system/ Other	Monitoring recommendations related to black box data[2]
Valproic acid and derivatives *(cont.)*	*Pancreatitis*: Occurs in children and adults after initial or long-term therapy.		
Zalcitabine	*Neuropathy*: Severe peripheral neuropathy; use with extreme caution in patients with pre-existing neuropathy. *Pancreatitis*: Rarely occurs. Monitor. *Lactic acidosis and hepatomegaly*: Reported with steatosis (including fatal cases) with the use of nucleoside analogs alone or in combination.	• Neuropathy • Pancreatitis • Hepatic • Lactic acidosis	• Patients with symptoms of hepatitis or pancreatitis should seek medical attention immediately and promptly discontinue drugs.
Zidovudine	*Hematological*: Neutropenia and severe anemia, particularly in patients with advanced HIV disease. *Myopathy*: Associated with prolonged use *Lactic acidosis and hepatomegaly*: Reported with steatosis (including fatal cases) with the use of nucleoside analogs alone or in combination.	• Hematological • Hepatic • Lactic acidosis • Myopathy	• Frequent blood counts strongly recommended during therapy in patients with advanced HIV disease. Periodic blood counts recommended for HIV-infected individuals who are asymptomatic or have early HIV disease. • Patients with prodromal symptoms of hepatitis should seek medical attention immediately and promptly discontinue drug.

1. Synopsis information presents a summary of black box data from the product information. Patient care decisions should not be made without reviewing the most recent product information insert.
2. Monitoring recommendations pertain only to the data that is presented in the black box. Some drugs may require additional monitoring for other safety issues. Always check the most recent and complete product information prior to making patient care decisions.

DRUG-INDUCED FECES DISCOLORATIONS

Orange/Red/Pink	Anticoagulants Aspirin Barium Heparin Phenazopyridine Rifampin
Yellow	Senna
Black	Acetazolamide Aluminum hydroxide Amphetamine Arsenicals Betamethasone Bismuth salts Charcoal Chlorpropamide Clindamycin Corticosteroids Cyclophosphamide Cytarabine Ethacrynic acid Ferrous salts Fluorouracil Hydralazine Indomethacin Levodopa Melphalan Mercury Compounds Methotrexate Phenylephrine Potassium salts Procarbazine Sulfonamides Tetracycline Thiotepa Warfarin

ANTACID DRUG INTERACTIONS

Antacid Drug Interactions

Drug	Antacid[1]				
	Aluminum salts	Calcium salts	Magnesium salts	Sodium bicarbonate	Magnesium-aluminum combinations
Allopurinol	↓				
Amphetamines				↑	
Benzodiazepines	↑		↓	↓	↓
Captopril					↓
Chloroquine	↓		↓		
Corticosteroids	↓		↓		↓
Dicumarol			↑		
Diflunisal	↓				
Digoxin	↓		↓		
Ethambutol	↓				
Flecainide				↑	
Fluoroquinolones		↓			↓
Histamine H_2 antagonists	↓		↓		↓
Hydantoins		↓	↓		↓
Iron salts	↓	↓	↓	↓	↓
Isoniazid	↓				
Ketoconazole				↓	↓
Levodopa					↑
Lithium				↓	
Methenamine				↓	
Methotrexate				↓	
Nitrofurantoin			↓		
Penicillamine	↓		↓		↓
Phenothiazines	↓		↓		↓
Quinidine		↑	↑	↑	↑
Salicylates		↓		↓	↓
Sodium polystyrene sulfonate					‡[2]
Sulfonylureas			↑	↓	↑
Sympathomimetics				↑	
Tetracyclines	↓	↓	↓	↓	↓
Thyroid hormones	↓				
Ticlopidine	↓		↓		↓
Valproic acid					↑

[1] Pharmacologic effect increased (↑) or decreased (↓) by antacids.
[2] Concomitant use may cause metabolic alkalosis in patients with renal impairment.

HISTAMINE H_2 ANTAGONIST DRUG INTERACTIONS

Histamine H_2 Antagonist Drug Interactions			
Precipitant drug	Object drug*		Description
Antacids Anticholinergics Metoclopramide	H_2 antagonists	↓	These agents may decrease the absorption of cimetidine. However, 1 study suggested cimetidine absorption is unaffected by concomitant multiple-dose antacid administration. Ranitidine absorption may be decreased by concurrent antacids; data conflict. Avoid simultaneous administration. Bioavailability of famotidine and nizatidine may be slightly decreased; no special precautions are necessary.
Cigarette smoking	Cimetidine	↓	Cigarette smoking reverses cimetidine-induced inhibition of nocturnal gastric secretion, hindering ulcer healing. Cigarette use is closely related to ulcer recurrence.
Cimetidine	Ferrous salts Indomethacin Ketoconazole Tetracyclines	↓	Pharmacologic effects of these agents may be decreased by cimetidine due to decreased absorption.
Cimetidine	Carmustine	↑	Bone marrow suppression (toxicity) of carmustine may be enhanced by cimetidine, possibly due to additive effect or inhibition of carmustine metabolism.
Cimetidine	Digoxin	↓	Serum digoxin concentrations may decrease during coadministration.
Cimetidine	Flecainide	↑	Pharmacologic effects of flecainide may be increased.
Cimetidine	Fluconazole	↓	Fluconazole plasma levels may be reduced, possibly due to decreased absorption.
Cimetidine	Fluorouracil	↑	Fluorouracil serum concentrations may be increased following chronic cimetidine use.
Cimetidine	Narcotic analgesics	↑	Toxic effects (eg, respiratory depression) may be increased.
Cimetidine Ranitidine	Procainamide	↑	Cimetidine may increase plasma levels of procainamide and its cardioactive metabolite n-acetyl-procainamide (NAPA) by decreasing renal tubular secretion. Ranitidine may decrease the renal clearance and increase AUC of procainamide. One study reported no effect of ranitidine on procainamide or NAPA elimination.
Cimetidine	Succinylcholine	↑	The neuromuscular blocking effects may be increased by cimetidine. Prolonged respiratory depression with extended periods of apnea may occur.
Cimetidine	Tocainide	↓	Cimetidine may decrease the pharmacologic effects of tocainide.
Nizatidine	Salicylates	↑	Increased serum salicylate levels occurred when nizatidine was administered to patients receiving very high doses of aspirin (3.9 g/day).
Ranitidine	Diazepam	↓	Diazepam's pharmacologic effects may be decreased due to decreased GI absorption by ranitidine. Staggering administration times may avoid this interaction.

continued

HISTAMINE H_2 ANTAGONIST DRUG INTERACTIONS—*continued*

Histamine H_2 Antagonist Drug Interactions—*continued*			
Precipitant drug	Object drug*		Description
Ranitidine	Sulfonylureas	↑	Ranitidine may increase the hypoglycemic effect of glipizide; 1 glyburide patient developed severe hypoglycemia after ranitidine. This did not occur in 2 studies with glyburide or tolbutamide. Glipizide dosage adjustment may be needed.
Ranitidine	Theophyllines	↔	Case reports indicate theophylline plasma levels may be increased by ranitidine, possibly increasing pharmacologic and toxic effects. However, controlled studies indicate an interaction does not occur. If this interaction occurs, it is rare.
Ranitidine	Warfarin	↑	Ranitidine may interfere with warfarin clearance (data conflict; significance not established). Hypoprothrombinemic effects may increase; may need adjustment.
H_2 antagonists	Ethanol	↑	Concurrent use may increase plasma ethanol levels and AUC. This interaction may have minimal clinical importance.

* ↑ = Object drug increased. ↓ = Object drug decreased. ↔ = Undetermined clinical effect.

PROTON PUMP INHIBITOR DRUG INTERACTIONS

Proton Pump Inhibitor Drug Interactions			
Precipitant drug	Object drug*		Description
Clarithromycin	Omeprazole	↑	Coadministration of omeprazole and clarithromycin may result in increases in plasma levels of omeprazole, clarithromycin, and 14-hydroxy-clarithromycin.
Omeprazole	Clarithromycin		
Sucralfate	Lansoprazole Omeprazole	↓	Coadministration delayed absorption and reduced proton pump inhibitor bioavailability by ≈ 17%. Therefore, take these agents ≥ 30 minutes prior to sucralfate.
Omeprazole	Benzodiazepines Diazepam Flurazepam Triazolam	↑	Omeprazole produced a 130% increase in the half-life of diazepam, probably caused by inhibition of oxidative metabolism. Plasma levels were also increased and total clearance of diazepam was decreased.
Omeprazole	Phenytoin	↑	Omeprazole reduced the plasma clearance of phenytoin by 15% and increased its half-life by 27%, probably caused by inhibition of oxidative metabolism.
Lansoprazole	Theophylline	↓	A 10% increase in theophylline clearance occurred. Additional titration of theophylline dosage may be required.
Omeprazole	Warfarin	↑	Omeprazole may prolong the elimination of warfarin via inhibition of oxidative metabolism.

* ↑ = Object drug increased. ↓ = Object drug decreased.

SUCRALFATE DRUG INTERACTIONS

Sucralfate Drug Interactions			
Precipitant drug	Object drug*		Description
Sucralfate	Antacids, aluminum-containing	↑	The total body burden of aluminum may be increased with sucralfate coadministration. See Warnings.
Sucralfate	Anticoagulants	↓	A decrease in the hypoprothrombinemic effect of warfarin may occur.
Sucralfate	Diclofenac	↓	The pharmacologic effects of diclofenac may be decreased.
Sucralfate	Digoxin	↓	Serum digoxin levels may be reduced, decreasing the therapeutic effects.
Sucralfate	Histamine H_2 antagonists Cimetidine Ranitidine	↓	Bioavailability of the histamine H_2 antagonists may be decreased. Administering the histamine H_2 antagonist ≥ 2 hours before sucralfate may eliminate the interaction.
Sucralfate	Hydantoins	↓	Phenytoin absorption may be decreased.
Sucralfate	Ketoconazole	↓	Ketoconazole bioavailability may be decreased.
Sucralfate	Levothyroxine	↓	The effects of levothyroxine may be decreased.
Sucralfate	Penicillamine	↓	Penicillamine's effectiveness may be lessened or negated.
Sucralfate	Quinidine	↓	Serum quinidine levels may be reduced, decreasing the therapeutic effects.
Sucralfate	Quinolones	↓	Bioavailability of the quinolones may be decreased. Administering the quinolone ≥ 2 hours before sucralfate may eliminate the interaction.
Sucralfate	Tetracycline	↓	Tetracycline bioavailability may be decreased.
Sucralfate	Theophylline	↓	Theophylline bioavailability may be decreased.

* ↑ = Object drug increased. ↓ = Object drug decreased.

GASTROINTESTINAL ANTICHOLINERGIC/ ANTISPASMODIC DOSAGE

Gastrointestinal Anticholinergic/Antispasmodic Dosage		
	Adult Dosage	
Drug	Oral	Parenteral
Anticholinergics		
Atropine	0.4-0.6 mg	0.4-0.6 mg
Scopolamine		0.32-0.65 mg
L-hyoscyamine	0.125-0.25 mg tid-qid (0.375 to 0.7 mg q 12 hrs – sustained release)	0.25-0.5 mg q 4 h
L-alkaloids of belladonna	0.25-0.5 mg tid	
Belladonna alkaloids	0.18-0.3 mg tid-qid	
Quaternary Anticholinergics		
Methscopolamine bromide	2.5 mg ac; 2.5-5 mg hs	
Clidinium bromide	2.5-5 mg tid-qid	
Glycopyrrolate	1-2 mg bid-tid	0.1-0.2 mg tid-qid
Mepenzolate bromide	25-50 mg qid	
Methantheline bromide	50-100 mg q 4-6 hrs	
Propantheline bromide	7.5-15 mg tid; 30 mg hs	
Tridihexethyl chloride	25-50 mg tid-qid	
Antispasmodics		
Dicyclomine HCl	20-40 mg qid	20 mg qid

FDA ORPHAN DRUGS WITH GI USES

Generic Name	Proposed Use	Sponsor/Manufacturer
4-aminosalicylic acid (*Pamisyl, Rezipas*)	Treatment of mild to moderate ulcerative colitis in patients intolerant to sulfasalazine	Parke-Davis Bristol-Myers Squibb Warren Beeken, MD, University of Vermont
Adeno-associated viral vector containing the gene for human coagulation factor IX (*Coagulin B*)	Intrahepatic treatment of patients with moderate to severe hemophilia	Avigen
Ammonium tetrathiomolybdate	Treatment of Wilson's disease	George J. Brewer, MD, University of Michigan Medical School
Bacitracin (*Altracin*)	Treatment of antibiotic-associated pseudo-membranous enterocolitis caused by toxins A and B elaborated by *Clostridium difficile*	A.L. Laboratories
Beclomethasone 17,21-dipropionate	Prevention of GI graft-vs-host disease	Enteron Pharmaceuticals
Beclomethasone dipropionate	For oral administration in the treatment of intestinal graft-vs-host disease	George B. McDonald, MD, Fred Hutchinson Cancer Research Center
Bovine colostrum	AIDS-related diarrhea	Donald Hastings, DVM
Bovine immunoglobulin concentrate, *Cryptosporidium parvum* (*Sporidin-G*)	Treatment of symptomatic relief of *Cryptosporidium parvum* infection of the GI tract in immunocompromised patients	GalaGen

continued

FDA ORPHAN DRUGS WITH GI USES—*continued*

Generic Name	Proposed Use	Sponsor/Manufacturer
Bovine whey protein concentrate (*Immuno-C*)	Treatment of cryptosporidiosis caused by the presence of *Cryptosporidium parvum* in the GI tract of patients who are immunodeficient, immunocompromised, or immunocompetent	Biomune Systems
CDP571	Treatment of Crohn's disease	Celltech Chiroscience Discovery
CY-1899	Chronic active hepatitis B infection in HLA-A2 positive patients	Cytel
Disaccharide tripeptide glycerol dipalmitoyl (*Immther*)	Treatment of pulmonary and hepatic metastases in patients with colorectal adenocarcinoma	ImmunoTherapeutics
Ethanolamine oleate (*Ethamolin*)	Esophageal varices that have recently bled, to prevent rebleeding	Block Drug
FIAU	Adjunctive treatment of chronic active hepatitis B	Oclassen Pharmaceuticals
Flumecinol (*Zixorn*)	Treatment of hyperbilirubinemia in newborn infants unresponsive to phototherapy	Farmacon
Glutamine	For use with human growth hormone in the treatment of short bowel syndrome (nutrient malabsorption from the GI tract resulting from an inadequate absorptive surface)	Nutritional Restart Pharmaceutical, L.P.
Hepatitis B immune globulin IV (*Nabi-HB*)	Prophylaxis against hepatitis B virus reinfection in liver transplant patients	NABI

continued

FDA ORPHAN DRUGS WITH GI USES—*continued*

Generic Name	Proposed Use	Sponsor/Manufacturer
Histrelin	Treatment of acute intermittent porphyria, hereditary coproporphyria, and variegata porphyria	Karl Anderson, MD, University of Texas Medical Branch at Galveston
Human growth hormone	For use with glutamine in the treatment of short bowel syndrome (nutrient malabsorption from the GI tract resulting from an inadequate absorptive surface)	Nutritional Restart Pharmaceutical, L.P.
Imatinib mesylate *(Gleevec)*	Treatment of GI stromal tumors	Novartis
Infliximab *(Remicade)*	Treatment of moderately to severely active Crohn's disease for the reduction of the signs and symptoms, in patients who have an inadequate response to con ventional therapy; and treatment of patients with fistulizing Crohn's disease for the reduction in the number of draining enterocutaneous fistula(s)	Centocor
Iodine I [123] murine monoclonal antibody to alpha-fetoprotein	Detection and treatment of hepatocellular carcinoma and hepatoblastoma	Immunomedics
Lactic acid bacteria *(Lactobacilli, Bifidobacteris*, and *Streptococci)*	Treatment of active chronic pouchitis and prevention of disease relapse in patients with chronic pouchitis	VSL Pharmaceuticals
Leucovorin calcium *(Wellcovorin)*	With 5-flluorouracil for the treatment of metastatic colorectal cancer	Glaxo Wellcome Research & Development

continued

FDA ORPHAN DRUGS WITH GI USES—*continued*

Generic Name	Proposed Use	Sponsor/Manufacturer
Monoclonal antibody to hepatitis B virus (human)	Prophylaxis of hepatitis B reinfection in patients undergoing liver transplantation secondary to end-stage chronic hepatitis B infection	Protein Design Labs
Monooctanoin *(Moctanin)*	Dissolution of cholesterol gallstones retained in common bile duct	Ethinek Pharm
MTC-DOX injection	Hepatocellular carcinoma	FeRx Inc
Nolatrexed *(Thymitaq)*	Treatment of hepatocellular carcinoma	Zarix
Nolatrexed	Treatment of hepatocellular carcinoma	Zarix
Oxandrolone *(Hepandrin)*	Treatment of moderate/severe acute alcoholic hepatitis in the presence of moderate protein calorie malnutrition	Bio-Technology General
Pegylated arginine deiminase *(Hepacid, Melanocid)*	Treatment of hepatocellular carcinoma	Phoenix Pharmacologics
Recombinant glycine2-human glucagon-like peptide-2	Treatment of short bowel syndrome	NPS Allelix
Recombinant human insulin-like growth factor-I *(PV802)*	Treatment of short bowel syndrome as a result of resection of the small bowel or as a result of congenital dysfunction of the intestines	GroPep Pty Ltd.

continued

FDA ORPHAN DRUGS WITH GI USES—*continued*

Generic Name	Proposed Use	Sponsor/Manufacturer
Short chain fatty acid enema (*Colomed*)	Treatment of the active phase of ulcerative colitis with involvement restricted to the left side of the colon	Orphan Medical
Somatostatin (*Zecnil*)	Adjunct to the nonoperative management of secreting cutaneous fistulas of the stomach, duodenum, small intestine (jejunum and ileum), or pancreas	Ferring Laboratories
Somatostatin	Bleeding esophageal varices	UCB Pharm
Somatropin (*Serostim*)	For use alone or in combination with glutamine in the treatment of short bowel syndrome	Serono Laboratories
Synthetic porcine secretin (*ChiRhoClin*)	For use in the diagnosis of gastrinoma associated with Zollinger-Ellison syndrome	ChiRhoClin
TAK-603	Crohn's disease	Tap Holdings Inc
Technetium Tc-99m murine monoclonal antibody to human AFP (*Immuraid*, *AFP-Scan*)	Detection of hepatocellular carcinoma and hepatoblastoma	Immunomedics
Thymalfasin (*Zadaxin*)	Treatment of chronic hepatitis B; treatment of hepatocellular carcinoma	SciClone Pharmaceuticals
Tri-antennary glycotripeptide derivative of 5-fluorodeoxyuridine monophosphate	Treatment for hepatocellular carcinoma	Cell Works

continued

FDA ORPHAN DRUGS WITH GI USES—*continued*

Generic Name	Proposed Use	Sponsor/Manufacturer
Trientine HCl (*Syprine*)	Treatment of patients with Wilson's disease who are intolerant, or inadequately responsive to penicillamine	Merck & Co.
Ursodiol (*URSO*)	Treatment of patients with primary biliary cirrhosis	Axcan Pharma
Ursodiol (*Actigall*)	Treatment of patients with primary biliary cirrhosis	Novartis
Vapreotide (*Octastatin*)	Treatment of GI and pancreatic fistulas	Debiopharm S.A.
Xenogeneic hepatocytes (*HepatAssist Liver Assist System*)	Treatment of severe liver failure	Circe Biomedical
Zinc acetate (*Glazin*)	Treatment of Wilson's disease	Teva Pharmaceuticals, USA

INVESTIGATIONAL GI DRUGS

Drug name:	Company:	Description:
5-HT-4 receptor antagonist LY-353433	Roberts Pharmaceutical Shire Pharmaceuticals Group	Treatment of functional bowel disorders to normalize GI motility
Esomeprazole proton pump inhibitor (IV formulation) ***Nexium***	AstraZeneca PLC	Proton pump inhibitor (PPI) for treatment of GI disorders (parenteral formulation)
Fedotozine	Pfizer/GlaxoSmithKline	Peripherally acting kappa selective opioid agonist for treatment of conditions involving hypersensitivity of the GI tract, including irritable bowel syndrome (IBS) and nonulcerative dyspepsia (NUD)
Interleukin-15	Immunex Corporation	Treatment of GI tract mucositis
Ion channel expression GI disease	ICAgen	Ion channel modulation for treatment of GI disease
Keratinocyte growth factor (KGF)	Amgen	Recombinant keratinocyte growth factor (KGF) for reduction of severity and duration of oral and GI mucositis induced by chemotherapy and radiation therapy in treatment of head and neck cancer
Lactoferrin, transgenic human	Pharming B.V.	Treatment of GI infections and infectious arthritis

continued

INVESTIGATIONAL GI DRUGS—*continued*

Drug name:	Company:	Description:
Motilides	Kosan Biosciences	Novel erythromycin-derived agonists of the motilin receptor for treatment of GI diseases including gastroparesis and gastroesophageal reflux disease unresponsive to antacids
Motilin agonist GM-611	Chugai Pharmaceuticals	Acid-stable erythromycin A derivative motilin agonist as a gastroprokinetic agent for treatment of GI motility disorders, such as gastroparesis, oral formulation
Neurotrophin-3 (NT-3)	Regeneron Pharmaceuticals	Naturally-occurring trophic protein for treatment of GI motility
Reversible acid pump inhibitor AR-H047108, RAPID	AstraZeneca PLC	Treatment of acid-related GI disease
Rifaximin ***Lumenax***	Salix Pharmaceuticals	GI-specific antibiotic for treatment of *Clostridium difficile* colitis, diverticulitis, small bowel overgrowth, traveler's diarrhea, and irritable bowel syndrome
Small molecule drug ***Apaza***	Nobex	Oral small molecule drug delivered via GI tract for treatment of inflammatory bowel disease
Vaccine *Escherichia coli*	MedImmune	Prevention of GI tract infections
Vaccine *Helicobacter pylori* **Helivax**	AntexBiologics	Vaccine/Adjuvant combination for prevention or treatment of peptic ulcers and GI disorders caused by *H. pylori*, oral formulation

INDEX

I

N